Behçet's Disease: An Integrated Approach

Erkan Alpsoy • Ayşe Boyvat
Tülin Ergun
Editors

Behçet's Disease: An Integrated Approach

Springer

Editors
Erkan Alpsoy
Dermatology and Venereology Department
Akdeniz University, School of Medicine
Antalya, Türkiye

Ayşe Boyvat
Dermatology and Venereology
Ankara University, Faculty of Medicine
Ankara, Türkiye

Tülin Ergun
Dermatology and Venereology
Marmara University Pendik Training and Research Hospital
Istanbul, Türkiye

ISBN 978-3-031-77250-4 ISBN 978-3-031-77251-1 (eBook)
https://doi.org/10.1007/978-3-031-77251-1

This Springer imprint is published by the registered company Springer Nature Switzerland AG
The registered company address is: Gewerbestrasse 11, 6330 Cham, Switzerland

Preface

This collaborative book, initiated by the Turkish Dermatological Society's Behçet's Disease Task Force, focuses on the optimal management of patients with Behçet's disease. Unlike previous works, it provides an in-depth exploration of mucocutaneous manifestations, which are commonly observed at disease onset or at any stage and are crucial for diagnosis. Additionally, this book aims to be inclusive by integrating the perspectives of various medical disciplines involved in the management of Behçet's disease. Our goal, in collaboration with authors who have extensive experience in the field, was to offer comprehensive and complete coverage of all aspects of Behçet's disease, adopting a holistic approach.

Each chapter thoroughly analyzes clinical symptoms and provides a detailed differential diagnosis. Controversies and nuances of the diagnostic process are explained comprehensively, ensuring that even clinicians who have never or only occasionally encountered these patients can confidently diagnose Behçet's disease. The incorporation of treatment algorithms and follow-up sections in the relevant chapters serves to promote a thorough approach to patient management. Additionally, typical and educational case presentations are included in some chapters to enhance the reader's understanding of the topics discussed. Throughout this book, there are visual elements, specifically highlighted in the chapters related to dermatology. The chapters on mucocutaneous Behçet's disease include original images that are believed to greatly aid in the process of diagnosis and differential diagnosis.

This book, with its authors' extensive knowledge of Behçet's disease, comprehensive content, and practical patient management approach, serves as a valuable guide for a wide range of medical specialties, including dermatology, rheumatology, ophthalmology, neurology, gastroenterology, cardiothoracic surgery, pathology, general practitioners, and students. As editors and contributors, our ultimate goal is for *Behçet's Disease: An Integrated Approach* to serve as a contemporary reference for clinicians and students dedicated to treating patients with Behçet's disease.

Antalya, Türkiye — Erkan Alpsoy
Ankara, Türkiye — Ayşe Boyvat
Istanbul, Türkiye — Tülin Ergun

Contents

Hulusi Behçet: Highlights from His Personal and Professional Life

1

Gülay Satar and Aysel Gürler

Contents

Hulusi Behçet was born on February 20, 1889, in Istanbul. During that time, an inspiring idea emerged among the enlightened minds to uplift Ottoman society by cultivating a new generation. This could only be accomplished through scientific and contemporary education, a viewpoint widely accepted among the educated. Hulusi Behçet's father, Ahmet Behçet, an Ottoman intellectual and education executive, was assigned to Lebanon at that time and he decided to send his son to a French boarding school [1–4] (Fig. 1.1).

Hulusi Behçet began his aspiring medical education in 1901 at the high school of military medicine. After graduating as a senior grade captain in 1910, he attended Gülhane Hospital, where he specialized in the field of dermatology and venereal diseases (Fig. 1.2). Hulusi Behçet developed his expertise by receiving training from highly regarded and competent dermatologists, bacteriologists and pathologists of that time [5]. These achievements formed the basis for his future studies in dermatopathology. Years later, when an e-book about the history of pathology was being written, Hulusi Behçet was included in the pioneers of this discipline [6].

In July 1914, he was appointed as the assistant of the chief physician at the Kırklareli Military Hospital. In addition to this duty, he worked as a specialist at Edirne Military Hospital. At the end of World War I, he worked as an honorary assisting physician first in Budapest and then at the Berlin Charité Hospital.

Hulusi Behçet had a short period of private practice upon his return to the homeland in 1923. Then, he was assigned to Hasköy Venereal Diseases Hospital as the chief physician. Six months later, he became head of the Dermatology and Venereology Clinic of Gureba Hospital. He worked together with Menahem Hodara (1869–1926) for 12 years, who integrated dermatology with histopathology and experimental studies. Hodara was a worldwide known figure as an author in medical literature with scrutinizing the diseases, his guidance in clinical studies, and

G. Satar (✉)
Dermatology and Venereology, Medical History and Ethics, Adana, Türkiye
e-mail: gsatar@cu.edu.tr

A. Gürler
Dermatology and Venereology, Ankara, Türkiye

E. Alpsoy et al. (eds.), *Behçet's Disease: An Integrated Approach*,
https://doi.org/10.1007/978-3-031-77251-1_1

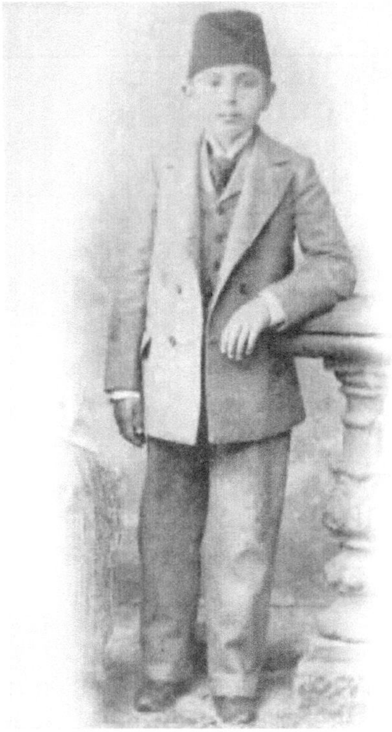

Fig. 1.1 Hulusi Behçet's childhood. Source: Satar G. Türk Tıbbının Sönmeyen Yıldızı Ord Prof Dr. Hulusi Behçet. Adana, Türkiye: Akademisyen Kitabevi; 2018

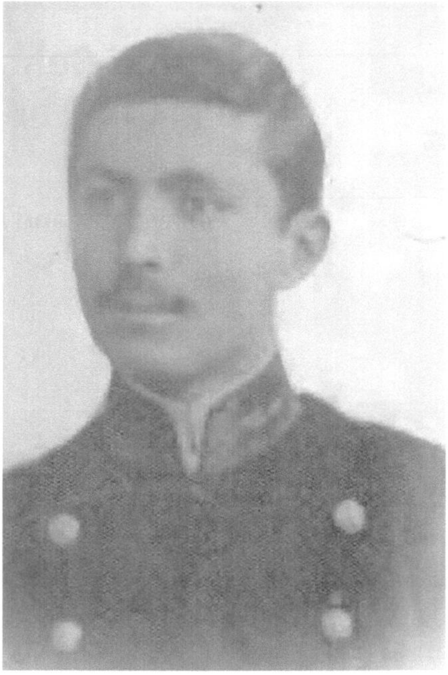

Fig. 1.2 Hulusi Behçet's graduation. Source: Satar G. Türk Tıbbının Sönmeyen Yıldızı Ord Prof Dr. Hulusi Behçet. Adana, Türkiye: Akademisyen Kitabevi; 2018

his creativity in treatment methods. Behçet and Hodara conducted more than 20 studies which were appreciated internationally [1].

A well-known French dermatologist, Gougerot, visited Hulusi Behçet at Gureba Hospital. He was impressed by the dermatopathology related works of his so much and requested these well-studied samples in order to present them at the French Dermatology and Venereology Society [2].

One of the most important cultural events during early years of the Republic of Türkiye was the renewal and modernization of higher education. This breakthrough is an important part and symbol of Mustafa Kemal Atatürk's cultural movement that started in 1924. By a historical coincidence, scientists who were under political pressure in Germany were invited to the existing and newly established Turkish universities. These faculty members immensely contributed to the development of Turkish universities [7].

Hulusi Behçet became a professor at Dermatology and Venereology Department of Istanbul University Faculty of Medicine during those times of the radical academic staff renewal operations in Türkiye (Fig. 1.3). He had already reached excellence in his professional endeavor and started his academic life in Istanbul University Faculty of Medicine where he had significant medical achievements. In the early days of university reform, Mustafa Kemal Atatürk seemed to encourage Hulusi Behçet by his words, "I want to see professors who do research at universities" and "Science is not through translation, but through study" [8]. He had chosen his father's middle name, Behçet, as his surname probably because he wanted his academic achievements to be recognized by a unique name in foreign publications.

Hulusi Behçet's one of the contributions to medical literature was the definition of the nail sign in cutaneous leishmaniasis, which scientists were already aware of but did not fully comprehend its diagnostic significance (Fig. 1.4).

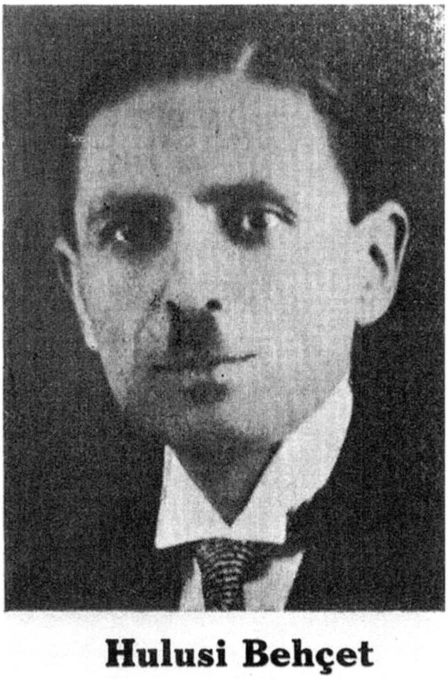

Fig. 1.3 Hulusi Behçet's assignment to Istanbul University. Source: Satar G. Türk Tıbbının Sönmeyen Yıldızı Ord Prof Dr. Hulusi Behçet. Adana, Türkiye: Akademisyen Kitabevi; 2018

His academic studies were mostly in the field of Behçet's disease during the last decade of his life. He spent great effort to get it accepted in the medical literature as a *sui generis* rather than a combination of a series of symptoms. The clinical appearance characterized by mouth and genital mucosal aphthae and ocular findings, was known since Hippocrates but not considered as a unique disease in the medical literature.

Hulusi Behçet's curiosity for research, careful observation, patience, and vast synthesis ability have gifted medicine a new and mysterious disease [2–4]. The characteristic feature of Hulusi Behçet's scientific approach was not to make the unknown things known but to appreciate the known things which were unrecognized or ignored. It can be defined as transforming empirical knowledge into scientific knowledge [2, 8].

Hulusi Behçet's studies on Behçet's disease started in 1917 and continued until 1937. As reported by him the basis of retarded identification of the disease was owing to individual standpoints of dermatologists, ophthalmologists and internists. The cause of the disease was unknown, the differences among the cases were remarkable. The involvement of multiple organs and systems made it difficult to reach the accurate diagnosis. He also indicated that the signs and symptoms included in the exacerbation period disappeared during the remission period. Close and meticulous observation of his three resembling cases led him to think about a distinctive disease [9].

The first case was a male patient who had been evaluated by the most well-known ophthalmology, dermatology and internal medicine physicians of Istanbul and Vienna for years with complaints of ulcers in his oral and genital mucosa, accompanying ocular symptoms, painful nodules in his legs, joint pains, and fever. Ophthalmologists tried to explain ocular problems with rheumatism, tuberculosis, syphilis, and leprosy, dermatologists attributed oral aphthae to digestive disorders, and painful swellings on the legs were diagnosed as erythema nodosum. Then the consultants decided to send him to Vienna. In Vienna, ophthalmologist Fuchs evaluated the ocular involvement, Riehl and Kyrle scrutinized the dermatological problems. All the investigations; biopsies, cultures, blood examinations and animal experiments performed for months yielded no results. Finally, Kyrle suggested that this might be a protozoan-borne disease unknown in Europe.

The second case was a 34-year-old woman who had painful ulcers in oral and genital areas, bloodshot eyes, and gave a story of having had several similar attacks before. No specific clinical condition was seen in histological and microbiological examinations performed during the attacks, and except for some conjunctival changes and episcleritis there were no severe ophthalmological findings.

The third case was a 41-year-old male patient who was sent to dermatology from dentistry and showed a similar clinical picture to the first two cases. Oral symptoms were as severe as the oral findings of pemphigus. There were acneiform lesions on his face and back, and widespread ulcerations in his genital area. One of his eyes

Fig. 1.6 Behçet's Disease first publication in German literature. Source: Satar G. Türk Tıbbının Sönmeyen Yıldızı Ord Prof Dr. Hulusi Behçet. Adana, Türkiye: Akademisyen Kitabevi; 2018

1152 Dermatologische Wochenschrift 1937 Nr. 36

Herpeseffloreszenzen bedingt. Was die Angina anlangt, so ist wohl anzunehmen, daß es sich um eine herpesbedingte, die mit Fieber einherging, handelte. Es könnte sich dabei um eine metastatische herpetische Angina bzw. um eine direkte Infektion durch den mutmaßlich infektiösen Speichel des Patienten (der auch an rezidivierendem Herpes labialis leidet) handeln; letzteres ist wahrscheinlicher. Anschr. d. Verf.: Reutlingen/Württbg., Karlstr. 30.

Aus der Dermatologischen Klinik (Hospital-Guraba) der Universität Istanbul
(Direktor: Professor Dr. Hulusi Behçet)

Über rezidivierende, aphthöse, durch ein Virus verursachte Geschwüre am Mund, am Auge und an den Genitalien

Von

Professor Hulusi Behçet

Mit 9 Abbildungen

Zahlreiche Arbeiten beschäftigen sich mit dem Ursprung der durch ein filtrierbares Virus hervorgerufenen Hauterkrankungen. Bekannt sind unter anderen auf diesem Gebiete die Arbeiten von Lipschütz, ebenso die Mitteilungen von Kummer und Nicolau auf dem Budapester Kongreß, ferner die Untersuchungen von Ravaut und Ferrand und schließlich die von P. Blum über Viruskrankheiten. Aus diesen Arbeiten geht hervor, daß manche Autoren, wie etwa Kummer, die Aphthen dem Herpes zugesellen. Andere wiederum teilen den Herpes der Gruppe der neuro-dermotropen Infektionen zu.

Es ist einigen Forschern gelungen, die Virusätiologie gewisser aphthöser Erscheinungen sicherzustellen, während andere zu keinen endgültigen Ergebnissen gelangten.

Die Fälle, die im folgenden erörtert werden sollen, wiesen folgendes klinische Bild auf: Läsionen am Mund, an den Genitalien und am Auge. Diese Schäden glichen jedoch nicht den Aphthoiden von Pospischil und den noch wenig erforschten Hautschädigungen, die man häufig bei Kindern antrifft.

Wenn man hinsichtlich ihrer Lokalisation die bei Rückfällen auftretenden Läsionen einzeln untersucht, so ergibt sich, daß sowohl die Mund- wie auch die Genitalsyndrome in jede Gruppe einreihbar sind. So treten beispielsweise in unserem zweiten Falle zuweilen die aphthösen Geschwüre an den Genitalien zuerst auf und lassen zunächst an Lipschütz-Geschwüre oder verschiedene Formen von Schleimhautgeschwüren (Esthiomène) denken. Bei den mehrmals im Jahre sich einstellenden Rückfällen treten indessen die Läsionen jeweils gleichzeitig oder nacheinander am Mund, an den Genitalien, an der Bindehaut, ja sogar als Entzündung der Regenbogenhaut auf. Diese Erscheinungen verdienen gesondert untersucht zu werden.

Bei einem der beiden Patienten, die wir seit 20 Jahren in Beobachtung haben, traten in den ersten Jahren anläßlich des Rezidivs sehr schmerzhafte, an Erythema nodosum erinnernde Erscheinungen auf. Sobald die aphthösen Läsionen an Mund und Genitalien im Abflauen waren, verschwanden gleichzeitig auch die Hautläsionen. Bei unseren beiden Fällen, die seit 20 bzw.

tion was accepted as a morbid entity, primarily in Belgium, Switzerland, Denmark, Austria and the United States.

Hulusi Behçet's decisive and insistent progress in his studies and publications broke the resistance of those who opposed this novel disease. Hulusi Behçet declared the support of ophthalmologists rather than dermatologists as a duty of conscience in the recognition period of this unique disease [9]. He respectfully commemorated the expelled German scientists who were assigned at universities in Istanbul and Ankara for their contribution to the process.

In fact, there was no consensus on naming of the disease in the days of definition and recognition, and it was often handled within the framework of syndrome. In 1946, the disease became known as Behçet's disease, especially in Europe, and was documented in medical records without any hesitation. There is an anecdote about that period. A university student was being followed up with the diagnosis of Behçet's tri-symptom in Ankara/Türkiye. He was referred to the ophthalmology clinic of Zurich University Faculty of medicine for a consultation. In the health report which was given to him after the examination, the diagnosis was mentioned as Behçet's disease, a disease known since 1938 and named after a Turkish physician.

Finally, during the dermatology congress convened in Geneva in 1947, Prof. Miescher from Zurich University Faculty of Medicine suggested to name the disease as Behçet's disease and with the approval of the other attending experts, a new name coined in the international medical literature: Morbus Behçet (Behçet's disease).

Hulusi Behçet insisted in supporting clinical studies not only by basic medical sciences but by basic sciences such as physics and chemistry as well. He successfully combined the basic scientific knowledge with his strong clinical experience and made many contributions to the medical literature.

Hulusi Behçet's professional interests included not only dermatology-specific diseases, but also the issues that have connections among dermatology and different disciplines. His publications were on bacteriological, mycological, parasitological, and pathological dimensions of dermatological problems. He also touched on issues such as allergy, hypersensitivity, autoimmunity, and skin findings related to hormonal conditions, which were extremely novel for that period. His propensity for interdisciplinary cooperation and teamwork was also remarkable. While investigating the etiology of pemphigus, he conducted experiments in collaboration with the Istanbul University General Experimental Pathology and Cancer Institute.

Hulusi Behçet was also a pioneer in applying dermatological treatment methods such as diathermy and the use of frozen carbon dioxide gas, in his routine practice which had not been included in classical books at that time. In one of his articles on diathermy, he mentioned that he first informed the female patient about the method he was treating then got approval for the application. This is remarkable in terms of medical ethics, and it is an indication of his foresightedness and the tendency to put the patient in the midpoint of his practice.

During most of his medical life penicillin and other antibiotic treatments were not available. In that period, syphilis had special importance among his professional interests. Syphilis was a serious public health problem worldwide. This catastrophic danger was passed from generation to generation and deeply affected the social structure because of its congenital form. Those days an official institution was established in Türkiye to combat syphilis and he did a lot for that organization along with the Dermatology and Venereal Diseases Association. Hulusi Behçet's efforts were great during those hard times, which included the preparation of the syphilis treatment guidelines and founding hospitals, dispensaries, and treatment units. He organized courses to train physicians to work in this field. He wrote books that can appeal to all physicians to raise awareness and sensitivity about the disease in the professional community.

He emphasized that the aim is not only to cure the patients but to prevent the transmission of the disease. He insisted that this disaster could be eliminated by conveying these ideas to the whole society with active propaganda and making treatment facilities accessible to everyone. Hulusi Behçet tried raising the awareness of society by the health education meetings and speeches on the radio, which was the most effective tool in the field of mass communication at that time.

Hulusi Behçet was not only a successful representative of this field of expertise but also a leader of the dermatology and venereology community. In this context, he has been active in continuous education; on the other hand, he has contributed a lot to the social connectedness of dermatologists. Hulusi Behçet was among the founder members of the expertise associations. He continued to support them at the management level. Hulusi Behçet's significant characteristic was to be the owner of the unique national dermatology and venereology journal for 14 years. He published this periodical mostly by his personal efforts supported by his close colleague Cevat Kerim İncedayı. In addition to original

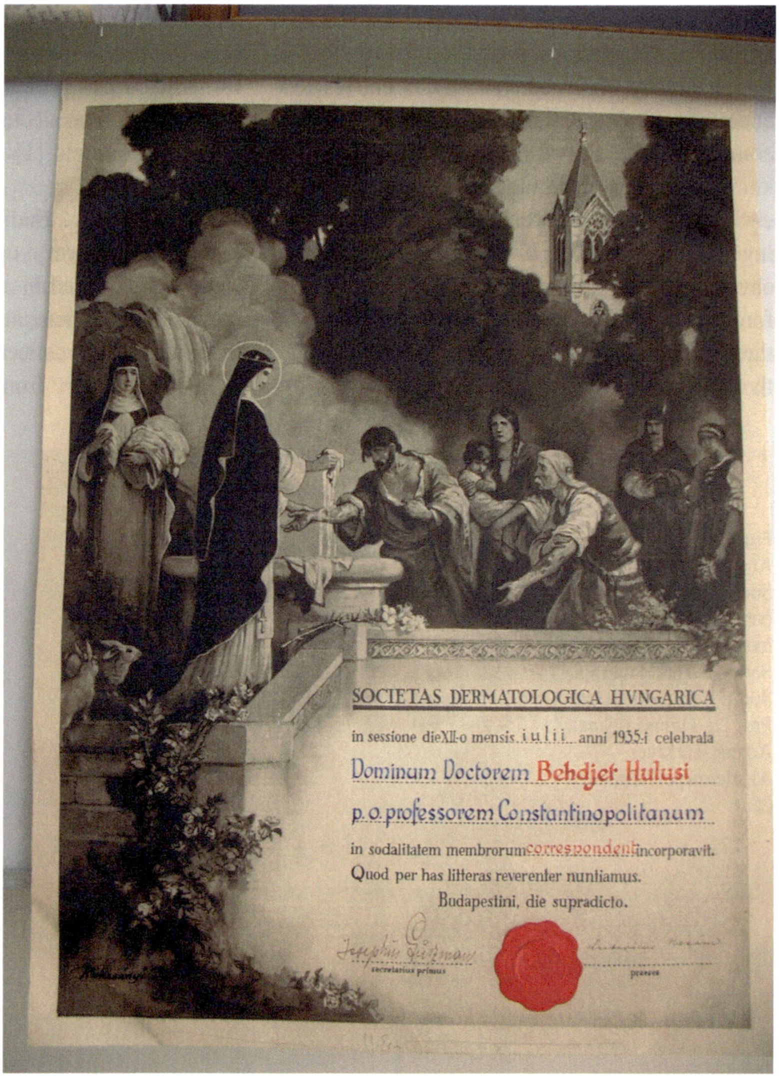

Fig. 1.9 The certificate correspondence membership of Hungary Dermatology Society. Source: Satar G. Türk Tıbbının Sönmeyen Yıldızı Ord Prof Dr. Hulusi Behçet. Adana, Türkiye: Akademisyen Kitabevi; 2018

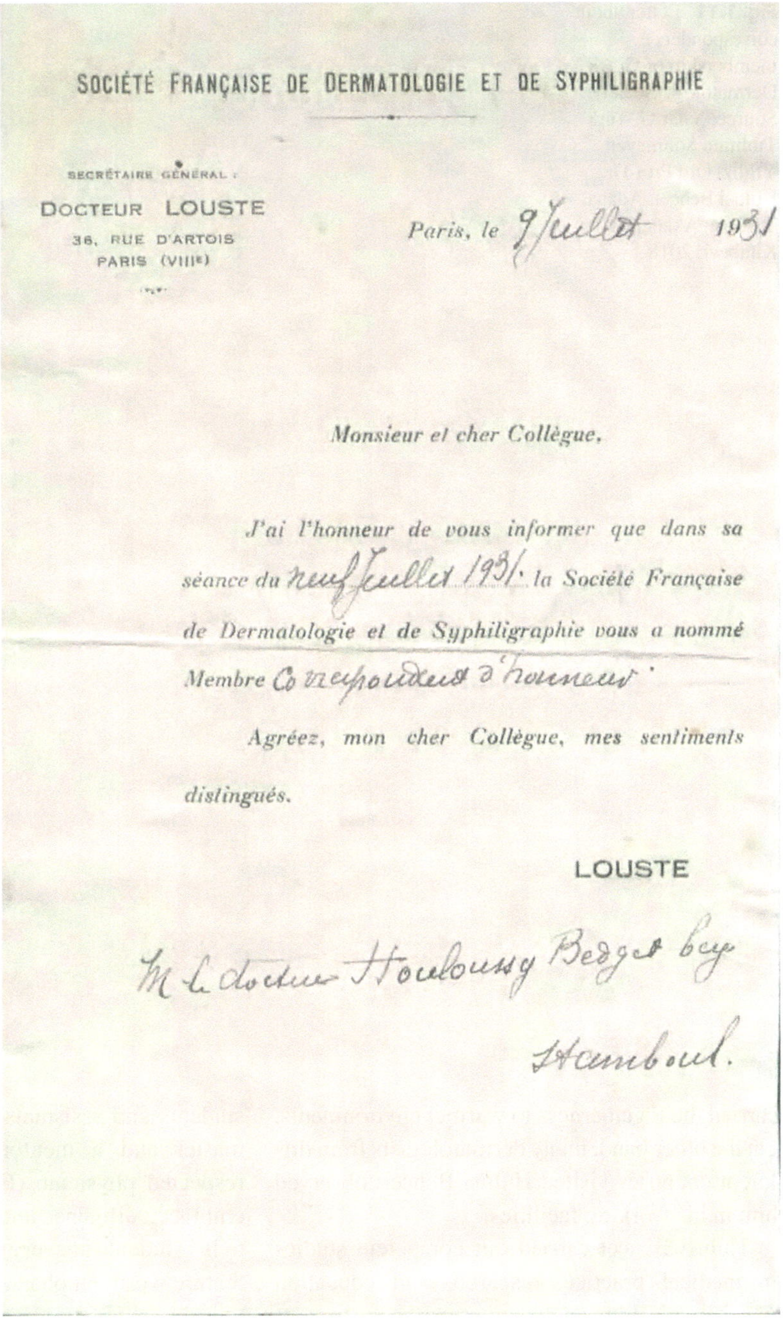

SOCIÉTÉ FRANÇAISE DE DERMATOLOGIE ET DE SYPHILIGRAPHIE

SECRÉTAIRE GÉNÉRAL :
DOCTEUR LOUSTE
36, RUE D'ARTOIS
PARIS (VIIIᴱ)

Paris, le 9 Juillet 1931

Monsieur et cher Collègue,

J'ai l'honneur de vous informer que dans sa séance du neuf Juillet 1931 la Société Française de Dermatologie et de Syphiligraphie vous a nommé Membre Correspondant d'honneur.

Agréez, mon cher Collègue, mes sentiments distingués.

LOUSTE

M. le docteur Houloussy Behçet bey

Stamboul.

Fig. 1.10 Letter about honorary correspondence membership of French Society of Dermatology and Syphiligraphy. Source: Satar G. Türk Tıbbının Sönmeyen Yıldızı Ord Prof Dr. Hulusi Behçet. Adana, Türkiye: Akademisyen Kitabevi; 2018

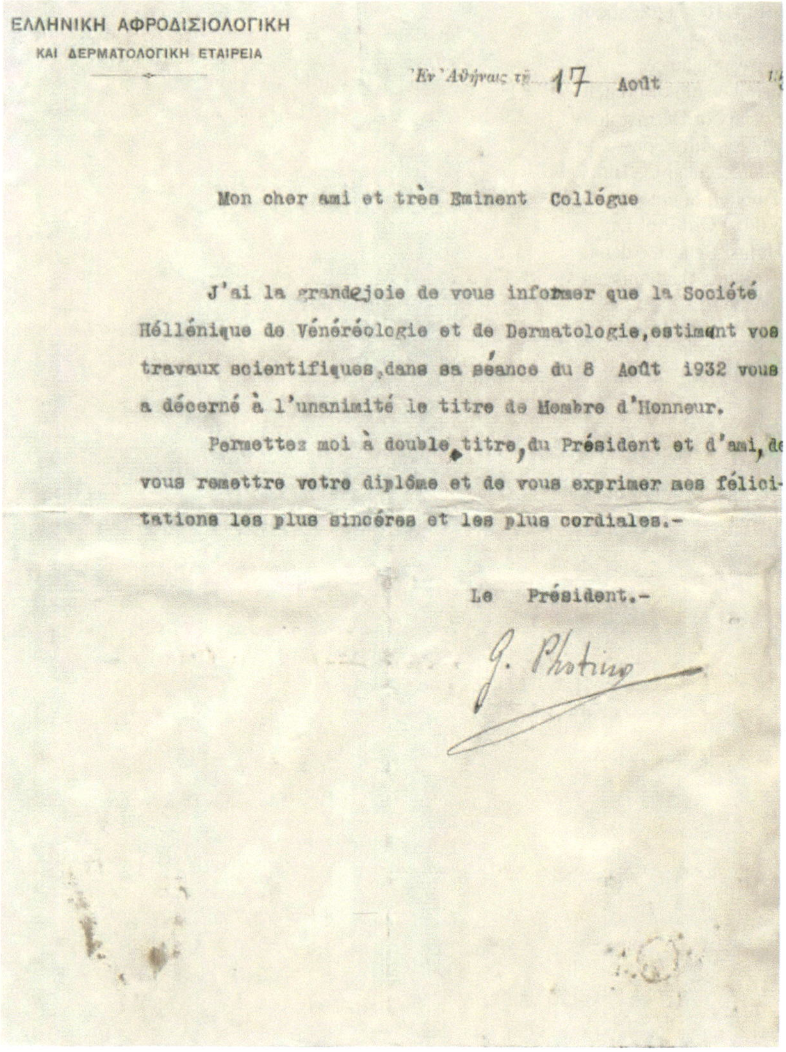

ΕΛΛΗΝΙΚΗ ΑΦΡΟΔΙΣΙΟΛΟΓΙΚΗ
ΚΑΙ ΔΕΡΜΑΤΟΛΟΓΙΚΗ ΕΤΑΙΡΕΙΑ

Ἐν Ἀθήναις τῇ 17 Août

Mon cher ami et très Eminent Collégue

J'ai la grande joie de vous informer que la Société Héllénique de Vénéréologie et de Dermatologie, estimant vos travaux scientifiques, dans sa séance du 8 Août 1932 vous a décerné à l'unanimité le titre de Membre d'Honneur.

Permettez moi à double titre, du Président et d'ami, de vous remettre votre diplôme et de vous exprimer mes félicitations les plus sincéres et les plus cordiales.-

Le Président.-

G. Photino

Fig. 1.11 Letter about correspondence membership of Greek Dermatology Society. Source: Satar G. Türk Tıbbının Sönmeyen Yıldızı Ord Prof Dr. Hulusi Behçet. Adana, Türkiye: Akademisyen Kitabevi; 2018

carried the togetherness to warmer environments. On the other hand, many dermatologists from different countries visited Hulusi Behçet; observed him in his working facilities.

Hulusi Behçet carried out competent studies in medical practice, research, and education which made him an inventor in the history of medicine. He won the appreciation of his patients and the society with his success in professional practices. He was sincerely appreciated by his students and assistants for his performance as a master and a mentor. He was a loved and respected physician (Fig. 1.12). He excessively embraced diligence and strongly recommended it to his students at every opportunity. An important feature worth emphasizing was his efforts to provide his students a broad perspective to enable them to see the sociocultural and historical dimensions of medicine [11].

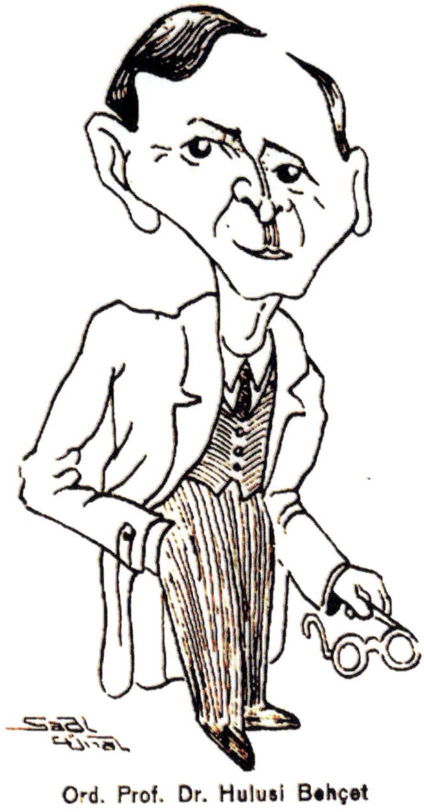

Fig. 1.12 Loved and respected master. Source: Satar G. Türk Tıbbının Sönmeyen Yıldızı Ord Prof Dr. Hulusi Behçet. Adana, Türkiye: Akademisyen Kitabevi; 2018

Despite the challenging historical circumstances of his time, he made significant scientific contributions throughout his relatively short life span of 59 years. Hulusi Behçet passed away on March 8, 1948, due to a heart attack, and the fact that this disease is named after him, Behçet's disease is a source of pride for the Turkish medical community [4] (Figs. 1.13 and 1.14).

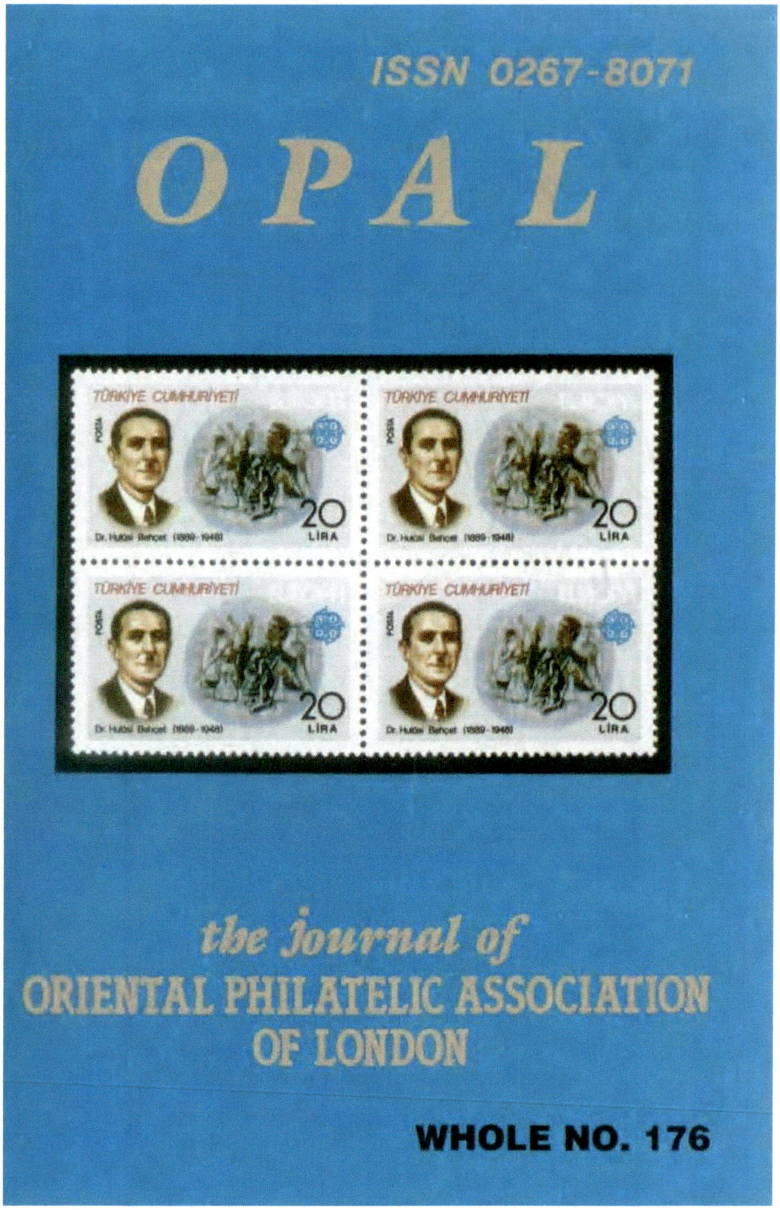

Fig. 1.13 A special issue and commemorative stamps from philatelic association of London. Source: Satar G. Türk Tıbbının Sönmeyen Yıldızı Ord Prof Dr. Hulusi Behçet. Adana, Türkiye: Akademisyen Kitabevi; 2018

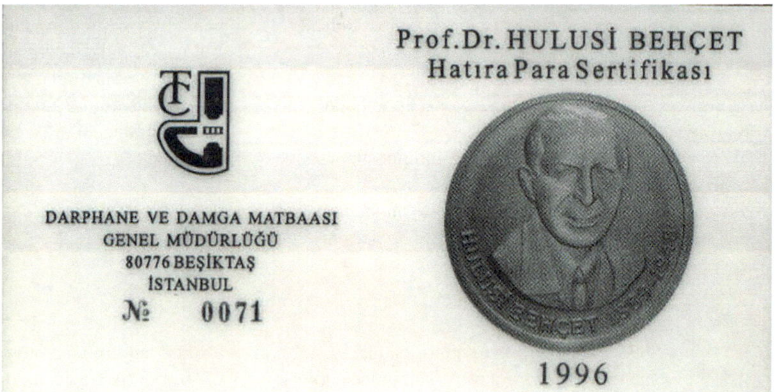

Fig. 1.14 The certificate of commemorative coin stamped in honor of Hulusi Behçet. Source: Satar G. Türk Tıbbının Sönmeyen Yıldızı Ord Prof Dr. Hulusi Behçet. Adana, Türkiye: Akademisyen Kitabevi; 2018

Conflicts of Interest The authors declare that they have no conflicts of interest.

References

1. Satar G. Türk Tıbbının Sönmeyen Yıldızı Ord Prof Dr Hulusi Behçet. Adana, Türkiye: Akademisyen Kitabevi; 2018.
2. Satar G, Kadıoğlu S. Bilim Adamı Kimliği ile Genel Olarak Kişilik İlişkisi Çerçevesinde Ord Prof Dr Hulusi Behçet. IX. Türk Tıp Tarihi Kongresi Bildiri Kitabı. Kahya E, Şar S, Ataç A, Mazıcıoğlu M, editörler. Ankara, Türkiye: Nobel Yayın Dağıtım; 2006. p. 408–411.
3. Saylan T. Life story of Dr Hulusi Behçet. Yonsei Med J. 1997;38(6):327–32. http://www.hulusibehcet.net/behcet.htm. Accessed 30 Mar 2006
4. Tüzün Y. Hulusi Behçet MD February 20, 1889 to March 8, 1948. Clinics in Dermatology. 2006;24:548–550.
5. Satar G, Kadıoğlu S. Hamdi Suat-Hulusi Behçet: an affective trainee-tutor relationship from Turkish medical history. Turk J Pathol. 2011;27(3):181–4.
6. Paksoy N. Behçet, Hulusi (1889–1948). In: van Krieken J. editor. Encyclopedia of Pathology. Springer; Cham, 2016.
7. Widmann H. Atatürk ve Üniversite Reformu. Çeviri: Kazancıgil A, Bozkurt S. İstanbul, Türkiye, Kabalcı Yayınevi, 1999.
8. Özata M. Atatürk Bilim ve Üniversite. 2.Basım, Ankara, Türkiye: Tübitak Yayınları; 2007.
9. Satar G, Kadıoğlu FG. Behçet Hastalığı ile ilgili isim tartışmaları. Türkiye Klinikleri J Med Ethics. 2014;22(1):23–32.
10. Behçet H. On relapsing, aphthous ulcers of the mouth, eye and genitalia caused by a virus. Clin Exp Rheumatol. 2010;28(Suppl. 60):S2–5.
11. Kadıoğlu S. Hulusi Behçet'ten Bir Açılış Dersi. Demirhan Erdemir A ve ark. I. Uluslararası Türk Tıp Tarihi Kongresi 10. Ulusal Türk Tıp Tarihi Kongresi. Bildiri Kitabı. Konya, Türkiye; 2008. p.768–782.

2 Historical Aspects and Description of Behçet's Disease

Selda Pelin Kartal and Erkan Alpsoy

Contents

Hulusi Behçet was born on February 20, 1889, in Istanbul. Due to his father's work, he received his primary education in Damascus, where he learned French, Latin, and German. His passion for knowledge and curiosity led him to pursue a career in medicine. He began his medical training at Gülhane Military Medical Academy in Istanbul and graduated from there in 1910 at the age of 21. After graduating, he began his dermatology training at Gülhane Dermatology and Venereology clinic and became a specialist in 1914. During this period and after his specialization, he actively collaborated with esteemed bacteriologists and pathologists of his era. With the aim of advancing his professional expertise, he journeyed to Europe in August 1918. He engaged in studies in Budapest and later pursued further education at the Charite Hospital in Berlin until October 1919. The University Reform, carried out under the leadership of Mustafa Kemal Atatürk in 1933, is a significant milestone in Turkish higher education during the Republican period. Istanbul University was established to fulfill the need for modern higher education, replacing Darülfünun. As part of this reform, Hulusi Behçet was appointed as a professor at the Dermatology and Venereology clinic. He was the first Turkish scientist to be awarded the title of professor in Turkish academic life [1, 2].

Hulusi Behçet has extensively studied various topics within the field of dermatology. Since 1920, Behçet has dedicated his attention to cutaneous leishmaniasis, wherein he documented "the nail sign" appearing nail-like extensions extending vertically by the removal of the crusts. His intense interest in syphilis propelled him to write numerous international articles and books, meticulously examining its diagnosis, treatment, hereditary qualities, serology, and societal implications. Hulusi Behçet's book, *Clinical and Practical Syphilis, Diagnosis and Related Diseases*, published in 1940, is considered one of his most significant studies. Each page of the book is divided into two sections: the upper half focuses on the clinical features of syphilis, while

S. P. Kartal (✉)
University of Health Sciences, Ankara Etlik City Hospital, Dermatology Clinic, Ankara, Türkiye

E. Alpsoy
Dermatology and Venereology Department, Akdeniz University, School of Medicine, Antalya, Türkiye
e-mail: ealpsoy@akdeniz.edu.tr

E. Alpsoy et al. (eds.), *Behçet's Disease: An Integrated Approach*,
https://doi.org/10.1007/978-3-031-77251-1_2

the lower half presents a differential diagnosis for other diseases exhibiting similar characteristics. Therefore, the reader had the opportunity to acquire knowledge about both syphilis and dermatology. Hulusi Behçet's extensive experience and knowledge of syphilis and his ability to recognize that the lesions of Behçet's disease are different from those of syphilis played an important role in the definition of Behçet's disease. He also identified the species and genera of the parasites responsible for "gale cereal" in Türkiye. By concentrating on fig dermatitis ("dermatitis Ficus carica"), he raised awareness of the disease in the Balkans and later in France and America. The first journal in the field of dermatology in Türkiye, titled *Turkish Archives of Dermatology and Venerology*, was published by Behçet in 1924. The publication of this journal is still ongoing. Starting in 1936, Behçet became a member of the editorial board of *Dermatologische Wochenschrift*, the most important journal of his time. In the same year, he was also elected to the editorial board of *Medizinische Welt*. Behçet's influential work in dermatology earned him the honor of becoming an honorary or associate member of various European national dermatology societies, including France, Austria, Hungary, and Greece. Hulusi Behçet was one of the rare dermatologists honored on a stamp. Turkey released three stamps on April 28, 1980, as part of the EUROPA/CEPT collection. One of them, a 20 lira stamp, was issued in memory of Behçet [3]. He passed away unexpectedly from a heart attack on March 8, 1948. His exceptional accomplishments in multiple fields within dermatology have positioned him as one of the most respected scientists worldwide. With his lifelong commitment to meticulous studies and producing new knowledge, Behçet left his mark on the scientific world by naming a disease after himself—Behçet's disease [1, 2, 4].

In this chapter, following a brief overview of Hulusi Behçet, we intend to summarize the steps he took to define Behçet's disease and how it gained acknowledgement in the medical community. Additionally, we discuss the historical chronology of the disease and the controversies surrounding its nomenclature, based on historical and scientific facts.

Hulusi Behçet identified the illness in three patients who exhibited comparable clinical characteristics and were under his long-term supervision, which is currently known all over the world as "Behçet's disease," "Behçet's syndrome," "Behçet's triad," "Trisymptom Behçet," or "Morbus Behçet" [1, 2, 4–8]. The first patient he saw, had recurrent oral and genital ulcers, painful leg nodules, fever, and joint pains. Specialists from various disciplines had examined him for his different symptoms and provided multiple diagnoses in Istanbul and Vienna. Some doctors thought of tuberculosis or syphilis while some other doctors said a microorganism which was not present in Europe might have caused the disease. Hulusi Behçet, who continued to examine the patient after his loss of vision, thought that the causative agent was a virus. In the next several years he met two more patients in 1932 and 1936 similar to that seen in the previous patient. Hulusi Behçet thought the symptoms of these three patients were the symptoms of a new disease with a follow-up of 21, 7, and 3 years [1, 2, 9].

The description of recurrent oral and genital ulcers together with hypopyon iritis that composed the new trisymptom complex disease was published at that time in one of the respected German journal *Dermatologische Wochenschrift* in 1937. "Über rezidivierende, Aphthöse, durch ein Virus verursachte Geschwüre amMund, am Auge und an den Genitalien" was the title [8]. In that same year, Hulusi Behçet presented his cases in a dermatology meeting in Paris. In this presentation he concluded that a dental infection might have played a role in the development of the disease [10, 11]. Much later in 1939 other similar results were published with the title "Tri-Symptomenkomplex" in another German journal *Medizinische Welt* [12]. And in 1940, his findings appeared in *Dermatologica* in English language with the title "triple symptom complex" [13]. In conclusion, the distinguishing feature of Hulusi Behçet from that of prior authors is his ability to combine three different symptoms and propose the existence of a new medical entity.

Jansen from Denmark was the first to use the name "Behçet syndrome" in the title of his report ["Sur les ulcérations aphteuses de la muqueuse de la bouche et de la peau génitale combinées avec les symptômes oculaires (=Syndrôme Behçet) [14] and "Ulcerous haemorrhagic colitis associated with Behçet's syndrome" [15]. In a similar case, Berlin used the phrase "Behçet syndrome" (Behçet's syndrome with involvement of the central nervous system. Report of a case, with necropsy, of lesions of the mouth, genitalia and eyes; review of the literature) [16]. Ephraim [17] once again gave "Behçet's triple symptom complex" an important place in history. From the United States, Ollendorf Curth [18, 19] published two separate articles introducing Behçet's syndrome's abortive form. In the latter article's title, the author emphasized Behçet's classic trio "recurrent oro-genital aphthae and hypopyon iritis" (Behçet syndrome). Hulusi Behçet's "three symptom complex" left a big impression on the medical community at that time. The term, Behçet's syndrome, was also coined and published extensively for the first time by Feigenbaum and Kornblueth [20]. With worldwide distribution, they paid respect to Dr. Behçet and his work by introducing "Behçet's syndrome" or "Behçet's disease." On September 13, 1947, international dermatologic societies came together in Zurich and named the disease as "Morbus Behçet," which honored the first describer of "triple symptom complex" [2–8].

As a dermatologist, Hulusi Behçet gave great importance to the recurrent oral ulcers. Today it is well known that oral ulcers are the most frequent, and the most common onset manifestation of the disease [21], which has been accepted as a "sine qua non" symptom. The diagnosis of Behçet's disease is based on clinical criteria because of the lack of a universally recognized pathognomonic laboratory test. Several sets of diagnostic criteria have been defined, and all of these criteria rely heavily on mucocutaneous manifestations. The International Study Group for Behçet's disease classification criteria has been widely accepted and used among clinicians worldwide since its description which requires the presence of recurrent oral ulcers for the diagnosis [22].

Hulusi Behçet also conducted significant research on the disease's etiology. In the third case, Behçet detected the presence of suppurate cysts and granulomas in the teeth through a detailed radiological examination, so he focused on a general microbial disease caused by a virus originating from the teeth. Professor Braun, an expert in this field, conducted virus studies on the second and third cases, and identified inclusion bodies that indicated the presence of a virus. Hulusi Behçet noticed a decrease in the frequency of attacks after the patients' teeth were extracted, which initially made him consider the teeth as the focal point of the disease. However, after reevaluating his opinion, he decided to abandon this idea as he believed that solely dental foci would not sufficiently explain a disease with systemic involvement [2, 5–11].

In the past, the disease has had several names such as "Gilbert's ophthalmia lenta" [23], "Gilbert–Behçet disease" [24, 25], "Gilbert–Adamantiades–Behçet disease" [26], "Adamantiades–Behçet disease" and "Hippocrates–Adamantiades–Behçet disease" [27].

Eponyms refer to a name, or noun formed after a person. Generally, they are used to labeling diseases in the field of medicine. As is the case with most diseases named after someone, the clinical features of Behçet's disease have been previously described by various scientists. The first clinical descriptions can be traced back to Hippocrates of Kos (460–377 BC). The treatise *Epidemics*, which is attributed to Hippocrates, comprises seven books. These records contain the observations of itinerant physicians who traveled in Northern Greece during the late fifth and early fourth centuries. In *Epidemics III*, one of these books, case histories, is organized in chronological order, documenting the progression of the disease day by day. In Case 7, there is a description of aphthous ulceration, genital ulceration, and iridocyclitis. Skin lesions (boils, sepsis, and "ectimata") are also mentioned. Feigenbaum reached the conclusion, based on this description, that the symptoms described in the case possibly caused an epidemic in ancient Greece [28, 29].

In 1772, the French Janin reported a male patient with recurrent hypopyon iritis [30]. Approximately 100 years later (1895) Neumann [31] from Austria and Christlieb from Würzburg [32], independent of each other, reported a total of 12 female patients with oral and genital aphthous ulcers. Reis [33] from Germany in 1906 found a recurrent eye inflammation together with erythema nodosum and arthritis in a male patient. Again in Germany in 1908, Blüthe [34] recorded his cases of four patients having recurrent hypopyon iridocyclitis and mucocutaneous symptoms together with arthritis. In addition, he confirmed iritis and optic atrophy histologically. Cases that carried similar symptoms were also recorded between 1920 and 1925 by Gilbert [35–38].

In 1930, Benediktos Adamantiades found hypopyon iritis together with mucocutaneous symptoms and arthritis in a 20-year-old male patient and much more concentrated on recurrent hypopyon iritis [39, 40] This case appeared in the 1931 *Ann Ocul (Paris)* journal with the heading of "Sur un cas d'iritis à hypopion récidivant" [41] Because of this publication, some authors called this illness "Adamantiades–Behçet disease." However, Benediktos Adamantiades was not the first author on this subject and cases that resembled the disease, especially with the heading "recurrent hypopyon iritis or iridocyclitis" took a place in history. Before Benediktos Adamantiades' writings, similar cases had already been reported by different authors in France, Austria, Germany, Greece, Holland, Japan, the Czech Republic, Poland, Belgium, and Switzerland. As indicated in history, similar notes, in fact, started in Hippocrates' days and continued from the eighteenth century through the last 300 years [28]. After Hippocrates encountered this endemic illness in the Middle East, until the beginning of 1900 years in the medical community's history very little information was found regarding this disease's individual symptoms. In all of the records, they emphasized known symptoms and especially "recurrent hypopyon iritis or iridocyclitis".

Benediktos Adamantiades considered recurrent hypopyon iritis as a separate clinical entity. It was well known that this clinical entity could have been caused by numerous eye illnesses and different illnesses such as tuberculosis, syphilis, leprosy, vasculitis, staphylococcal infections, sepsis, and local bacterial infections [8]. Indeed, Benediktos Adamantiades had thought that the cause of this clinical entity was syphilis, tuberculosis, and/or bacteremia. Likewise, he started to cure his patient with an antisyphilitic treatment, but he could not produce a successful result [41, 42]. Again, Benediktos Adamantiades cited Drs. Reis [33], Gilbert [35], and Weve's [43] similar cases in his respected paper, and concluded that staphylococcal infection and local eye disease could have played a role as the cause in the development of the disease. Between 1930 and 1940, similar cases such as "recurrent eye lesions" and/or "recurrent mucocutaneous lesions" were also reported by Dascalopoulos (1932) [44], von Hippel (1932) [45], Matras (1932) [46], Urbanek (1932, 1934) [47, 48], Whitwell (1934) [49], Nishimura (1936) [50], Blobner (1937) [51], Weekers-Reginster (1938) [52, 53], Knabb (1938) [54], and Schmidt (1938) [55, 56]. With the given information on Table 2.1 [30–38, 43, 57–64] today we can declare that all of the symptoms that were recorded before Benediktos Adamantiades' single case report are concordant with Behçet's disease. The authors who informed people of the above cases had tried to claim other illnesses with the symptoms that these patients showed. They tried to explain these symptoms with septic metastasis, tuberculosis, syphilis, focal bacterial infections, allergies or coincidental combination of the respected symptoms. Not one of the authors above could claim their findings as a new and single illness or syndrome. Benediktos Adamantiades in an article written much later (12 years after Hulusi Behçet's original publication), actually chose to use Behçet's name in describing the disease [65].

By the work which the Editor Hasan Yazıcı brought us today the English translation of the original work of Hulusi Behçet, the article can be reached [11] and readers can clearly understand that Hulusi Behçet demonstrated the lesions of

Table 2.1 Case reports considered today to be concordant with Behçet's disease before Dr. Adamantiades' single case report

Date	Author(s)	Findings	Journal/congress
1772	Janin [30]	Recurrent hypopyon iritis	Fréres Périsse, Lyon-PF Didot, Paris
1895	Neumann [31]	Recurrent oral and genital ulcers	*Wien Klin Rundsch*
1895	Christlieb [32]	Recurrent oral and genital ulcers	Inaugural dissertation. Universität Würzburg
1906	Reis [33]	Recurrent eye inflammation together with erythema nodosum and arthritis	*Klin Monatsbl Augenheilkd*
1908	Blüthe [34]	Recurrent hypopyon iritis–iridocyclitis, mucocutaneous findings and arthritis. Histologic findings of uveitis and optic atrophy	Inaugural thesis, D Strauss, Heidelberg
1920–1925	Gilbert [35–38]	Recurrent hypopyon iritis–iridocyclitis, recurrent arthritis, mucocutaneous findings and histologic findings of uveitis	*Arch Augenheilkd* (1920); *Arch Augenheilkd* (1921); *Klin Monatsbl Augenheilkd* (1923); *Arch Augenheilkd* (1925)
1922	Planner and Remenowsky [57]	Iritis and genital lesion	*Arch Dermatol Syphil (Berlin)*
1923	Weve [43]	Recurrent hypopyon iritis–iridocyclitis, mucocutaneous findings, arthritis, periodontitis, and neurologic findings	*Arch Augenheilkd*
1924	Shigeta [58]	Recurrent mucocutaneous ulcers, recurrent hypopyon iritis, and histologic findings of uveitis and optic atrophy	*Acta Soc Ophthalmol Jpn*
1925	Pils [59]	Mucocutaneous findings, thrombophlebitis, and arthralgia	*Arch Dermatol Syphil (Berlin)*
1926	Grütz [60]	Recurrent genital lesion and arthralgia	*Zbl Haut*
1928	Carol and Ruys [61]	Recurrent genital lesion and arthralgia	*Ned Tschr Genek*
1929	Samek and Fisher [62]	Recurrent mucocutaneous lesions, erythema nodosum, and first introduction of skin pathergy test	*Arch Dermatol Syphil (Berlin)*
1930	Walter and Roman [63]	Recurrent mucocutaneous lesions (histologic findings of leukocytoclastic vasculitis in genital ulcer and skin lesion)	*Dermatol Wochenschr*
1930	Kumer [64]	Mucocutaneous lesions (histologic findings of leukocytoclastic vasculitis in genital ulcer and erythema nodosum) and neurologic findings	*Dermatol Z*

the mouth, the genitalia, and the eye together. Although scientific discoveries often reflect a group effort over time, they usually refer to one person [66, 67]. The man behind the eponym "Behçet's disease" is Hulusi Behçet.

The term "Silk Road disease" started being used occasionally following the first international congress for Behcet's disease patients in Japan in 2000. Authors mostly of Far Eastern origin used this expression as a synonym for Behçet's disease. The disease's name, Silk Road disease, was derived from its high occurrence in countries bordering the Mediterranean and the Far East. These countries are all situated between the 30th and 45th parallel north. The occurrence of the disease and HLA-B_{51} carriage is infrequent in the northern or southern part of this parallel. The disease is believed by Silk Road defenders to have spread along its trade route. However, it is more scientifically sound to explain gene distribution through ancient demographic movements, rather than trade routes. Another important point worth considering is the time difference between the period when the disease is identified and the period when the Silk Road is active [68].

In conclusion, the authors who meticulously documented the clinical signs and symptoms of the disease throughout history undoubtedly had a significant impact on defining the disease. However, it is important to acknowledge that describing a clinical picture is not equivalent to initially perceiving it as a distinct disease. Hulusi Behçet took the observed symptoms described throughout history and by grouping the symptoms he tried to explain them with one illness; as a result, he deserved to take a place in modern medicine. This is the distinguishing characteristic of Hulusi Behçet compared to other authors.

References

1. Saylan T. Life story of Dr. Hulusi Behçet. Yonsei Med J. 1997;38:327–32.
2. Tüzün Y. Hulusi Behçet, MD: February 20, 1889 to March 8, 1948. Clin Dermatol. 2006;24(6):548–50.
3. Shampo MA, Davis MD. Dermatologists honored on stamps. Arch Dermatol. 2006;142(11):1489–92.
4. Paksoy N. Behçet, Hulusi (1889–1948). In: van den Tweel JG, editor. Pioneers in pathology. Encyclopedia of pathology. Cham: Springer; 2017. https://doi.org/10.1007/978-3-319-41995-4_4037.
5. Ustün C. A famous Turkish dermatologist, Dr. Hulusi Behçet. Eur J Dermatol. 2002;12(5):469–70.
6. Alpsoy E. Behçet disease. Turkderm. 2009;43(Suppl 2):21–3.
7. Dilsen N. History and development of Behçet's disease. Rev Rhum Engl Ed. 1996;63:512–9.
8. Kartal Durmazlar SP, Kandi B. Naming dilemma of Behçet's disease. J Turk Acad Dermatol. 2011;5(1):jtad1151r1.
9. Evereklioglu C. Behcet's disease or Adamantiades-Behcet disease? An evidence-based historical survey. Med Sci Monit. 2010;16(6):RA136-42.
10. Behçet H. Ü ber rezidivierende, Aphthöse, durch ein Virus verursachte Geschwüre am Mund, am Auge und an den Genitalien. Dermatol Wochenschr. 1937;105:1152–7.
11. Behçet H, Matteson EL. On relapsing, aphthous ulcers of the mouth, eye and genitalia caused by a virus. 1937. Clin Exp Rheumatol. 2010;28(4 Suppl 60):S2–5.
12. Behçet H. Einige Bemerkungen zu meinen Beobachtungen über den Tri-Symptomenkomplex. Med Welt. 1939;13:1222–7.
13. Behçet H. Some observations on the clinical picture of the so-called triple symptom complex. Dermatologica. 1940;81:73–83.
14. Jensen T. Sur les ulcérations aphteuses de la muqueuse de la bouche et de la peau génitale combinées avec les symptômes oculaires (=Syndrôme Behçet). Acta Dermatol Venereol. 1941;22:64–79.
15. Jensen T. Ulcerous haemorrhagic colitis associated with Behçet's syndrome. Ugeskrift För Laeger. 1941;106:176–80.
16. Berlin C. Behçet's syndrome with involvement of central nervous system. Report of a case, with necropsy, of lesions of the mouth, genitalia and eyes; review of the literature. Arch Dermatol Syphil (Chicago). 1944;49:227–33.
17. Ephraim H. Triple symptom complex of Behçet. Arch Dermatol Syphil (Chicago). 1944;50:37–8.
18. Ollendorff CH. Behçet's syndrome, abortive form (?) (recurrent genital ulcerations). Arch Dermatol Syphil (Chicago). 1946;54:481–3.
19. Ollendorff CH. Recurrent genito-oral aphthosis and uveitis with hypopyon (Behçet's syndrome). Arch Dermatol Syphil (Chicago). 1946;54:179–96.
20. Feigenbaum A, Kornblueth W. Behçet's disease as manifestation of a chronic septic condition connected with a constitutional disorder. With a report of 4 cases. Acta Med Orient. 1946;5:139–51.
21. Alpsoy E, Donmez L, Onder M, Gunasti S, Usta A, Karincaoglu Y, Kandi B, Buyukkara S, Keseroglu O, Uzun S, Tursen U, Seyhan M, Akman A. Clinical features and natural course of Behcet's disease in 661 cases: a multicentre study. Br J Dermatol. 2007;157(5):901–6.
22. International Study Group for Behçet's Disease. Criteria for diagnosis of Behçet's disease. Lancet. 1990;335:1078–80.
23. Unger L. The Behçet syndrome (Gilbert's ophthalmia lenta). Med Klin (Munich). 1957;52:1346–7.
24. Ito K, Ishii T, Mizuno A. Acneiform eruption of syphilis, Gilbert-Behçet's disease and papulonecrotic dermatophytid. Bull Pharm Res Inst. 1961;32:15–27.
25. Wollensak J, Frenger W. Observations on Gilbert-Behçet disease. Ber Zusammenkunft Dtsch Ophthalmol Ges. 1965;66:418–25.
26. Lemke L. The differential diagnosis of recurrent hypopyoniritis (Gilbert-Adamantiadis-Behçet disease). Acta Ophthalmol. 1965;43:487–95.
27. Cheng TO. Behçet disease, Adamantiades-Behçet disease or Hippocrates-Adamantiades-Behçet disease? Chest. 2002;122:381–2.
28. Adams F. The genuine works of Hippocrates, translated from the Greek. London: The Sydenham Society; 1849. p. 403–4.
29. Feigenbaum A. Description of Behçet's syndrome in the Hippocratic third book of endemic diseases. Br J Ophthalmol. 1956;40:355–7.
30. Janin J. Mémoires et observations anatomiques, physiologiques et physiques sur l'oeil, et sur les maladies qui affectent cet organe. Avec un précis des opérations et des remédies qu'on doit pratiquer pour les guerres. Fréres Périsse, Lyon-PF Didot, Paris, 1772. p. 412–4.
31. Neumann I. Die Aphthen am weiblichen Genitale. Wien Klin Rundsch. 1985;9:289–307.
32. Christlieb O. Über Stomatitis und Vulvitis aphthosa. Inaugural Dissertation. Universität Würzburg 1895.

33. Reis W. Augenerkrankung und Erythema nodosum. Klin Monatsbl Augenheilkd. 1906;44(203):6.
34. Blüthe L. Zur Kenntnis des rezidivierenden Hypopyons. Inauguralthesis, D Strauss, Heidelberg, 1908.
35. Gilbert W. Ü ber die rezidivierende eitrige Iridozyklitis (I.septica) und ihre Beziehungen zur septischen Allgemeinerkrankung. Arch Augenheilkd. 1920;86:29–49.
36. Gilbert W. Über den pathologisch-anatomischen Befund bei Iridocyclitis septica (Iritis mit rezidivierendem Hypopyon). Arch Augenheilkd. 1921;87:27–34.
37. Gilbert W. Zur Frage der Iridozyklitis mit rezidivierendem Hypopyon ("Iritis septica"). Klin Monatsbl Augenheilkd. 1923;71:409–14.
38. Gilbert W. Ü ber eine chronische Verlaufsformen der metastatischen Ophthalmie ("Ophthalmia lenta"). Arch Augenheilkd. 1925;96:119–30.
39. Adamantiades B. Sur un cas d'iritis à hypopion récidivant. Ann Ocul (Paris). 1931;168:271–8.
40. Adamantiades B. A case of recurrent hypopyon iritis. Proc Med Soc Athens. 1930:586–93.
41. Adamantiades B. La thrombophlébite comme quatrie'me symptôme de l'iritis récidivante à hypopyon. Ann Ocul (Paris). 1946;179:143–8.
42. Adamantiades B. Le symptôme complexe de l'uvéite récidivante à hypopyon. Ann Ocul (Paris). 1953;186:846.
43. Weve H. Über rezidivierende allergische Staphylokokkenuveitis. Arch Augenheilkd. 1923;93:14–39.
44. Dascalopoulos N. Sur deux cas d'uvéite récidivante. Ann Ocul (Paris). 1932;169:387–9.
45. von Hippel E. Ein Fall von Iridocyclitis mit rezidivierendem Hypopyon mit anatomischem Befund. Graefes Arch Clin Exp Ophthalmol. 1932;128:272–9.
46. Matras A. Über aphthenartige Mundschleimhautveränderungen beim Ulcus vulvae acutum mit positivem Bac. Crassus-Befund Arch Dermatol Syphil (Berl). 1932;166:491–7.
47. Urbanek J. Zur Frage der Entstehung und Ätiologie der periodisch rezidivierenden Hypopyon-Uveitis. Zeitschr Augenheilkd. 1932;79:145–58.
48. Urbanek J. Fall von rezidivierender Hypopyon-Uveitis. Zeitschr Augenheilkd. 1934;83:357–64.
49. Whitwell GP. Recurrent buccal and vulvar ulcers with associated embolic phenomenon in skin and eye. Br J Dermatol. 1934;46:414–9.
50. Nishimura M. A case of ulcus vulvae acutum with aphthae-like lesions in the mucous membranes of the mouth associated with acute iritis. Arch Dermatol Syphil (Chicago). 1936;34:900.
51. Blobner F. Zur rezidivierenden Hypopyoniritis. Z Augenheilkd. 1937;91:129–39.
52. Weekers L, Reginster H. Contribution à l'étude de l'iritis récidivante à hypopion (uvéite allergique récidivante à hypopion). Bull Soc Belg Ophthalmol. 1938;76:31–44.
53. Weekers L, Reginster H. Un nouveau syndrome: iritis, ulce'res aigus de la bouche et de la vulve. Sa parenté avec l'iritis récidivante à hypopion. Arch Ophthalmol (Paris). 1938;2:697–705.
54. Knapp P. Rezidivierende Hypopyoniritis. Ophthalmologica (Basel). 1938;96:297.
55. Schmidt R. Diskussionsbemerkung zu Stromburg: Zur Frage der rezidivierenden Hypopyoniritis. Vereinigung Rhein-Mainischer Augenärzte. Klin Monatsbl Augenheilkd. 1938;100:615.
56. Schmidt R. Zum Krankheitsbild der rezidivierenden Hypopyon-Uveitis. Graefes Arch Clin Exp Ophthalmol. 1940;142:185–202.
57. Planner H, Remenowsky F. Beiträge zur Kenntnis der Ulcerationen am außeren weiblichen Genitale. Arch Dermatol Syphil (Berlin). 1922;140:162–88.
58. Shigeta T. Recurrent iritis with hypopyon and its pathological findings. Acta Soc Ophthalmol Jpn. 1924;28:516–22.
59. Pils H. Ein Beitrag zur Aphthosis. Arch Dermatol Syphil (Berlin). 1925;149:4–8.
60. Grütz O. Stomatitis et vulvitis aphthosa chronica rezidivans (blastomycetica)? Zbl Haut. 1926;20:415–6.
61. Carol WL, Ruys SC. Over aphthosis en ulcus vulvae acutum. Ned Tschr Genek. 1928;1:396–406.
62. Samek J, Fischer E. Erythema nodosum als bakterielle Metastase eines Ulcus vulvae acutum. Arch Dermatol Syphil (Berlin). 1929;158:729–33.
63. Walter F, Roman I. Beitrag zur Kenntnis der hämatogenen Hautmetastasen bei Ulcus vulvae acutum. Dermatol Wochenschr. 1930;90:705–9.
64. Kumer L. Über Haut-und Mundschleimhauterscheinungen beim Ulcus vulvae acutum. Dermatol Z. 1930;57:401–11.
65. Adamantiades B, Lorando N. Sur le syndrome complexe de uvéite récidivante ou soi-distant syndrome complexe de Behçet. Presse Med. 1949;57:501.
66. Woywodt A, Matteson E. Should eponyms be abandoned? Yes. BMJ. 2007;335(7617):424.
67. Whitworth JA. Should eponyms be abandoned? No. BMJ. 2007;335(7617):425.
68. Satar G, Kadıoğlu FG. Disagreement on the nomination of the Behçet's disease; review. Turkiye Klinikleri J Med Ethics. 2014;22:1.

Behçet's Disease Epidemiology and Geographical Variations

3

Murat Borlu and Eda Öksüm Solak

Contents

3.1 Introduction

Behçet's disease (BD) occurs in individuals with a genetic predisposition and is triggered by various factors such as the environment and infection. Considering the regions where the disease is common, it reflects a distribution that supports that the disease occurs under the influence of both genetic and environmental factors. The disease was first defined by Prof. Hulusi Behçet who described it as a "triple symptom complex" disease in 1937 [1, 2]. The triple symptom complex refers to oral ulcers, genital ulcers, and eye involvement, which are the most common presentations of the disease; however, today it is known that many different organs and systems are involved. Its underlying pathology is primarily vasculitis, which significantly contributes to morbidity and, in severe cases, mortality. The prevalence of BD varies substantially across different regions worldwide. This chapter delves into the epidemiology and geographical distribution of BD, drawing upon current knowledge.

3.2 Incidence and Geographical Distribution

Epidemiological studies conducted to date and publications on the disease show that the disease is most frequently seen in Türkiye, the Middle East, and the Far East regions extending to

M. Borlu (✉) · E. Öksüm Solak
Dermatology and Venereology Department, Erciyes University Medical School, Kayseri, Türkiye

E. Alpsoy et al. (eds.), *Behçet's Disease: An Integrated Approach*,
https://doi.org/10.1007/978-3-031-77251-1_3

Japan, followed by European and African countries neighboring the Mediterranean Sea. Because a long and wide region from the Mediterranean to the Far East is affected by the disease, the disease was also named "Silk Road disease" in the past, referring to the historical "Silk Road." Studies indicate that in countries situated along the Silk Road, the prevalence of BD ranges between 14 and 20 per 100,000 people [3]. However, this definition does not fully reflect the distribution of the disease, and patients with signs of BD were mentioned even in the Hippocratic period when the historical Silk Road was not yet defined.

In the first prevalence study conducted in Türkiye by Demirhindi et al., patients were evaluated based on O'Duffy's diagnostic criteria resulting in a prevalence of 80 per 100,000 [4]. Similarly, Azizlerli et al. conducted a study in a similar region employing the International Study Group (ISG) Criteria for 23,986 individuals over 12 years old. The study found a BD prevalence of 420 per 100,000 [5].

In a study by İdil et al. in Ankara, an inland province of Türkiye, 17,256 individuals over 10 years old were included, and the BD prevalence was reported as 11 per 10,000 [6]. In the study conducted by Çölgeçen et al. in Kayseri province, a two-stage approach was undertaken. Individuals over 10 years old were included, with the first phase aimed at identifying individuals with recurrent oral ulcers (ROUs) through home visits, and the second phase aimed to further examine individuals with ROUs in hospital settings for the presence of other symptoms associated with BD. The study employed the ISG criteria established by the International Study Group for Behçet's Disease Group, revealing a BD prevalence of 170 per 100,000 [7].

A comprehensive two-stage cross-sectional study conducted in Türkiye involved the random selection of adults aged 20 and older from 52 urban and 33 rural family medicine offices. These individuals were invited to family medicine units and examined by three dermatologists. In the second stage, patients with symptoms suggestive of BD underwent pathergy tests, ophthalmologic examinations, and blood tests at the regional university hospital. This study reported a remarkably high prevalence of 600 per 100,000 in the sample population [8].

Other countries have presented different data regarding the prevalence of BD. For instance, in a multiethnic study conducted in France, the prevalence of BD was reported as 7.1 per 100,000 [9]. In Senegal, where the disease was expected to have a low incidence among black populations, an estimated annual incidence of 3.84 per 100,000 was reported [10]. The prevalence rate in the Kyushu region in the south of Japan stands at 1 per 100,000, whereas it increases significantly to 30 per 100,000 in the Hokkaido region in the north. In the UK, the prevalence rate was reported as 0.64 per 100,000, while in the United States, it falls within the range of 0.12–0.33 per 100,000 [11]. Remarkably, a study conducted in Jordan reported a much higher prevalence of BD, at 664 per 100,000, exceeding expectations [12]. Figure 3.1 and Table 3.1 show the prevalence of BD in different countries around the world.

The fact that the frequency of the disease and disease findings varies greatly can be explained by the use of different criteria to define the disease, differences in the application of the pathergy test, whether the studies are community based or hospital based, and in which specialty clinic the study was conducted. When reporting disease frequency, it is extremely important to include the method used in the studies in which these numbers were obtained. For these reasons, the scope and method of studies on disease frequency should be taken into consideration.

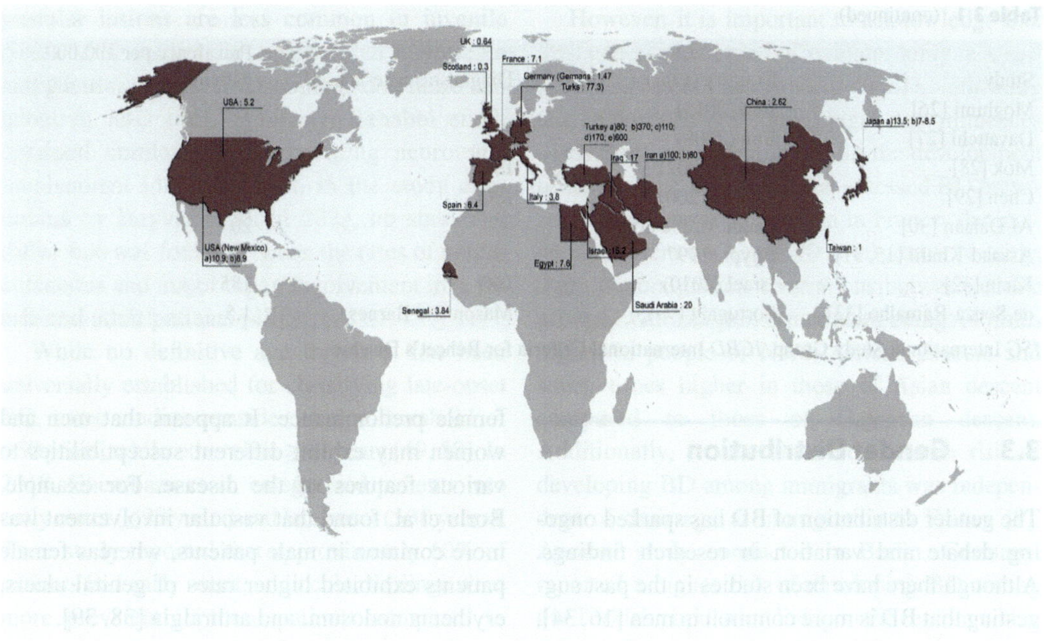

Fig. 3.1 The prevalence of Behçet's disease in the World

Table 3.1 Prevalences of Behçet's disease observed in different countries in the world

Study	Country (year)	Diagnostic criteria used	Prevalence per 100,000 patients
Demirhindi [4]	Türkiye (1981)	O'Duffy's	80
Yurdakul [13]	Türkiye (1988)	O'Duffy's	370
İdil [6]	Türkiye (2002)	ISG	110
Azizlerli [5]	Türkiye (2003)	ISG	421
Çölgeçen [7]	Türkiye (2015)	ISG	170
Yalçın [8]	Türkiye (2016)	ISG	600
Nakae [14, 15]	Japan (1993)		13.5
Yamamoto [16]	Japan (1974)		7–8.5
Mahr [9]	France (2003)	ISG	7.1
Papoutsis [17]	Germany (2006)		1.47 77.3
Altenburg [18]	Germany (2006)	ISG	4.16 (past 10 years)
Gonzalez-Gay [19]	Spain (2000)	ISG	6.4
Chamberlain [20]	UK (1977)	–	0.64
Salvarani [21]	Italy (2007)	ISG	3.8
Jankowski [22]	Scotland (1992)	ISG	0.3
Krause [23]	Israel (2007)	ISG	15.2
Ndiaye [10]	Senegal (2015)	ISG	3.84
Calamia [24]	United States (2009)	ISG	5.2
Muruganandam [25]	United States (2019)	ISG ICBD	10.9 8.9

(continued)

changing environmental factors can reduce the frequency of the disease even in the same race. It is important to consider how long ago and to what extent the environmental factors changed, and also in which generation these studies were carried out.

Studies conducted in various countries have shown variability in the familial prevalence of BD. Familial history was more frequently observed in Turkish (18.2%), Korean (15.4%), and Israeli (13.2%) patients with BD, compared to Chinese (2.6%), Japanese (2.2%), and European (ranging from 0% to 4.5%) patients with BD. Notably, the frequency of familial cases was significantly higher in pediatric patients (12.3%) than in adult patients (2.2%) [58].

The disease is more common in certain races, but it can vary depending on environmental changes even in the same race. Considering international migration and epigenetic factors, the frequency of BD may increase over time in countries where it is less common today.

3.6 Geographical Distribution of Clinical Findings

The clinical manifestations of BD also exhibit variations by geographic region. For instance, data collected in New York in 2005 indicated that patients of northern European descent had a higher incidence of gastrointestinal disease compared to patients from ethnically endemic regions. In contrast, fewer cases of eye disease and vascular involvement were reported in this population compared to other centers in Türkiye and Japan [40, 59]. Japan and Korea show a higher prevalence of gastrointestinal involvement than other countries [60]. The prevalence of ocular involvement in patients with BD varies between 28.9% and 79% in different reports, with a notably lower occurrence of ocular involvement (14.1%) in a study conducted in China compared to other countries [61].

Likewise, the pathergy test used in the diagnosis of BD exhibits geographical differences. While there is no standard consensus among clinicians on the most appropriate method to perform the test, studies have suggested that positive rates can be increased by making at least two needle punctures with a large hypodermic needle (21G or less) in the hairless skin of the forearm. The highest prevalence of pathergy positivity has been found in Silk Road countries, where BD also has the highest prevalence [62]. However, a recent study in Iran indicates that over the years, the sensitivity of the pathergy test has decreased, while its specificity has increased [63]. Studies from Türkiye and Japan also show a decrease in pathergy positivity over the years [41]. For instance, in a study conducted in Türkiye in the 1980s, pathergy positivity was 74%, whereas this rate was 37.8% in a 2007 study [42, 64] and 44.4% in a 2014 study [7]. These differences in pathergy test results may be attributed to variations in the test application methodology and ethnic characteristics. Furthermore, the widespread use of disposable needles instead of blunt, reusable, sterilized needles in recent years may have contributed to the decrease in the prevalence of positive test results [42]. In contrast to the 75% pathergy positivity rate in the 1975 study by Sakane et al. in Japan, this rate decreased to approximately 50% in the 2011 study [65, 66]. The incidence of the disease and the rate of pathergy positivity are gradually decreasing in Japan. However, the most significant decreasing symptom appears to be gastrointestinal involvement. This shows us that changing environmental factors, especially diet, may affect the frequency of the disease.

3.7 Conclusion

Genetic predisposition plays a significant role in determining the prevalence of BD. Notably, even among individuals sharing the same living environment, differences in prevalence due to ethnic origin are evident. Furthermore, varying prevalence rates are observed among communities of the same ethnic origin when environmental factors change, often due to migration. This highlights that not only ethnicity but also environmental disparities may influence disease prevalence. Over time, the prevalence of BD can change within the same populations, particularly in countries where the condition is common. Generally, the prevalence of BD has decreased over the last two decades in such regions. Additionally, the frequency of clinical manifestations of BD has evolved over time, leading to multiple revisions of diagnostic criteria. Therefore, it is imperative to periodically update studies on disease prevalence and continuously refresh our knowledge about BD.

References

1. Behçet H. Uber rezidivierende apthose, durch ein virüs verursachte Geschwure am Mund, am Auge und an den Genitalien. Dermatol Wochenschr. 1937;105:1152–7.
2. Acar A, Gerçeker TB. Etiology and pathogenesis. Behçet Hastalığı. Turkiye Klinikleri J Dermatol-Special Topics. 2017;10(4):271–7.
3. Alpsoy E, Zouboulis CC, Ehrlich GE. Mucocutaneous lesions of Behcet's disease. Yonsei Med J. 2007;48(4):573–85. https://doi.org/10.3349/ymj.2007.48.4.573.
4. Demirhindi O, et al. Silivri Fener koyu ve yoresinde Behçet hastaligi sikligi ve bu hastaligin toplum icinde taranabilmesinde kullanabilecek bir yontem. Cerrahpasa Tip Fak Derg. 1981;12(1):509–14.
5. Azizlerli G, Köse AA, Sarica R, et al. Prevalence of Behçet's disease in Istanbul. Turkey Int J Dermatol. 2003;42(10):803–6. https://doi.org/10.1046/j.1365-4362.2003.01893.x.
6. Idil A, Gürler A, Boyvat A, et al. The prevalence of Behçet's disease above the age of 10 years. The results of a pilot study conducted at the Park Primary Health Care Center in Ankara, Turkey. Ophthalmic Epidemiol. 2002;9(5):325–31. https://doi.org/10.1076/opep.9.5.325.10338.
7. Çölgeçen E, Özyurt K, Ferahbaş A, et al. The prevalence of Behçet's disease in a city in Central Anatolia in Turkey. Int J Dermatol. 2015;54(3):286–9. https://doi.org/10.1111/ijd.12173.
8. Baş Y, Seçkin HY, Kalkan G, et al. Investigation of Behçet's disease and recurrent Aphthous stomatitis frequency: the highest prevalence in Turkey. Balkan Med J. 2016;33(4):390–5. https://doi.org/10.5152/balkanmedj.2016.15101.
9. Mahr A, Belarbi L, Wechsler B, et al. Population-based prevalence study of Behçet's disease: differences by ethnic origin and low variation by age at immigration. Arthritis Rheum. 2008;58(12):3951–9. https://doi.org/10.1002/art.24149.
10. Ndiaye M, et al. Behçet's disease in black skin. A retrospective study of 50 cases in Dakar. J Dermatol Case Rep. 2015;9:98–102.
11. Sakane T, Takeno M, Suzuki N, et al. Behçet's disease. N Engl J Med. 1999;341(17):1284–91. https://doi.org/10.1056/NEJM199910213411707.
12. Madanat WY, Alawneh KM, Smadi MM, et al. The prevalence of Behçet's disease in the north of Jordan: a hospital-based epidemiological survey. Clin Exp Rheumatol. 2017;35(Suppl 108(6)):51–4.
13. Yurdakul S, Günaydin I, Tüzün Y, Tankurt N, Pazarli H, Ozyazgan Y, Yazici H. The prevalence of Behçet's syndrome in a rural area in northern Turkey. J Rheumatol. 1988;15(5):820–2.
14. Nakae K, Masaki F, Hashimato T, Inaba G, Mochizuki M, Sakane T. Recent epidemiological features of Behçet's disease in Japan. In: Wechsler B, Godeau P, editors. Behçet's disease. Amsterdam: Excerpta Medica; 1993. p. 145–51.
15. Yurdakul S, Yazıcı Y. Epidemiology of Behçet's syndrome and regional differences in disease expression. In: Yazıcı Y, Yazıcı H, editors. Behçet's Syndrome. Springer Science+Business Media.
16. Yamamoto Sİ. A nation-wide survey of Behcet's disease in Japan-1-epidemiological survey. Jpn J Ophthalmol. 1974;18(3):282–90.
17. Papoutsis NG, Abdel-Naser MB, Altenburg A, et al. Prevalence of Adamantiades-Behçet's disease in Germany and the municipality of Berlin: results of a nationwide survey. Clin Exp Rheumatol. 2006;24(5 Suppl 42):S125. Erratum in: Clin Exp Rheumatol. 2007 May-Jun;25(3):507–8
18. Altenburg A, Papoutsis N, Orawa H, et al. Epidemiologie und Klinik des Morbus Adamantiades-Behçet in Deutschland—Aktuelle pathogenetische Konzepte und therapeutische Möglichkeiten [epidemiology and clinical manifestations of Adamantiades-Behçet disease in Germany—current pathogenetic concepts and therapeutic possibilities]. J Dtsch Dermatol Ges. 2006;4(1):49–64; quiz 65-6. German. https://doi.org/10.1111/j.1610-0387.2006.05841.x.
19. González-Gay MA, García-Porrúa C, Brañas F, López-Lázaro L, Olivieri I. Epidemiologic and clinical aspects of Behçet's disease in a defined area of Northwestern Spain, 1988–1997. J Rheumatol. 2000;27(3):703–7.
20. Chamberlain MA. Behcet's syndrome in 32 patients in Yorkshire. Ann Rheum Dis. 1977;36(6):491–9. https://doi.org/10.1136/ard.36.6.491.
21. Salvarani C, Pipitone N, Catanoso MG, Cimino L, Tumiati B, Macchioni P, Bajocchi G, Olivieri I, Boiardi L. Epidemiology and clinical course of Behçet's disease in the Reggio Emilia area of Northern Italy: a seventeen-year population-based study. Arthritis Rheum. 2007;57(1):171–8. https://doi.org/10.1002/art.22500.
22. Jankowski J, Crombie I, Jankowski R. Behçet's syndrome in Scotland. Postgrad Med J. 1992;68(801):566–70. https://doi.org/10.1136/pgmj.68.801.566.
23. Krause I, Yankevich A, Fraser A, et al. Prevalence and clinical aspects of Behcet's disease in the north of

Israel. Clin Rheumatol. 2007;26(4):555–60. https://doi.org/10.1007/s10067-006-0349-4.
24. Calamia KT, Wilson FC, Icen M, Crowson CS, Gabriel SE, Kremers HM. Epidemiology and clinical characteristics of Behçet's disease in the US: a population-based study. Arthritis Rheum. 2009;61(5):600–4. https://doi.org/10.1002/art.24423.
25. Muruganandam M, Rolle NA, Sibbitt WL Jr, et al. Characteristics of Behcet's disease in the American Southwest. Semin Arthritis Rheum. 2019;49(2):296–302. https://doi.org/10.1016/j.semarthrit.2019.03.003.
26. Moghimi N, Davatchi F, Rahimi E, et al. WHO-ILAR COPCORD study (stage 1, urban study) in Sanandaj. Iran Clin Rheumatol. 2015;34(3):535–43. https://doi.org/10.1007/s10067-013-2430-0.
27. Davatchi F, Jamshidi AR, Banihashemi AT, et al. WHO-ILAR COPCORD study (stage 1, urban study) in Iran. J Rheumatol. 2008;35(7):1384.
28. Mok CC, Cheung TC, Ho CT, Lee KW, Lau CS, Wong RW. Behçet's disease in southern Chinese patients. J Rheumatol. 2002;29(8):1689–93.
29. Chen YC, Chang HW. Clinical characteristics of Behçet's disease in southern Taiwan. J Microbiol Immunol Infect. 2001;34(3):207–10.
30. Al-Dalaan A, Bahabri S, Al-Balla SR, Al-Sheikh AA, Al-Humidan E, Al-Sedairy ST. Abnormalities of T cell subsets in Behcet disease. Ann Saudi Med. 1993;13(3):275–9. https://doi.org/10.5144/0256-4947.1993.275.
31. Assaad-Khalil SH, Kamel FA, Ismail EA. Starting a regional registry for patients with Behçet's disease in north West Nile Delta region in Egypt. Behçet's Disease. 1997:173–6.
32. Klein P, Weinberger A, Altmann VJ, Halabi S, Fachereldeen S, Krause I. Prevalence of Behcet's disease among adult patients consulting three major clinics in a Druze town in Israel. Clin Rheumatol. 2010;29(10):1163–6. https://doi.org/10.1007/s10067-010-1472-9. Epub 2010 May 14
33. de Souza-Ramalho P, D'Almeida MF, Freitas JP, Pinto J. Behçet's disease in Portugal. Acta Medica Port. 1991;4(2):79–82.
34. Yazici H, Tüzün Y, Pazarli H, et al. Influence of age of onset and patient's sex on the prevalence and severity of manifestations of Behcet's syndrome. Ann Rheum Dis. 1984;43(6):783–9.
35. Alpsoy E, Bozca BC, Bilgic A. Behçet disease: an update for dermatologists. Am J Clin Dermatol. 2021;22(4):477–502.
36. Cho SB, Cho S, Bang D. New insights in the clinical understanding of Behçet's disease. Yonsei Med J. 2012;53:35–42.
37. Davatchi F, Chams-Davatchi C, Shams H, et al. Behcet's disease: epidemiology, clinical manifestations, and diagnosis. Expert Rev Clin Immunol. 2017;13(1):57–65.
38. Borlu M, Demırel B, Kartal D, et al. The effects of epidemiological and clinical findings in Behçet's disease on the course and prognosis of the disease. Acta Med Mediterr. 2016;32:843.
39. Mahr A, Maldini C. Épidémiologie de la maladie de Behçet [Epidemiology of Behçet's disease]. Rev Med Interne. 2014;35(2):81–9. French. https://doi.org/10.1016/j.revmed.2013.12.005.
40. Yazici H, Seyahi E, Hatemi G, Yazici Y. Behçet syndrome: a contemporary view. Nat Rev Rheumatol. 2018;14(2):107–19. https://doi.org/10.1038/nrrheum.2017.208.
41. Cansu DÜ, Kaşifoğlu T, Korkmaz C. Do clinical findings of Behçet's disease vary by gender?: a single-center experience from 329 patients. Eur J Rheumatol. 2016;3(4):157–60. https://doi.org/10.5152/eurjrheum.2016.038.
42. Alpsoy E, Donmez L, Onder M, et al. Clinical features and natural course of Behçet's disease in 661 cases: a multicentre study. Br J Dermatol. 2007;157(5):901–6. https://doi.org/10.1111/j.1365-2133.2007.08116.x.
43. Borlu M, Ukşal U, Ferahbaş A, et al. Clinical features of Behçet's disease in children. Int J Dermatol. 2006;45(6):713–6. https://doi.org/10.1111/j.1365-4632.2006.02754.x.
44. Koné-Paut I. Behçet's disease in children, an overview. Pediatr Rheumatol Online J. 2016;14(1):10. https://doi.org/10.1186/s12969-016-0070-z.
45. Karincaoglu Y, Borlu M, Toker SC, et al. Demographic and clinical properties of juvenile-onset Behçet's disease: a controlled multicenter study. J Am Acad Dermatol. 2008;58(4):579–84. https://doi.org/10.1016/j.jaad.2007.10.452.
46. Krause I, Uziel Y, Guedj D, et al. Childhood Behçet's disease: clinical features and comparison with adult-onset disease. Rheumatology (Oxford). 1999;38(5):457–62. https://doi.org/10.1093/rheumatology/38.5.457.
47. Bahabri SA, al-Mazyed A, al-Balaa S, el-Ramahi L, al-Dalaan A. Juvenile Behçet's disease in Arab children. Clin Exp Rheumatol. 1996;14(3):331–5.
48. Boyvat A, Oktem A, Kalay Yildizhan I, Ates A, Yalcindag N, Koksoy C, Yucesan C. A comparison of adult and juvenile Behcet patients and a look at clinical trends: retrospective data from a Turkish follow-up cohort study. Dermatology. 2023;239(6):958–65. https://doi.org/10.1159/000534316.
49. Sungur G, Hazirolan D, Hekimoglu E, et al. Late-onset Behçet's disease: demographic, clinical, and ocular features. Graefes Arch Clin Exp Ophthalmol. 2010;248(9):1325–30. https://doi.org/10.1007/s00417-010-1399-5.
50. Güzelant ÖG. Late-Onset Behçet's Disease. In: Seyahi E, editor. Behçet's disease. 1st ed. Ankara: Türkiye Klinikleri; 2020. p. 85–8.
51. Ghembaza MEA, Lounici A. Relationship between age at onset and clinical characteristics of Behçet's disease. Acta Dermatovenerol Alp Pannonica Adriat. 2018;27(4):175–7.
52. Ishido T, Horita N, Takeuchi M, et al. Clinical manifestations of Behçet's disease depending on sex and

age: results from Japanese nationwide registration. Rheumatology (Oxford). 2017;56(11):1918–27. https://doi.org/10.1093/rheumatology/kex285.
53. Akkoç N. Update on the epidemiology, risk factors and disease outcomes of Behçet's disease. Best Pract Res Clin Rheumatol. 2018;32(2):261–70. https://doi.org/10.1016/j.berh.2018.08.010.
54. Dalvi SR, Yildirim R, Yazici Y. Behcet's Syndrome. Drugs. 2012;72(17):2223–41. https://doi.org/10.2165/11641370-000000000-00000.
55. Mohammad A, Mandl T, Sturfelt G, et al. Incidence, prevalence and clinical characteristics of Behcet's disease in southern Sweden. Rheumatology (Oxford). 2013;52(2):304–10. https://doi.org/10.1093/rheumatology/kes249.
56. Kappen JH, van Dijk EH, Baak-Dijkstra M, et al. Behçet's disease, hospital-based prevalence and manifestations in the Rotterdam area. Neth J Med. 2015;73(10):471–7.
57. Hirohata T, Kuratsune M, Nomura A, et al. Prevalence of Behçet's syndrome in Hawaii. With particular reference to the comparison of the Japanese in Hawaii and Japan. Hawaii Med J. 1975;34(7):244–6.
58. Koné-Paut I, Geisler I, Wechsler B, et al. Familial aggregation in Behçet's disease: high frequency in siblings and parents of pediatric probands. J Pediatr. 1999;135(1):89–93. https://doi.org/10.1016/s0022-3476(99)70333-1.
59. Yazici Y, Filopoulos MT, Schimmel E, et al. Clinical characteristics, treatment and ethnic/racial differences in the manifestations of 518 Behcet's syndrome patients in the United States [abstract]. Arthritis Rheum. 2010;62(Suppl):1284.
60. Tursen U, Gurler A, Boyvat A. Evaluation of clinical findings according to sex in 2313 Turkish patients with Behçet's disease. Int J Dermatol. 2003;42(5):346–51. https://doi.org/10.1046/j.1365-4362.2003.01741.x.
61. Wang LY, Zhao DB, Gu J, et al. Clinical characteristics of Behçet's disease in China. Rheumatol Int. 2010;30(9):1191–6. https://doi.org/10.1007/s00296-009-1127-9.
62. International Team for the Revision of the International Criteria for Behçet's Disease (ITR-ICBD). The international criteria for Behçet's disease (ICBD): a collaborative study of 27 countries on the sensitivity and specificity of the new criteria. J Eur Acad Dermatol Venereol. 2014;28(3):338–47. https://doi.org/10.1111/jdv.12107.
63. Davatchi F, Chams-Davatchi C, Ghodsi Z, et al. Diagnostic value of pathergy test in Behcet's disease according to the change of incidence over the time. Clin Rheumatol. 2011;30:1151–5.
64. Alpsoy E. Behçet's disease. Epidemiol Turkiye Klinikleri J Dermatol-Special Topics. 2017;10(4):265–70.
65. Yazici H, Tüzün Y, Tanman AB, et al. Male patients with Behçet's syndrome have stronger pathergy reactions. Clin Exp Rheumatol. 1985;3(2):137–41.
66. Ideguchi H, Suda A, Takeno M, et al. Behçet disease: evolution of clinical manifestations. Medicine (Baltimore). 2011;90(2):125–32. https://doi.org/10.1097/MD.0b013e318211bf28.

What Do the Genetic Studies Tell Us About Behçet Disease?

4

Ahmet Gül

Contents

4.1 Introduction

Behçet disease (BD) is an inflammatory disorder with a multifactorial etiology, and a complex genetic tendency plays an important role in its pathogenesis [1, 2]. Familial aggregation had long been noted, and analysis of families in Turkey revealed high sibling recurrence risk ratio (λs) values ranging between 11.4 and 52.5, which suggests a strong genetic contribution [3]. Ortiz-Fernandez and Sawalha analyzed the Immunochip genotyping data of a large case–control cohort from Türkiye and estimated the narrow sense heritability (h^2) of BD as 0.36 (SE = 0.03) on the observed scale based on the proportion of variance in case–control status. However, they calculated the liability scale as 0.16 (SE = 0.02) after a correction for the ascertainment bias [4]. BD has several monogenic mimics, but typical cases are multifactorial, and heritability analyses also support an important contribution of environmental factors to the pathogenesis [1, 5, 6].

BD is much more prevalent in the Eastern Mediterranean populations and along the Silk Road up to China, Korea, and Japan compared to the northern European and American populations, and the contribution of genetics may also show variations in different ethnic groups [4]. The geographic distribution of BD overlaps greatly with the frequency of Human Leukocyte Antigen (HLA)-B51 allele in the healthy

A. Gül (✉)
Division of Rheumatology, Department of Internal Medicine, Istanbul Faculty of Medicine, Istanbul University, Istanbul, Türkiye
e-mail: agul@istanbul.edu.tr

E. Alpsoy et al. (eds.), *Behçet's Disease: An Integrated Approach*,
https://doi.org/10.1007/978-3-031-77251-1_4

4.4 Phenotype and Genetics

The clinical presentation of BD is heterogeneous, and factor analysis or hierarchical cluster analysis methods have revealed different disease subsets, such as those characterized mainly by mucocutaneous only, mucocutaneous and arthritis, uveitis, vascular, gastrointestinal, and neurologic manifestations [33, 34]. The distribution of these phenotypic features may show ethnic or time-dependent changes, and the role of genetics in the determination of disease subsets has not been clarified so far. HLA-B*51 has been associated with the characteristic features of BD with the complete phenotype including uveitis, and HLA-A*26 has also been associated with uveitis in Japanese patients [12, 13, 35]. On the other hand, HLA-B*51 has not been associated with gastrointestinal involvement, which may explain the decreasing frequency of HLA-B*51 in Japanese patients along with a decrease in the frequency of patients with the complete type of BD manifestations and an increase in the frequency of those patients with gastrointestinal manifestations [36].

Available genetic studies lack enough power to explore the heterogeneity of clinical presentations by subgroup analyses. Uveitis has usually been the largest subset in endemic areas, and a recent study screening the uveitis group reported novel associations with ZMIZ1, RPS6KA4, IL10RA, SIPA1-FIBP-FOSL1, and VAMP1 in Chinese patients [37], but none of them was replicated in other populations. Another study investigated manifestation-specific variations by conducting a case–case association study and reported novel associations in the ocular subset with SLCO4A1 and in the neurologic subset with DDX60L [38]. Further studies are required to clarify whether the phenotypic heterogeneity and disease subsets are associated with manifestation-specific genes, or different environmental triggers are responsible for the activation of organ-specific inflammatory responses in a shared genetic background.

4.5 Epigenetic Changes

Epigenetic changes may also contribute to the genetic susceptibility to BD, and some of them may even be resolved with the treatment. An epigenome-wide study of DNA methylation revealed aberrant gene expressions in cytoskeletal genes in monocytes and CD4 T cells of Turkish BD patients, and a reversal of the DNA methylation was observed with the treatment of BD manifestations [39]. Lower methylation of the HLA-B locus and a relatively higher expression of HLA-B*51 were observed in familial and sporadic BD cases compared to their unaffected relatives or healthy controls [40]. Another epigenome-wide study in Han Chinese patients with BD uveitis revealed hypomethylation of four genes, namely FKBP5, FLJ43663, RUNX2, and NFIL3, and it was most significantly different for FKBP5 [41].

Analysis of the circulating miRNAs showed the deregulation of miR-224-5p, miR-206, and miR-653-5p, and the annotation analyses suggested an associated functional role in thrombo-inflammatory mechanisms [42].

Overall, epigenetic studies have several limitations, and the significance of the reported findings should be evaluated with further replication and functional studies.

4.6 Genetics and Diagnosis

As discussed in the introduction, BD is a multifactorial disease, and there is no place for genetic testing in the diagnosis. There are only preliminary approaches for the calculation of polygenic risk scores, and there is no study documenting the use of these scores in the initial evaluation of BD patients or prediction of their prognosis [4].

HLA-B*51 has been the strongest genetic factor described so far; however, it could not be used as a diagnostic test [36]. The frequency of HLA-B*51 may be as high as 29% in some healthy populations, and its pathogenic role has been affected by the contributions of the ERAP1 variants, other genetic polymorphisms, and environmental triggers. Further studies are being awaited for the development of novel methods, which could be used for the prediction of disease prognosis or treatment responses.

4.7 Conclusions

Genetics play an important role in the pathogenesis of BD, and GWAS conducted in relatively large samples of patients and controls revealed several genetic variations, which affect the innate and adaptive immune responses to yet unidentified environmental triggers. Some of these susceptibility genes are shared with disorders characterized by aphthous ulcers and some are with SpA and IBD (Fig. 4.1). However, HLA-B*51 is still the most significant risk factor defining the characteristic phenotype of BD among all others, and ERAP1 haplotype 10-driven peptidome contributes to the pathogenesis by affecting the proper folding of HLA-B*51 molecule in the endoplasmic reticulum and also activation of cytotoxic T-cell and NK cell responses.

References

1. Gul A. Genetics of Behcet's disease: lessons learned from genomewide association studies. Curr Opin Rheumatol. 2014;26(1):56–63. https://doi.org/10.1097/BOR.0000000000000003.
2. Gul A. Pathogenesis of Behcet's disease: autoinflammatory features and beyond. Semin Immunopathol. 2015;37(4):413–8. https://doi.org/10.1007/s00281-015-0502-8.
3. Gul A, Inanc M, Ocal L, Aral O, Konice M. Familial aggregation of Behcet's disease in Turkey. Ann Rheum Dis. 2000;59(8):622–5. https://doi.org/10.1136/ard.59.8.622.
4. Ortiz-Fernandez L, Sawalha AH. Genetics of Behcet's disease: functional genetic analysis and estimating disease heritability. Front Med (Lausanne). 2021;8:625710. https://doi.org/10.3389/fmed.2021.625710.
5. Papadopoulou C, Omoyinmi E, Standing A, Pain CE, Booth C, D'Arco F, et al. Monogenic mimics of Behcet's disease in the young. Rheumatology (Oxford). 2019;58(7):1227–38. https://doi.org/10.1093/rheumatology/key445.
6. Burleigh A, Omoyinmi E, Papadopoulou C, Al-Abadi E, Hong Y, Price-Kuehne F, et al. Genetic testing of Behcet's disease using next-generation sequencing to identify monogenic mimics and HLA-B*51. Rheumatology (Oxford). 2023; https://doi.org/10.1093/rheumatology/kead628.
7. Verity DH, Marr JE, Ohno S, Wallace GR, Stanford MR. Behcet's disease, the Silk Road and HLA-B51: historical and geographical perspectives. Tissue Antigens. 1999;54(3):213–20. https://doi.org/10.1034/j.1399-0039.1999.540301.x.
8. Abi-Rached L, Jobin MJ, Kulkarni S, McWhinnie A, Dalva K, Gragert L, et al. The shaping of modern human immune systems by multiregional admixture with archaic humans. Science. 2011;334(6052):89–94. https://doi.org/10.1126/science.1209202.
9. Ohno S, Aoki K, Sugiura S, Nakayama E, Itakura K, Aizawa M. Letter: HL-A5 and Behcet's disease. Lancet. 1973;2(7842):1383–4. https://doi.org/10.1016/s0140-6736(73)93343-6.
10. Ohno S, Asanuma T, Sugiura S, Wakisaka A, Aizawa M, Itakura K. HLA-Bw51 and Behcet's disease. JAMA. 1978;240(6):529.
11. de Menthon M, Lavalley MP, Maldini C, Guillevin L, Mahr A. HLA-B51/B5 and the risk of Behcet's disease: a systematic review and meta-analysis of case-control genetic association studies. Arthritis Rheum. 2009;61(10):1287–96. https://doi.org/10.1002/art.24642.
12. Maldini C, Lavalley MP, Cheminant M, de Menthon M, Mahr A. Relationships of HLA-B51 or B5 genotype with Behcet's disease clinical characteristics: systematic review and meta-analyses of observational studies. Rheumatology (Oxford). 2012;51(5):887–900. https://doi.org/10.1093/rheumatology/ker428.
13. Gul A, Uyar FA, Inanc M, Ocal L, Tugal-Tutkun I, Aral O, et al. Lack of association of HLA-B*51 with a severe disease course in Behcet's disease. Rheumatology (Oxford). 2001;40(6):668–72. https://doi.org/10.1093/rheumatology/40.6.668.
14. Ombrello MJ, Kirino Y, de Bakker PI, Gul A, Kastner DL, Remmers EF. Behcet disease-associated MHC class I residues implicate antigen binding and regulation of cell-mediated cytotoxicity. Proc Natl Acad Sci USA. 2014;111(24):8867–72. https://doi.org/10.1073/pnas.1406575111.
15. Kirino Y, Bertsias G, Ishigatsubo Y, Mizuki N, Tugal-Tutkun I, Seyahi E, et al. Genome-wide association analysis identifies new susceptibility loci for Behcet's disease and epistasis between HLA-B*51 and ERAP1. Nat Genet. 2013;45(2):202–7. https://doi.org/10.1038/ng.2520.
16. Takeuchi M, Ombrello MJ, Kirino Y, Erer B, Tugal-Tutkun I, Seyahi E, et al. A single endoplasmic reticulum aminopeptidase-1 protein allotype is a strong risk

factor for Behcet's disease in HLA-B*51 carriers. Ann Rheum Dis. 2016;75(12):2208–11. https://doi.org/10.1136/annrheumdis-2015-209059.
17. Guasp P, Barnea E, Gonzalez-Escribano MF, Jimenez-Reinoso A, Regueiro JR, Admon A, Lopez de Castro JA. The Behcet's disease-associated variant of the aminopeptidase ERAP1 shapes a low-affinity HLA-B*51 peptidome by differential subpeptidome processing. J Biol Chem. 2017;292(23):9680–9. https://doi.org/10.1074/jbc.M117.789180.
18. Chen L, Shi H, Koftori D, Sekine T, Nicastri A, Ternette N, Bowness P. Identification of an unconventional subpeptidome bound to the Behcet's disease-associated HLA-B*51:01 that is regulated by endoplasmic reticulum aminopeptidase 1 (ERAP1). Mol Cell Proteomics. 2020;19(5):871–83. https://doi.org/10.1074/mcp.RA119.001617.
19. Cavers A, Kugler MC, Ozguler Y, Al-Obeidi AF, Hatemi G, Ueberheide BM, et al. Behcet's disease risk-variant HLA-B51/ERAP1-Hap10 alters human CD8 T cell immunity. Ann Rheum Dis. 2022;81(11):1603–11. https://doi.org/10.1136/ard-2022-222277.
20. Remmers EF, Cosan F, Kirino Y, Ombrello MJ, Abaci N, Satorius C, et al. Genome-wide association study identifies variants in the MHC class I, IL10, and IL23R-IL12RB2 regions associated with Behcet's disease. Nat Genet. 2010;42(8):698–702. https://doi.org/10.1038/ng.625.
21. Lee YJ, Horie Y, Wallace GR, Choi YS, Park JA, Choi JY, et al. Genome-wide association study identifies GIMAP as a novel susceptibility locus for Behcet's disease. Ann Rheum Dis. 2013;72(9):1510–6. https://doi.org/10.1136/annrheumdis-2011-200288.
22. Hou S, Yang Z, Du L, Jiang Z, Shu Q, Chen Y, et al. Identification of a susceptibility locus in STAT4 for Behcet's disease in Han Chinese in a genome-wide association study. Arthritis Rheum. 2012;64(12):4104–13. https://doi.org/10.1002/art.37708.
23. Xavier JM, Shahram F, Sousa I, Davatchi F, Matos M, Abdollahi BS, et al. FUT2: filling the gap between genes and environment in Behcet's disease? Ann Rheum Dis. 2015;74(3):618–24. https://doi.org/10.1136/annrheumdis-2013-204475.
24. Kappen JH, Medina-Gomez C, van Hagen PM, Stolk L, Estrada K, Rivadeneira F, et al. Genome-wide association study in an admixed case series reveals IL12A as a new candidate in Behcet disease. PLoS One. 2015;10(3):e0119085. https://doi.org/10.1371/journal.pone.0119085.
25. Ortiz-Fernandez L, Carmona FD, Montes-Cano MA, Garcia-Lozano JR, Conde-Jaldon M, Ortego-Centeno N, et al. Genetic analysis with the immunochip platform in Behcet disease. Identification of residues associated in the HLA class I region and new susceptibility loci. PLoS One. 2016;11(8):e0161305. https://doi.org/10.1371/journal.pone.0161305.
26. Takeuchi M, Mizuki N, Meguro A, Ombrello MJ, Kirino Y, Satorius C, et al. Dense genotyping of immune-related loci implicates host responses to microbial exposure in Behcet's disease susceptibility. Nat Genet. 2017;49(3):438–43. https://doi.org/10.1038/ng.3786.
27. Ortiz Fernandez L, Coit P, Yilmaz V, Yentur SP, Alibaz-Oner F, Aksu K, et al. Genetic association of a gain-of-function IFNGR1 polymorphism and the intergenic region LNCAROD/DKK1 with Behcet's disease. Arthritis Rheumatol. 2021;73(7):1244–52. https://doi.org/10.1002/art.41637.
28. Dudding T, Haworth S, Lind PA, Sathirapongsasuti JF, andMe Research T, Tung JY, et al. Genome wide analysis for mouth ulcers identifies associations at immune regulatory loci. Nat Commun. 2019;10(1):1052. https://doi.org/10.1038/s41467-019-08923-6.
29. Manthiram K, Preite S, Dedeoglu F, Demir S, Ozen S, Edwards KM, et al. Common genetic susceptibility loci link PFAPA syndrome, Behcet's disease, and recurrent aphthous stomatitis. Proc Natl Acad Sci USA. 2020;117(25):14405–11. https://doi.org/10.1073/pnas.2002051117.
30. Kirino Y, Zhou Q, Ishigatsubo Y, Mizuki N, Tugal-Tutkun I, Seyahi E, et al. Targeted resequencing implicates the familial Mediterranean fever gene MEFV and the toll-like receptor 4 gene TLR4 in Behcet disease. Proc Natl Acad Sci USA. 2013;110(20):8134–9. https://doi.org/10.1073/pnas.1306352110.
31. Burillo-Sanz S, Montes-Cano MA, Garcia-Lozano JR, Ortiz-Fernandez L, Ortego-Centeno N, Garcia-Hernandez FJ, et al. Mutational profile of rare variants in inflammasome-related genes in Behcet disease: a next generation sequencing approach. Sci Rep. 2017;7(1):8453. https://doi.org/10.1038/s41598-017-09164-7.
32. Burillo-Sanz S, Montes-Cano MA, Garcia-Lozano JR, Olivas-Martinez I, Ortego-Centeno N, Garcia-Hernandez FJ, et al. Behcet's disease and genetic interactions between HLA-B*51 and variants in genes of autoinflammatory syndromes. Sci Rep. 2019;9(1):2777. https://doi.org/10.1038/s41598-019-39113-5.
33. Tunc R, Keyman E, Melikoglu M, Fresko I, Yazici H. Target organ associations in Turkish patients with Behcet's disease: a cross sectional study by exploratory factor analysis. J Rheumatol. 2002;29(11):2393–6.
34. Soejima Y, Kirino Y, Takeno M, Kurosawa M, Takeuchi M, Yoshimi R, et al. Changes in the proportion of clinical clusters contribute to the phenotypic evolution of Behcet's disease in Japan. Arthritis Res Ther. 2021;23(1):49. https://doi.org/10.1186/s13075-020-02406-6.
35. Kato H, Takeuchi M, Horita N, Ishido T, Mizuki R, Kawagoe T, et al. HLA-A26 is a risk factor for Behcet's disease ocular lesions. Mod Rheumatol. 2021;31(1):214–8. https://doi.org/10.1080/14397595.2019.1705538.
36. Takeno M. The association of Behcet's syndrome with HLA-B51 as understood in 2021. Curr Opin Rheumatol. 2022;34(1):4–9. https://doi.org/10.1097/BOR.0000000000000846.

37. Su G, Zhong Z, Zhou Q, Du L, Ye Z, Li F, et al. Identification of novel risk loci for Behcet's disease-related uveitis in a Chinese population in a genome-wide association study. Arthritis Rheumatol. 2022;74(4):671–81. https://doi.org/10.1002/art.41998.
38. Casares-Marfil D, Esencan D, Alibaz-Oner F, Cefle A, Yazici A, Duzgun N, et al. Clinical trait-specific genetic analysis in Behcet's disease identifies novel loci associated with ocular and neurological involvement. Clin Immunol. 2023;253:109657. https://doi.org/10.1016/j.clim.2023.109657.
39. Hughes T, Ture-Ozdemir F, Alibaz-Oner F, Coit P, Direskeneli H, Sawalha AH. Epigenome-wide scan identifies a treatment-responsive pattern of altered DNA methylation among cytoskeletal remodeling genes in monocytes and CD4+ T cells from patients with Behcet's disease. Arthritis Rheumatol. 2014;66(6):1648–58. https://doi.org/10.1002/art.38409.
40. Ozkilinc Onen M, Everest E, Demirci T, Koprulu Sen P, Kiziltepe Kisakesen E, Ozguler Y, et al. HLA-B gene methylation and expression in Behcet's syndrome: a potential role of epigenetics in the pathogenesis. Clin Exp Rheumatol. 2024; https://doi.org/10.55563/clinexprheumatol/1sf43v.
41. Yu H, Du L, Yi S, Wang Q, Zhu Y, Qiu Y, et al. Epigenome-wide association study identifies Behcet's disease-associated methylation loci in Han Chinese. Rheumatology (Oxford). 2019;58(9):1574–84. https://doi.org/10.1093/rheumatology/kez043.
42. Emmi G, Bagni G, Lastraioli E, Di Patti F, Bettiol A, Fiorillo C, et al. A unique circulating miRNA profile highlights thrombo-inflammation in Behcet's syndrome. Ann Rheum Dis. 2022;81(3):386–97. https://doi.org/10.1136/annrheumdis-2021-220859.

How Behçet's Disease Occurs: Disease Mechanisms

5

Başak Yalçın and Erkan Alpsoy

Contents

5.1 Introduction

Behçet's disease [BD) is a chronic, immuno-inflammatory disease with multisystemic involvement. The exact cause of BD is unknown. Some environmental factors are suspected to trigger an abnormal immune response in genetically predisposed patients [1]. The genes that contribute to genetic predisposition can be categorized into two groups: HLA-associated genetic factors and non-HLA-associated genetic factors. Genetic factors predispose individuals to immune dysregulation, which is a crucial mechanism in the pathogenesis of diseases [2]. Therefore, individuals with a genetic predisposition may experience immune dysregulation, leading to the development of BD, due to various environmental factors such as bacterial and viral infections, as well as microbiota [3].

The pathogenesis of the disease is not fully understood, which complicates its classification within a specific group. While BD is classified as an inflammatory disease, it was inevitably influenced by the prevailing explanations for

B. Yalçın (✉)
Private Practice, Dermatology and Venereology, Ankara, Türkiye

E. Alpsoy
Dermatology and Venereology Department, Akdeniz University, School of Medicine, Antalya, Türkiye
e-mail: ealpsoy@akdeniz.edu.tr

E. Alpsoy et al. (eds.), *Behçet's Disease: An Integrated Approach*,
https://doi.org/10.1007/978-3-031-77251-1_5

5.4 Dysregulation of the Immune System

BD is predominantly considered an autoinflammatory disease in which dysfunction of the innate immune system plays a crucial role in pathogenesis. Unprovoked inflammatory episodes without signs of antigen-specific T cells or autoantibodies, increased neutrophil granulocyte activity, and elevated interleukin-1β (IL-1β) levels suggest an autoinflammatory background to the disease [1, 24].

Autoinflammatory diseases are a group of hereditary conditions characterized by recurrent inflammation attacks, particularly involving innate immunity, without any apparent cause and the absence of a clear autoimmune pathology. Unlike classical autoimmune diseases, there are no high levels of autoantibodies or antigen-specific T cells. Inflammatory attacks often affect the skin, serous membranes, joints, gastrointestinal tract, and eyes. Acute phase reactants are elevated. Familial Mediterranean fever is one of the most well-known autoinflammatory diseases. In recent years, in parallel with the advancements in genetics and molecular biology, autoinflammatory diseases have become better understood, and an increasing number of diseases have begun to be classified within this group. The definition of autoinflammatory diseases has been revised to include diseases in which innate immunity is the main element along with individual predisposition in their development, but in which adaptive immunity also contributes. McGonagle and McDermott classified BD as a mixed (complex) pattern disease, bridging polygenic autoimmune diseases and polygenic autoinflammatory diseases. One of the main reasons for this is the strong association of BD with MHC class I antigens [25].

The presence of autoantibodies and antigen-specific T cells in the pathogenesis of the disease, as well as the amelioration of the disease by classical immunosuppressive drugs, indicated the involvement of autoimmune mechanisms. However, it is now widely accepted that these incidents are mainly associated with tissue injury and do not directly contribute to the pathogenesis of the disease. Again, features such as the lack of anti-nuclear antibodies, female predominance, or an increased risk of autoimmunity do not support autoimmunity in BD [2].

The concept of seronegative spondyloarthropathy first emerged in 1974 to describe a group of diseases with shared genetic, epidemiological, clinical, and radiological features. Seronegative spondyloarthropathies are a heterogeneous group of diseases that primarily affect the sacroiliac joints and spine. They can cause organ involvement as well as joint symptoms. BD shares common features with seronegative spondyloarthropathies, such as eye and joint involvement, as well as skin and mucosal manifestations. However, the ocular involvement observed in BD differs from that seen in ankylosing spondylitis (AS), which is the prototype of spondyloarthropathies. While a mild anterior uveitis is commonly observed in AS, panuveitis is characteristic of BD, which can lead to blindness if not treated. Sacroiliitis is a highly specific clinical finding for AS; It is rarely observed in BD, at least its frequency is not increased compared to the general population. Skin/mucosal and genitourinary involvements that can be observed in reactive arthritis or Reiter syndrome, which is another important seronegative spondyloarthropathy, are also different from those seen in BD. Urethritis or circinate balanitis, which can be observed in reactive arthritis, are not found in BD, and genital ulcers, one of the most common clinical symptoms in BD, are not observed in reactive arthritis. BD is closely related to HLA-B*51 and has no obvious association with the HLA-B*27 antigen, which is detected with high frequency in AS [26].

In recent years, McGonagle et al. proposed that BD be defined as an "MHC-I-opathy" along with spondyloarthropathies such as AS, reactive arthritis, psoriatic arthritis (PsA) and inflammatory bowel disease-associated arthritis. In developing this definition, it is important to determine that the IL-17/IL-23 pathway, which is an active pathway in AS and PsA, is also significant in BD [8, 27]. On the other hand, BD is often associated with acne-like papulopustular lesions and arthritis, as well as enthesitis, which is a significant phenotypic feature of spondyloarthropathies. These observations have also contributed to the characterization of BD as an MHC-I-opathy. Common features of MHC-I-opathies include genetic associations linked to MHC-I-associated adaptive immunity, the initiation of typical innate immune-related inflammatory symptoms by tissue-specific factors (like injury, microdamage, and barrier dysfunction in environmentally exposed organs), and the significant involvement of unconventional lymphocytes like innate lymphoid cells in lymphoid stress monitoring through the IL-23–IL-17 axis at specific tissue sites [2, 28]. Other common features of MHC-I-opathies include the absence of female predominance, fluctuating disease activity, genetic associations with ERAP 1/2 and IL-23–IL-17 axis genes in addition to MHC-I genes, and a positive response to anticytokine therapies rather than B cells. From this perspective, BD can be considered a disease within the spectrum of MHC-I-opathies [8, 28]. However, it should be emphasized that HLA-B*51 or another MHC-I allele is not present in a large proportion of patients, even in the endemic areas of the disease [29].

5.4.1 Dysregulation of the Innate Immune System

Dysregulation of the innate immune system, particularly an exaggerated innate immune response, plays a crucial role in the immunopathogenesis of BD, especially in the early stages of the disease. Neutrophil hyperactivity is the main feature of BD and contributes to inflammation and tissue damage. High levels of pro-inflammatory cytokines, including IL-8, interferon (INF) γ, and tumor necrosis factor (TNF)- α activate neutrophils. Neutrophils have an increased capacity for migration, phagocytosis, and the production of reactive oxygen species (ROS). Neutrophil infiltration and the release of ROS from these cells contribute to inflammation, tissue damage, and thrombosis [30]. Another concept related to neutrophils that may play a role in the immunopathogenesis of BD is neutrophil extracellular traps (NET)osis. NETosis is a unique form of cell death in neutrophils. In this process, the neutrophil nuclei decondense, the cell membrane ruptures, and a web-like structure of cellular DNA, histones, and some antimicrobial proteins, known as NETs, is released. In BD, spontaneous NETosis can play a crucial role in enhancing tissue injury, inflammation, and thrombosis. Although the primary function of NETs is to trap and neutralize pathogens for infection control, excessive NETosis in BD can release potential autoantigens extracellularly and trigger autoimmunity [15].

In addition to neutrophils, various other subsets of the innate immune system, such as mast cells, monocytes, natural killer (NK) cells and γδ T cells also contribute to the innate immune response in BD. Mast cells have been frequently observed in BD lesions, indicating that the consumption of foods high in histamine may serve as a potential trigger for oral lesions [31]. NK cells increase in the peripheral blood and in the lesions of BD during the acute phase. They contribute to triggering the Th1 response. In BD, proinflammatory cytokines of the innate immune system, such as TNF-α, IL-1, and IL-6, increase [32]. These cytokines play an important role in regulating the inflammatory process. Pattern recognition receptors (PRRs) are another crucial component of the innate immune system. In BD, some alterations in the function and expression of PRRs, including Toll-like receptors (TLRs), pathogen-associated molecular patterns (PAMPs) and damage-associated molecular patterns (DAMPs), have been identified. These alterations may be involved in inappropriate activation of the innate immune response in the disease [15, 30].

5.4.2 Dysregulation of the Adaptive Immune System

While the innate immune system initiates the disease, the adaptive immune system contributes to the chronicity and severity of the condition. In BD, there is abnormal activation of CD4+ T helper cells (Th) and cytotoxic CD8+ T cells (Tc), which trigger various immune responses and direct cellular attacks on perceived pathogens and affected tissues, respectively, via their cytokines [1, 2]. In BD, there is a Th shift toward Th1/

Th17, which is favored by antigen-presenting cells (APCs) of the innate immune system. Increased production and secretion of pro-inflammatory Th1 cytokines such as TNF-α, IFN-γ and the Th17 cytokine IL-17 play a crucial role in maintaining inflammation. Pro-inflammatory cytokines promote inflammation, and IL-17 is involved in autoinflammatory processes. IL-17 levels increase in the blood of BD patients during active disease [27]. CD8+ T cells, via IL-17, also enhance the intensity, scope, and chronicity of innate and adaptive immune responses, leading to sustained neutrophilic inflammation. CD8+ T cells are the primary source of IL-8 and granulocyte–macrophage colony-stimulating factor (GM-CSF), which are crucial in the biology of neutrophils and neutrophilic inflammation. In contrast to effector T cells, Treg cells are suppressed in BD [30].

Although T cells play the primary role in the adaptive immune response, B cells and autoantibodies can also be significant. Anti-endothelial cell antibodies (AECAs) have been described in BD. The production of autoantibodies can trigger inflammation and cause vasculitis through complement- or antibody-dependent cell toxicity [33].

5.5 Vasculitis in BD

BD vasculitis can affect blood vessels of all sizes, including both arteries and veins. It is a unique form of vasculitis in which the role of immune complexes or autoantibodies in the pathogenesis is of limited significance [8]. These autoantibodies appear to develop as a result of endothelial cell damage and are not primarily pathogenic. Among the autoantibodies described in BD, serum anti-endothelial antibodies such as IgM anti-human α-enolase and IgA anti-heterogeneous nuclear ribonucleoprotein (hnRNP)A2/B1 antibodies are the most important. They accumulate on the endothelium, stimulate the expression of adhesion molecules, and subsequently cause the recruitment of neutrophils to the endothelium. Prohibitin, HSP27, and annexin are additional targets for anti-endothelial antibodies [34]. However, as mentioned above, the main mechanism of vasculitis does not depend on immune complexes or autoantibodies [8]. Activation of vascular endothelial cells due to chronic inflammation, which is involved in the pathogenesis of the disease, leads to endothelial damage and thrombosis, thereby exacerbating inflammation. The main event here is the activation of endothelial cells, resulting in thrombosis. Immunothrombosis is the term used to describe this concept. Immunothrombosis is the primary cause of vasculitis in BD [35].

Hyperreactive neutrophils adhering to endothelial cells are another crucial factor in the vasculitic process in BD. The excessive production of ROS by neutrophils destroys the endothelial structure and causes thrombosis. In addition to ROS, NETs also play an important role in thrombosis by predisposing to thrombophilia [30, 36].

In summary, BD is a complex condition that shares common characteristics with autoimmune diseases, autoinflammatory diseases, and MHC-I-opathies. It is not possible to explain the pathogenesis of the disease with a single mechanism since several environmental and genetic factors play important roles (Table 5.1). The fact that the disease has been known since the time of Hippocrates (460–370 BC) and that the factors involved in the pathogenesis (environmental, genetic, epigenetic, etc.) have changed significantly during this period makes the pathogenesis of the disease more complex.

Table 5.1 Shared and non-shared features of autoimmune diseases, autoinflammatory diseases, and "MHC-I-opathy" with Behçet's disease (BD)

Autoimmune diseases	
Features shared with BD	**Features not shared with BD**
1. Antigen specific T cells (T-cell responses to heat shock proteins of Streptococcus species and *Mycobacterium tuberculosis*)* **2.** Presence of autoantibodies against endothelial cells, enolase and retinal S-antigen* **3.** Amelioration of the disease by immunosuppressive drugs **It is generally acknowledged that these incidents are primarily connected to tissue injury and do not play a direct role in the disease's pathogenesis*	**1.** No female predominance **2.** Lack of anti-nuclear antibodies **3.** Lack of concomitant autoimmune diseases **4.** No signs of antigen-specific T cells or autoantibodies in inflammatory episodes **5.** No classical MHC Class II association
Autoinflammatory diseases	
Features shared with BD	**Features not shared with BD**
1. Unprovoked recurrent inflammatory attacks **2.** Involvement of the skin, serous membranes, joints, GI tract, and eyes in inflammatory attacks **3.** Elevated acute phase reactants **4.** Increased neutrophil granulocyte activity **5.** Elevated IL-1β	**1.** Most autoinflammatory diseases start in childhood, but BD starts after puberty **2.** Vasculitis is uncommonly seen in autoinflammatory diseases **3.** IL-1β blockade is effective for autoinflammatory diseases, but not convincingly successful in BD
MHC-I-opathies	
Features shared with BD	**Features not shared with BD**
1. Absence of female predominance **2.** Fluctuating disease activity **3.** Genetic association with MHC-I genes **4.** Genetic associations with ERAP 1/2 and IL-23/IL-17 genes **5.** Positive response to anti-cytokine therapy rather than B cells	**1.** Absence of HLA-B*51 or another MHC-I allele in a significant number of BD patients **2.** Absence of sacroiliac joint or spine involvement in BD **3.** Presence of prominent ocular involvement in BD **4.** Presence of genital ulcer in BD

References

1. Leccese P, Alpsoy E. Behçet's disease: an overview of etiopathogenesis. Front Immunol. 2019;10:1067.
2. Mattioli I, Bettiol A, Direskeneli GS, et al. Pathogenesis of Behçet's syndrome: genetic, environmental and immunological factors. Front Med. 2021;8:713052.
3. Cheng L, Zham H, Liu Y, et al. Infectious agents and pathogenesis of Behçet's disease: an extensive review. Clin Immunol. 2023;251:109631.
4. Wright V. A unifying concept for spondyloarthropathies. Clin Orthop Relat Res. 1979;143:8–14.
5. Frassanito MA, Dammacco R, Cafforio P, et al. Th1 polarization of the immune response in Behcet's disease: a putative pathogenetic role of interleukin-12. Arthritis Rheum. 1999;42:1967–74.
6. Yazici H, Fresko I. Behcet's disease and other autoinflammatory conditions: what's in a name? Clin Exp Rheumatol. 2005;23:S1–2.
7. Direskeneli H. Autoimmunity vs autoinflammation in Behcet's disease: do we oversimplify a complex disorder? Rheumatology. 2006;45:1461–5.
8. McGonagle D, Aydin SZ, Gul A, et al. 'MHC-I-opathy'-unified concept for spondyloarthritis and Behçet's disease. Nat Rev Rheumatol. 2015;11:731–4.
9. Ilgen U. Clusters in Behcet's syndrome. Arthritis Res Ther. 2022;24:242.
10. Jo YG, Ortiz-Fernandez L, Coit P, et al. Sex-specific analysis in Behcet's disease reveals higher genetic risk in male patients. Autoimmunity. 2022;132:102882.
11. Hatemi G, Yazici Y. Outcome measures in Behcet syndrome. Clin Immunol. 2023;251:109341.
12. Khoshbakht S, Baskurt D, Vural A, Vural S. Behçet's disease: a comprehensive review on the roleof HLA-B*51, antigen presentation, and inflammatory cascade. Int J Mol Sci. 2023;24:16382.
13. de Menthon M, Lavalley MP, Maldini C, Guillevin L, Mahr A. HLA-B51/B5 and the risk of Behçet's disease: a systematic review and meta-analysis of case-control genetic association studies. Arthritis Rheum. 2009;61:1287–96.
14. Mahmoudi M, Aslani S, Meguro A, et al. A comprehensive overview on the genetics of Behcet's disease. Int Rev Immunol. 2022;41:84–106.
15. Joubert M, Andre M, Barnich N, et al. Microbiome and Behçet's disease: a systematic review. Clin Exp Rheumatol. 2023;41:2093–104.

16. Kaneko F, Oyama N, Yanagihori H, et al. The role of streptococcal hypersensitivity in the pathogenesis of Behçet's disease. Eur J Dermatol. 2008;18:489–98.
17. Kaneko F, Togashi A, Nomura E, et al. A new diagnostic way for Behçet's disease: skin prick with self-saliva. Genet Res Int. 2014;2014:581468.
18. Kim DY, Cho S, Choi MS, et al. Immunopathogenic role of Herpes simplex virus in Behçet's disease. Genet Res Int. 2013;2013:638273.
19. Jun JB, Kim HJ, Kazmi SZ, et al. Significant decline in the incidence of Behcet's disease in South Korea: a nationwide population-based study (2002–2017). Arthritis Care Res. 2021;73:1689–96.
20. Behçet H. Ü ber rezidivierende, Aphthöse, durch ein Virus verursachte Geschwüre am Mund, am Auge und an den Genitalien. Dermatol Wochenschr. 1937;105:1152–7.
21. Seoudi N, Bergmeier LA, Drobniewski F, et al. The oral mucosal and salivary microbial community of Behçet's syndrome and recurrent aphthous stomatitis. J Oral Microbiol. 2015;7:2715.
22. Ogunkolade W, Senusi AA, Desai P, et al. Profiling the microbiome of oral and genital mucosal surfaces in Behcet's disease. Clin Immunol. 2023;253:109654.
23. Kim JC, Park MJ, Lee ES. Alteration of the fecal but not salivary microbiome in patients with Behcet's disease according to disease activity shift. Microorganisms. 2021;9:1449.
24. Gul A. Pathogenesis of Behçet's disease: autoinflammatory features and beyond. Semin Immunopathol. 2015;37:413–8.
25. McGonagle D, McDermott MF. A proposed classification of the immunological diseases. PLoS Med. 2006;8:e297.
26. Moll JM, Haslock IF, Wright V. Associations between ankylosing spondylitis, psoriatic arthritis, Reiter's disease, the intestinal arthropathies, and Behcet's syndrome. Medicine. 1974;53:343–64.
27. Ekinci NS, Alpsoy E, Karakas AA, Yilmaz SB, Yegin O. IL-17A has an important role in the acute attacks of Behçet's disease. J Invest Dermatol. 2010;130:2136–8.
28. Kuiper JJ, Prinz JC, Stratikos E, et al. EULAR study group on 'MHC-I-opathy': identifying disease-overarching mechanisms across disciplines and borders. Ann Rheum Dis. 2023;82:887–96.
29. Hatemi G, Karatemiz G, Yazici H. Behçet's disease: an MHC-I-opathy? Clin Exp Rheumatol. 2017;104:5.
30. Perazzio LE, Andrade LE, Souza AW. Understanding Behçet's disease in the context of innate immunity activation. Front Immunol. 2020;11:586558.
31. Volle G, Fraison JB, Gobert D, Goulenok T, Dhote R, Fain O, et al. Dietary and nondietary triggers of oral ulcer recurrences in Behçet's disease. Arthritis Care Res. 2017;69:1429–36.
32. Alpsoy E, Bozca BC, Bilgic A. Behçet disease: an update for dermatologists. Am J Clin Dermatol. 2021;22:477–502.
33. Kim D, Nakamura K, Kaneko F, et al. Mucocutaneous manifestations of Behçet's disease: pathogenesis and management from perspective of vasculitis. Front Med. 2022;9:987393.
34. Chen P, Zhang C, Chang L. HnRNP A1 is involved in deep vein thrombosis patients with Behcet's disease. EBioMedicine. 2016;6:215–21.
35. Emmi G, Becatti M, Bettiol A, et al. Behçet's syndrome as a model of thrombo-inflammation: the role of neutrophils. Front Immunol. 2019;10:01085.
36. Jancour A, Cacoub P, Boulaftali Y, et al. Neutrophil, NETs and Behçet's disease: a review. Clin Immunol. 2023;250:109318.

Microbiota: Does it Have a Role in the Development and Severity of the Disease?

6

Tülin Ergun

Contents

6.1 Introduction

Hulusi Behçet, in his initial description of the disease, "recurrent aphthous ulcers caused by a virus on the mouth, eye, and genitals" postulated microbial involvement in its etiology [1]. Thereafter many investigators from different parts of the world have delved into the role of microorganisms in disease processes. Identification of microorganisms from BD patients by cultures, in vitro assays to discover the microorganism-immune system interactions, identification of gut, oral, genital microbiota and lastly metagenomic studies have all aimed to address the potential role of microorganisms and their products in the etiology. While no single microorganism has been pinpointed as the sole cause of the key pathogenesis and the mechanisms by which microorganisms participate in

T. Ergun (✉)
Dermatology and Venereology, Marmara University Pendik Training and Research Hospital, Istanbul, Türkiye
e-mail: tulin@marmara.edu.tr

E. Alpsoy et al. (eds.), *Behçet's Disease: An Integrated Approach*,
https://doi.org/10.1007/978-3-031-77251-1_6

lipid profiles following intensive periodontal treatment, has been demonstrated. Thus the impact of microbiota-based therapies as adjuncts in BD may be an interesting area for further research [21, 22, 31].

6.5 Intestinal Dysbiosis and BD

The gut microbiota, often considered a metabolic organ, serves multiple homeostatic functions crucial for maintaining human health. Microbial metabolites, including short chain fatty acids(SCFAs) such as acetate, propionate, butyrate, as well as bile acids, indoles, lipopolysaccharides, trimethylamine N-oxide, and others, possess various biological functions and can either activate or dampen immune responses. Consequently, gut dysbiosis may lead to pro-inflammatory responses, and has been linked to allergy, cancer, various autoimmune, metabolic, and neuropsychiatric diseases [2, 5, 32, 33].

Several studies aimed to uncover the role of microbiota in BD. Consolandi et al. were first studying the fecal microbiome and SCFAs in 22 patients with BD and 16 age-matched healthy controls. They found reduced total diversity for the gut microbial community, a remarkable depletion of butyrate producing bacteria such as Roseburia and Subdoligranulum genera and a significant decrease of butyrate production in BD patients compared to healthy individuals. Given the key role of butyrate in maintenance of the host immune homeostasis, with its systemic and local immuno-modulating properties that inhibit intestinal proinflammatory cytokines and promote T-cell differentiation into regulatory T cells (Tregs) lineage, investigators proposed decreased butyrate production could lead to reduced Tregs responses and activation of immuno-pathological T-effector responses in BD [34].

Shimizu et al. investigated the fecal microbiota of 12 Japanese BD patients and 12 healthy individuals, showing no significant difference in species numbers and bacterial diversity of each sample between groups. However BD patients exhibited a significant increase in Bifidobacterium and Eggerthella, lactate-producing bacteria, as well as a decrease in Megamonas and Prevotella, compared to healthy individuals. Although no relationships were found among gut bacterial taxonomic abundance and clinical activity, serum CRP, and cumulative steroid doses, the investigators hypothesized that dysregulated SCFA production of gut microbiota may occur in BD patients [35].

In another study, Shimuzu et al. analyzed fecal samples of 13 BD patients and 27 normal individuals, revealing significantly increased relative abundances of Lactobacillus, Bifidobacterium, and Streptococcus spp., and a reduction in propionate and butyrate-producing bacteria such as *Megamonas hypermegale* and Butyrivibrio species. Such decreases in butyrate can skew T cells toward Th17 and lead to reductions in Tregs. Additionally, metagenomic study identified altered gene functions of lipid/nucleic acid metabolism, postulated to be related to the immune aberrations observed in patients with BD [36].

van der Houwen compared gut microbiota of 19 Dutch and 14 Italian BD patients with 32, age, gender and ethnicity-matched healthy controls, finding no significant differences in microbial alpha-diversity between groups. However, a significant segregation of beta-diversity, which quantifies the number of different communities, based on the country of origin was reported with a significant decrease in Barnesiellaceae and an increase in Lactobacillaceae limited to Italian BD patients. Further investigations at genus level revealed a significant decrease of relative abundance in unclassified Barnesiellaceae and in Lachnospira in BD patients compared with healthy controls, which was more prominent in Italian cohort [25]. The authors proposed a possible link between decreased abundance of Barnesiellaceae and an increased tumor necrosis factor (TNF)-α levels in BD. Also decreased abundance of Lachnospira may be related to the decreased production of SCFAs, eventually leading to dysfunction of Tregs and activation of the NF kappa β-pathway in BD [37].

Another study by Kim et al. investigated fecal microbiota of nine patients with BD, seven with RAS, 16 healthy controls, finding no differences in alpha diversity among groups, although alterations were observed according to disease activity.

Patients with active BD had *B. uniformis* as the most abundant taxon, although its relationship to the inflammatory process is not known [27].

In their study, Bilge et al. analyzed fecal microbiota in 27 patients with BD and ten healthy controls, finding the genera Actinomyces, Libanicoccus, Collinsella, Eggerthella, Enterorhabdus, Catenibacterium, and Enterobacter to be more abundant in BD patients than in healthy controls. In contrast, Bacteroides, Cricetibacter, Alistipes, Lachnospira, Dielma, Akkermansia, Sutterella, Anaerofilum, Ruminococceae UCG007, Acetanaerobacterium, and Copropaacter were significantly lower in patients with BD group. Also composition of microbiota differed among various disease phenotypes in BD patients. For instance, Lachnospiraceae NK4A136 was related to uveitis, Dialister, Intestinomonas, and Marvinbryantia to the mucocutaneous and Gemella to the vascular phenotypes [38].

In another study, Oezguen et al. investigated intestinal microbiota of 14 healthy controls, 13 BD patients with neurological involvement and 13 multiple sclerosis patients, reporting a significant decrease in Prevotella in BD group, which was associated with increased tendency toward inflammatory disorders [39].

Recently, Wang et al. analyzed 695 fecal samples of patients with BD uveitis (n: 24), Vogt–Koyanagi–Harada disease, inflammatory bowel diseases, rheumatoid arthritis, ankylosing spondylitis and healthy controls. Although microbial diversity of BD patients were comparable to healthy controls, patients with BD had an increased abundance of Bilophila, Alistipes and Stenotrophomonas as well as lower abundances of Dorea, Blautia, Coprococcus, Erysipelotrichaceae, and Lachnospiraceae. In BD patients, SteTDR, a peptide of Stenotrophomonas, which is an opportunistic pathogen capable of triggering innate inflammatory response via TLRs, was able to stimulate peripheral blood mononuclear cells to produce more IFN-γ and IL-17. Further functional analysis revealed a relationship between these strains and proteins of immune-related pathways including Th1 and Th2 cell differentiation, natural killer cell-mediated cytotoxicity, TNF signaling pathway and hypoxia inducible factor signaling pathways. One enriched protein specific for BD was in the Toll and Imd signaling pathway. The gut microbiome of BD patients was enriched in L-methionine and L-threonine biosynthesis. Since methionine is a well-known potent neutrophil chemoattractant and threonine is able to activate the MAPK pathway, the authors claimed that they might be involved in BD pathogenesis by enhancing neutrophil activation and inflammatory responses [40]. Wang et al. also transplanted fecal samples from 20 patients with active ocular BD to mice, and reported decreases of three short chain fatty acids, including butyric acid, propionic acid, and valeric acid as well as a damage in intestinal barrier integrity. Single cell RNA sequencing revealed an enrichment of genes associated with innate immune responses in the neutrophils and CD4+ T cells. In addition, functional analysis of neutrophils and T cells exhibited an enhanced Th1 and Th17 cell differentiation as well as down-regulation of Tregs in association with activation of neutrophils [41].

Recently, Ye et al. performed a metagenomic study of the gut microbiome in 32 ocular BD patients receiving no systemic medications and 74 matched controls and found significant differences in the relative abundances of 97 genera and 23 species between groups. At the species level, 23 microbes were enriched in BD patients, including opportunistic pathogens, such as Stenotrophomonas spp., Actinomyces spp., and Corynebacterium spp. Further analysis revealed that, sulfate-reducing bacteria (SRB) and opportunistic pathogens were enriched in patients with BD and methanogens and butyrate-producing bacteria were enriched in healthy controls. The investigators transplanted the feces of active BD patients to mice and reported the emergence of severe uveitis in the BD recipient group as compared to the healthy recipient group. The authors proposed the mechanism by which these changes may contribute to the pathogenesis. Accordingly, shortage of butyrate, which protects intestinal barrier and serves homeostasis by inducing differentiation of Treg cells, may facilitate the expression of inflammatory molecules with subsequent invasion by Th1 and Th17 cells. Also, higher hydrogen sulfide, produced by SRB, may damage intestinal barrier by pro-inflammatory effects and relative lack of methane may increase oxidative stress-related barrier injury, thereby triggering inflammatory response [28].

The immune changes observed in patients with BD encompass various aspects, such as the activation of neutrophils, elevation in circulating Th17 cells and Th1 cytokines, alongside a reduction in Tregs [42, 43]. Given that the aforementioned microbial disruptions are thought to trigger neutrophil activation, Tregs suppression, enhanced Th1 and Th17 cell differentiation, and elevated levels of TNF-α, IFN-γ, and IL-17, it suggests a notable involvement of the microbiota in the development of BD.

6.6 Microbial Dysbiosis and Immune Dysregulation in Behçet's Disease: Exploring Potential Mechanisms

Disturbances in the oral and intestinal microbiota can lead to immune dysregulation through several mechanisms (Fig. 6.1). Here are some examples:

6.6.1 Bacterial Translocation

Current research highlights the pathogenetic role of bacterial translocation in various disorders, including cardiovascular and central nervous system diseases. Pathogenic bacteria causing periodontitis are capable of inducing neuroinflammation by entering into the bloodstream, crossing blood-brain barrier and damaging central nervous tissues [42, 43, 44, 45]. Translocation of oral microbiome into the peripheral blood has also been linked to endothelial dysfunction and cardiovascular diseases [46]. In patients with BD, recurrent oral and genital ulcers may enable microorganisms to reach distant organs like the eye, central nervous system, subcutaneous tissue, and trigger innate inflammatory responses. Notably, the presence of antibodies against bacterial heat shock protein 65 in the cerebrospinal fluid of neuro-Behçet patients suggests a possible role of translocation in BD [47].

6.6.2 Molecular Mimicry

BD patients have antibodies against middle neurofilament (NF-M) constituting filamentous neuronal compounds in the brain, retina, and skin,

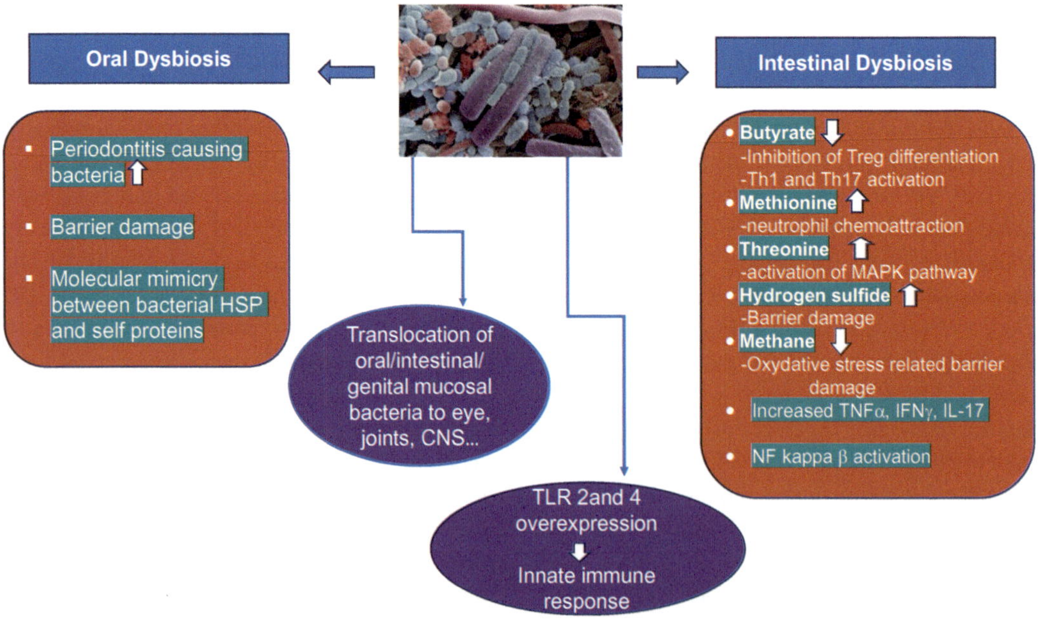

Fig. 6.1 Potential Mechanisms of Immune Dysregulation due to Microbial Dysbiosis in BD [53]. (Picture adapted from https://www.nature.com/articles/nature.2012.10299). *CNS* central nervous system, *NF kappa β* nuclear factor kappa β, *TNF-α* tumor necrosing factor-α, *IL-17* interleukin-17, *IFN-γ* interferon γ, *MAPK* mitogen-activated protein kinase, *TLR* toll-like receptor, *HSP* heat shock protein

which shares significant homology with bacterial HSP-65 [48]. Oral bacteria causing periodontitis express HSP60 family proteins, which can trigger T-cell responses in BD patients [49].

6.6.3 Immune Dysregulation Related to Microbial Metabolites

SCFAs, particularly butyrate, play crucial immunomodulatory roles, primarily promoting tolerance under steady-state conditions. Reduced butyrate levels due to intestinal dysbiosis in BD may contribute to the generation of Th1 and Th17 cells, whereas lack of methane may increase oxidative stress-related barrier injury [50].

6.6.4 Overexpression of Toll like Receptors

Microbial dysbiosis due to damaged intestinal barrier may trigger overexpression of TLR 2 and 4 which may induce an inflammatory reaction [51].

6.7 Clinical Significance of Microbiota Modulation

The modification of the microbiota in the treatment of various diseases has been a subject of great interest and extensive research by researchers in recent years. An Italian study investigated the impact of microbiota composition through dietary modifications on BD features. Seventeen omnivore BD patients on stable treatment were randomized to either a habitual diet supplemented with oral butyrate or a lacto-ovo-vegetarian diet, that increases butyrate production. Both interventions led to a significant reduction in leukocyte reactive oxygen species production, plasma lipid peroxidation, and an increase in plasma total antioxidant capacity as well as an improvement in fibrin susceptibility to plasmin-induced lysis. Furthermore both interventions led to a significant reduction in disease activity and corticosteroids use [52]. These findings are promising, indicating that further research in this area would be beneficial.

6.8 Microbial Dysbiosis: Causative or Epiphenomenon?

Although current data suggests a possible link between microbial dysbiosis and BD, several unresolved issues persist. The composition of the microbiota is influenced by numerous factors, including dietary habits, smoking, hormonal factors, lifestyle, medications, coexisting diseases, and geographical factors, which vary among study populations. Moreover, most patients enrolled in studies receive heterogeneous treatment modalities that may impact the microbiota. Additionally, evidence regarding perturbations of fungi, algae, and viruses is lacking, and there is an absence of uniformity in sampling and sequencing methodology across studies. Lastly, different bacterial species have been identified in different studies, leading to inconsistency among findings and making it challenging to establish causality and understand pathogenesis.

6.9 Conclusion

Studies focusing on gut microbiota of patients with BD have revealed decrease in the abundance of SCFA-producing bacteria and fecal butyrate levels. Similar alterations have been observed in patients with inflammatory bowel disease and diabetes mellitus. These alterations could potentially impact immune responses by promoting Th1 and Th17 responses while impairing the function of Tregs. Moreover, increased abundances of opportunistic pathogens like sulfate-reducing bacteria may trigger innate immune responses by disrupting intestinal barrier and upregulating the expression of TLRs. Nevertheless, the temporal relation between these alterations and the disease process remains unclear. Further comprehensive studies, encompassing BD patients from diverse geographic regions and focusing on the analysis of microbial metabolites' impact on immune function, can provide insights for microbiota-based treatment approaches. These may involve administering appropriate probiotics, implementing dietary modifications rich in prebiotics to promote the release of beneficial bacterial metabolites, or utilizing postbiotics such as SCFAs.

References

1. Behçet H. Über rezidivierende, Aphtöse, durch Ein Virus verursachte Geschwüre am Mund, am Augeund an den Genitalien. Derm Wschr. 1937;105(36):1152–7.
2. Grice EA, Segre JA. The human microbiome: our second genome. Annu Rev Genom Hum Genet. 2012;13:151–70.
3. Wikoff WR, Anfora AT, Liu J, Schultz PG, Lesley SA, Peters EC, et al. Metabolomics analysis reveals large effects of gut microflora on mammalian blood metabolites. Proc Natl Acad Sci USA. 2009;106(10):3698–703. https://doi.org/10.1073/pnas.0812874106.
4. Thomas S, Izard J, Walsh E, Batich K, Chongsathidkiet P, Clarke G, et al. The host microbiome regulates and maintains human health: a primer and perspective for non-microbiologists. Cancer Res. 2017;77:1783–812.
5. Levy M, Kolodziejczyk AA, Thaiss CA, Elinav E. Dysbiosis and the immune system. Nat Rev Immunol. 2017;17:219–32.
6. Gürler A, Boyvat A, Tursen U. Clinical manifestations of Behçet's disease. An analysis of 2147 patients. Yonsei Med J. 1997;38:423–7.
7. Alpsoy E, Bozca BC, Bilgic A. Behçet disease: an update for dermatologists. Am J Clin Dermatol. 2021;22(4):477–502. https://doi.org/10.1007/s40257-021-00609-4.
8. Kurauchi T, Yokota K, Matsuo T, Fujinami Y, Isogai H, Isogai E, Ohtsuki H, Oguma K. Neutrophil and lymphocyte responses to oral streptococcus in Adamantiades-Behçet's disease. FEMS Immunol Med Microbiol. 2006; https://doi.org/10.1016/j.femsim.
9. Yay M, Çelik Z, Aksoy A, Alibaz-Öner F, Inanç N, Ergun T, Direskeneli H, Mumcu G. Oral health is a mediator for disease severity in patients with Behçet's disease: a multiple mediation analysis study. J Oral Rehabil. 2019;46(4):349–54. https://doi.org/10.1111/joor.12750.
10. Mizushima YMT, Hoshl K, Ohno S. Induction of Behçet's disease symptoms after dental treatment and streptococcal antigen skin test. J Rheumatol. 1988;15:1029–30.
11. Karacayli U, Mumcu G, Simsek I, Pay S, Kose O, Erdem H, Direskeneli H, Gunaydin Y, Dinc A. The close association between dental and periodontal treatments and oral ulcer course in behcet's disease: a prospective clinical study. J Oral Pathol Med. 2009;38(5):410–5. https://doi.org/10.1111/j.1600-0714.2009.00765.x.
12. Inaba Y, Kurosawa M, Nishibu A, Kaneko F, Kawakami Y, Tamakoshi A, Kawamura T. Epidemiologic and clinical characteristics of Behçet disease in Japan:results from nationwide survey in 2003. Clin Exp Rheumatol. 2004;22(4 Suppl 34):S84.
13. Direskeneli H, Mumcu G. A possible decline in the incidence and severity of Behçet's disease: implications for an infectious etiology and oral health. Clin Exp Rheumatol. 2010;28(4 Suppl 60):S86–90.
14. Kaneko F, Oyama N, Nishibu A. Streptococcal infection in the pathogenesis of Behçet's disease and clinical effects of minocycline on the disease symptoms. Yonsei Med J. 1997;38(6):444–54. https://doi.org/10.3349/ymj.1997.38.6.444.
15. Mumcu G, Ergun T, Elbir Y, Eksioglu-Demiralp E, Yavuz S, et al. Clinical and immunological effects of azithromycin in Behcet's disease. J Oral Pathol Med. 2005;34:13–6.
16. Çalgüneri M, Ertenli I, Kiraz S, Erman B, Çelik I. Effect of prophylactic benzathine penicillin on mucocutaneous symptoms of Behcet's disease. Dermatology. 1996;192(2):125–8. 29
17. Çalgüneri M, Kiraz S, Ertenli I, Benekli M, Karaaslan Y, Çelik I. The effect of prophylactic penicillin treatment on the course of arthritis episodes in patients with Behcet's disease. A randomized clinical trial. Arthritis Rheum. 1996;39(12):2062–5.
18. Human Oral Microbiome Database. Available online: https://www.homd.org/. Accessed 31 Aug 2023.
19. Lee YH, Chung SW, Auh QS, Hong SJ, Lee YA, Jung J, Lee GJ, Park HJ, Shin SI, Hong JY. Progress in oral microbiome related to oral and systemic diseases: an update. Diagnostics. 2021;11:1283.
20. Bacali C, Vulturar R, Buduru S, Cozma A, Fodor A, Chis A, Lucaciu O, Damian L, Moldovan ML. Oral microbiome:getting to know and befriend neighbors, a biological approach. Biomedicines. 2022;10:671.
21. Morrison AG, Sarkar S, Umar S, Lee STM, Thomas SM. The contribution of the human oral microbiome to oral disease: a review. Microorganisms. 2023;11:318.
22. Huang X, Huang X, Huang Y, Zheng J, Lu Y, et al. The oral microbiome in autoimmune diseases: friend or foe? J Transl Med. 2023;21:211. https://doi.org/10.1186/s12967-023-03995-x.
23. Coit P, Mumcu G, Ture-Ozdemir F, Unal AU, Alpar U, Bostanci U, Ergun T, Direskeneli H, Sawalha AH. Sequencing of 16S rRNA reveals a distinct salivary microbiome signature in Behçet's disease. Clin Immunol. 2016;169:28–35. https://doi.org/10.1016/j.clim.2016.06.002.
24. Seoudi N, Bergmeier LA, Drobniewski F, Paster B, Fortune F. The oral mucosal and salivary microbial community of Behçet's syndrome and recurrent aphthous stomatitis. J Oral Microbiol. 2015;7:27150. https://doi.org/10.3402/jom.v7.27150.
25. van der Houwen TB, van Laar JAM, Kappen JH, van Hagen PM, de Zoete MR, van Muijlwijk GH, et al. Behçet's disease under microbiotic surveillance? A combined analysis of two cohorts of Behçet's disease patients. Front Immunol. 2020;11:1192. https://doi.org/10.3389/fimmu.2020.01192.
26. Habibagahi Z, Khorshidi H, Hekmati S. Periodontal health status among patients with Behçet's dis-

ease. Scientifica. 2016:7506041. https://doi.org/10.1155/2016/7506041.
27. Kim JC, Park MJ, Park S, Lee ES. Alteration of the fecal but not salivary microbiome in patients with Behçet's disease according to disease activity shift. Microorganisms. 2021;9(7):1449. https://doi.org/10.3390/microorganisms9071449.
28. Ye Z, Zhang N, Wu C, Zhang X, Wang Q, Huang X, Du L, et al. A metagenomic study of the gut microbiome in Behcet's disease. Microbiome. 2018;6(1):135. https://doi.org/10.1186/s40168-018-0520-6.
29. Balt J, Uehara O, Abiko Y, Jamyanjav B, Jav S, Nagasawa T, et al. Alteration of oral flora in Mongolian patients with Behçet's disease: a multicentre study. Clin Exp Rheumatol. 2020;38(Suppl 127(5)):80–5.
30. Ogunkolade W, Senusi AA, Desai P, Sacoor S, Bibi A, Gokani B, Sandionigi A, Fortune F. Profiling the microbiome of oral and genital mucosal surfaces in Behçet's disease. Clin Immunol. 2023;253:109654. https://doi.org/10.1016/j.clim.2023.
31. D'Aiuto F, Parkar M, Nibali L, Suvan J, Lessem J, Tonetti MS. Periodontal infections cause changes in traditional and novel cardiovascular risk factors: results from a randomized controlled clinical trial. Am Heart J. 2006;151:977–84.
32. de Vos WM, Tilg H, Van Hul M, Cani PD. Gut microbiome and health: mechanistic insights. Gut. 2022;71(5):1020–32. https://doi.org/10.1136/gutjnl-2021-326789.
33. Smith PM, Howitt MR, Panikov N, Michaud M, Gallini CA, Bohlooly YM, Glickman JN. Garrett WS the microbial metabolites, short-chain fatty acids, regulate colonic Treg cell homeostasis. Science. 2013;341:569–73.
34. Consolandi C, Turroni S, Emmi G, Severgnini M, Fiori J, Peano C, et al. Behçet's syndrome patients exhibit specific microbiome signature. Autoimmun Rev. 2015;14:269–76.
35. Shimizu J, Kubota T, Takada E, Takai K, Fujiwara N, Arimitsu N, et al. Bifidobacteria abundance-featured gut microbiota compositional change in patients with Behçet's disease. PLoS One. 2016;11:e0153746. https://doi.org/10.1371/journal.pone.0153746.
36. Shimizu J, Ubota T, Takada E, Takai K, Fujiwara N, Arimitsu N, et al. Relative abundance of Megamonas hypermegale and Butyrivibrio species decreased in the intestine and its possible association with the T cell aberration by metabolite alteration in patients with Behçet's disease. Clin Rheumatol. 2019;38:1437–45.
37. Richards JL, Yap YA, McLeod KH, Mackay CR, Mariño E. Dietary metabolites and the gut microbiota: an alternative approach to control inflammatory and autoimmune diseases. Clin Transl Immunol. 2016;5:e82. https://doi.org/10.1038/cti.2016.29.
38. Yasar Bilge NS, Brocal VP, Kasifoglu T, Bilge U, Kasifoglu N, Moya A, Dinleyici EC. Intestinal microbiota composition of patients with Behçet's disease: differences between eye, mucocutaneous and vascular involvement. The Rheuma-BIOTA study. Clin Exp Rheumatol. 2020;38(Suppl 127(5)):60–8.
39. Oezguen N, Yalcınkaya N, Kucukalı CI, Dahdouli M, Hollister MEB, Luna R, Türkoglu R, et al. Microbiota stratification identifies disease-specific alterations in neuro-Behçet's disease and multiple sclerosis. Clin Exp Rheumatol. 2019;37(Suppl. 121):S58–66.
40. Wang Q, Wu S, Ye X, Tan S, Huang F, Su G, Kijlstra A, Yang P. Gut microbial signatures and their functions in Behcet's uveitis and Vogt-Koyanagi-Harada disease. J Autoimmun. 2023;137:103055. https://doi.org/10.1016/j.jaut.2023.103055.
41. Wang Q, Yi S, Su G, Du Z, Pan S, Huang X, Cao Q, et al. Changes in the gut microbiome contribute to the development of Behcet's disease via adjuvant effects. Front Cell Dev Biol. 2021;9:716760. https://doi.org/10.3389/fcell.2021.716760.
42. Ahmed MB, Houman H, Miled M, Dellagi K, Louzir H. Involvement of chemokines and Th1 cytokines in the pathogenesis of mucocutaneous lesions of Behçet's disease. Arthritis Rheum. 2004;50:2291–5. https://doi.org/10.1002/art.20334.
43. Sonmez C, Yucel AA, Yesil TH, Kucuk H, Sezgin B, Mercan R, Yucel AE, et al. Correlation between IL-17A/F, IL-23, IL35 and IL-12/-23 (p40) levels in peripheral blood lymphocyte cultures and disease activity in Behcet's patients. Clin Rheumatol. 2018;37:2797–804.
44. Bello-Corral L, Alves-Gomes L, Fernández-Fernández JA, Fernández-García D, Casado-Verdejo I, Sánchez-Valdeón L. Implications of gut and oral microbiota in neuroinflammatory responses in Alzheimer's disease. Life Sci. 2023;333:122132. https://doi.org/10.1016/j.lfs.2023.122132.
45. Dioguardi M, Crincoli V, Laino L, Alovisi M, Sovereto D, Mastrangelo F, lo Russo L, lo Muzio L. The role of periodontitis and periodontal bacteria in the onset and progression of Alzheimer's disease: a systematic review. J Clin Med. 2020:9. https://doi.org/10.3390/jcm9020495.
46. Gualtero DF, Lafaurie GI, Buitrago DM, Castillo Y, Vargas-Sanchez PK, Castillo DM. Oral microbiome mediated inflammation, a potential inductor of vascular diseases: a comprehensive review. Front Cardiovasc Med. 2023;10:1250263. https://doi.org/10.3389/fcvm.2023.1250263.
47. Taşçi B, Direskeneli H, Serdaroglu P, Akman-Demir G, Eraksoy M, Saruhan-Direskeneli G. Humoral immune response to mycobacterial heat shock protein (hsp)65 in the cerebrospinal fluid of neuro-Behçet patients. Clin Exp Immunol. 1998;113(1):100–4. https://doi.org/10.1046/j.1365-2249.1998.00620.x.
48. Lule S, Colpak AI, Balci-Peynircioglu B, Gursoy-Ozdemir Y, Peker S, Kalyoncu U, Can A, et al. NF-M immunoreactive sera cross-reacted with bacterial HSP-65 (Behçet disease serum is immunoreactive to neurofilament medium which share common epitopes to bacterial HSP-65, a putative trigger). J Autoimmun. 2017;84:87–96. https://doi.org/10.1016/j.jaut.2017.08.002.
49. Cho SB, Zheng Z, Ahn KJ, Choi MJ, Cho S, Kim DY, Lee HS, Bang D. Serum IgA reactivity against GroEL

is OUs. GUs and EN-like lesions could also be the initial symptoms of the disease [3, 8, 9]. Mucocutaneous manifestations may be the only clinical spectrum observed in some patients. Organ involvement can occur in some patients months or years later [3, 10, 11]. Hamuryudan et al. [12] suggested that OU activity is a predictive factor for the development of major organ involvement in young male patients. In a recent study, Mumcu et al. [13] reported that increased mucocutaneous activity may be associated with new major organ involvement in young female BD patients.

Therefore, given the significance of mucocutaneous manifestations, particularly in diagnosing the disease, and the potential for these symptoms to indicate major organ involvement in most patients, it is crucial for physicians managing BD to have a comprehensive knowledge of the mucocutaneous manifestations and their differential diagnosis. Early and effective disease management may prevent serious organ involvement with beneficial outcomes [14]. A collaborative approach involving multiple disciplines should be employed for the follow-up of patients with BD, with dermatologists playing a pivotal role in this team [1]. The aim of this chapter is to provide an in-depth overview of the clinical spectrum of mucocutaneous manifestations and their differential diagnosis.

7.2 Oral Ulcers

Oral ulcers are painful aphthous lesions that occur on the oral mucosa. Ranging in size from a few millimeters to larger than 1 cm, the OU can present as either a single or multiple lesions. They start as erythematous, vesiculopustular lesions and eventually transform into oval or round ulcers within 24–48 h. They are surrounded by an erythematous halo and have a grayish yellow necrotic base [6, 15]. These ulcers commonly appear on non-keratinizing mucosal surfaces, such as the lips, buccal mucosa, ventral and lateral surfaces of the tongue, floor of the mouth, and soft palate. However, they are less frequently found in keratinized areas like the hard palate, gingiva, and dorsal side of the tongue. Although rare, ulcers can also be found in the tonsils and pharynx [1].

OUs can be categorized into three types: minor, major, or herpetiform, based on their size and number. Minor OUs, which are the most common, make up 80–85% of cases. These ulcers are characterized by their small size, measuring less than 1 cm, and their shallow nature (Fig. 7.1). They typically heal within 1–2 weeks without leaving any scars. Major OUs, accounting for 10–15% of cases, are less frequently observed. They share similarities with minor OUs in terms of appearance, but they are larger, measuring more than 1 cm in diameter. Additionally, they are deeper and cause more intense pain (Fig. 7.2). These ulcers take longer to heal and often result in scarring and tissue loss. Herpetiform OUs, the rarest form, constitute only 5% of cases. They are characterized by their small size, measuring 1–3 mm, and their high number, ranging from 10 to 100 (Fig. 7.3). Of note, at any given time, there can be more than one type of aphthae present [1, 15].

In general, OUs resolve spontaneously within a period of 1–3 weeks. However, major OUs can take up to 6 weeks to heal [6, 15, 16]. Recurrences of OUs can happen unpredictably, ranging from days to months apart. Local traumas can trigger these recurrences through a mucosal pathergy reaction [16–18]. Volle et al. found that the majority of patients are able to recognize triggers for recurring BD-related OUs, with fatigue/stress and food being the most prevalent triggers. The most commonly reported foods were nuts, pineapple, peanuts, Emmental cheese, almonds, lemons, and other cheeses. The commonly cited OU-triggering foods, with their histamine-rich or -liberating properties, indicate a hyperreactivity mechanism [19]. Smoking cessation and menstruation may play a role in the recurrence of OUs in BD. Additionally, patients with BD often have conditions associated with poor oral hygiene, such as periodontitis, chronic tonsillitis, and dental caries. The occurrence of OUs and disease attacks in these patients might be associated with unusual streptococcal strains, particularly *S. sanguinis* [7].

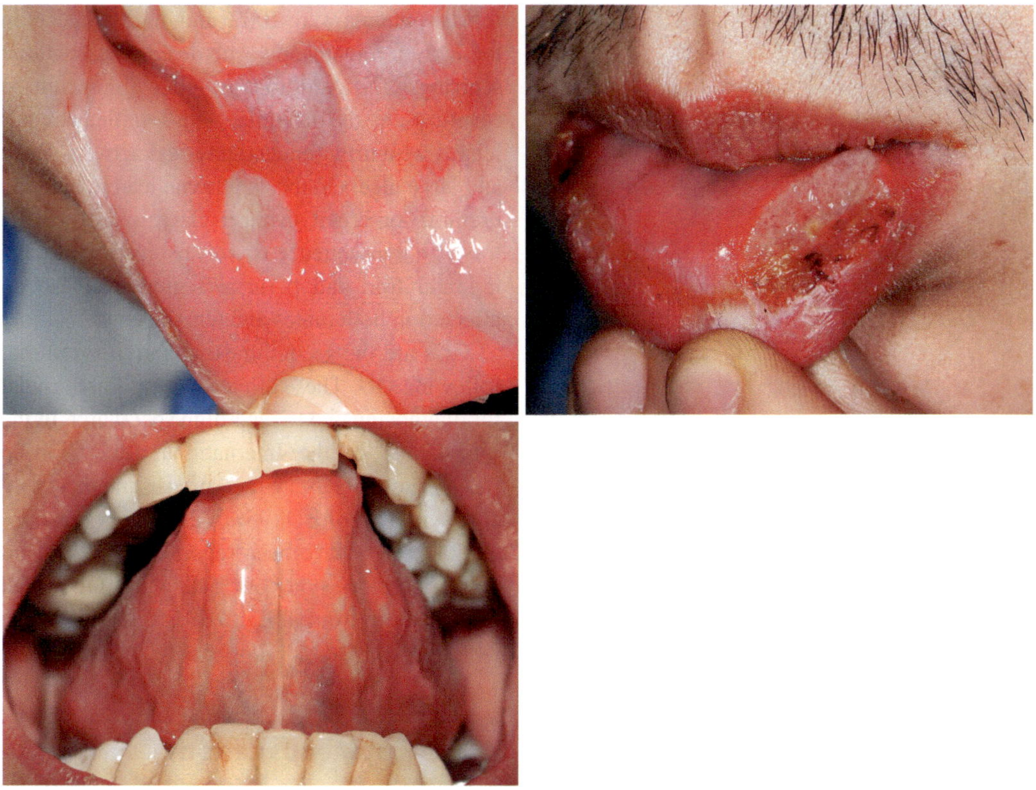

Figs. 7.1–7.3 Oral ulcers can be classified into three categories: minor (Fig. 7.1), major (Fig. 7.2), or herpetiform (Fig. 7.3), depending on their size and number

OUs can be extremely painful and can cause difficulties with eating, drinking, speaking, swallowing, and maintaining oral hygiene [13]. While the frequency and severity of mucocutaneous symptoms decrease with age, OUs can persist throughout the course of the disease [20]. They are observed in almost all cases of the disease [7]. In different populations such as Türkiye, Greece, Italy, Egypt, and Japan, OUs have been reported as the initial manifestation in a significant percentage of cases (63.4–88.7%) [21–25]. Additional symptoms required for the diagnosis of the disease typically appear around 4 years after the onset of OUs [3, 9]. The morphology and course of OUs seen in BD are similar to recurrent aphthous stomatitis (RAS), making it difficult to distinguish between the two clinically. However, a comparative study found that major OUs and involvement of multiple oral mucosa sites were more common in BD patients compared to RAS patients [26].

7.3 Genital Ulcers

Their clinical presentation is similar to OUs but has a lower frequency of recurrence. GUs are typically oval or round in shape and covered with a necrotic or yellowish membrane. They can be either solitary or multiple in nature, with a higher prevalence in the scrotum (89%) (Fig. 7.4) in males and labia majora (71%) (Fig. 7.5) in females [27]. GUs can be observed on various parts of the male genitalia, including the penis shaft, glans, and even the meatal urethra. Ulcers in female patients can present in labia minora, vagina, and, rarely, in the cervix, leading to a potential bloody purulent discharge in the latter two sites [6, 13]. The average healing time for GUs is approximately 2–4 weeks. Scarring is a frequent consequence resulting from their deeper location. Hence, it is imperative to examine both the residual scars of past ulcers and the current

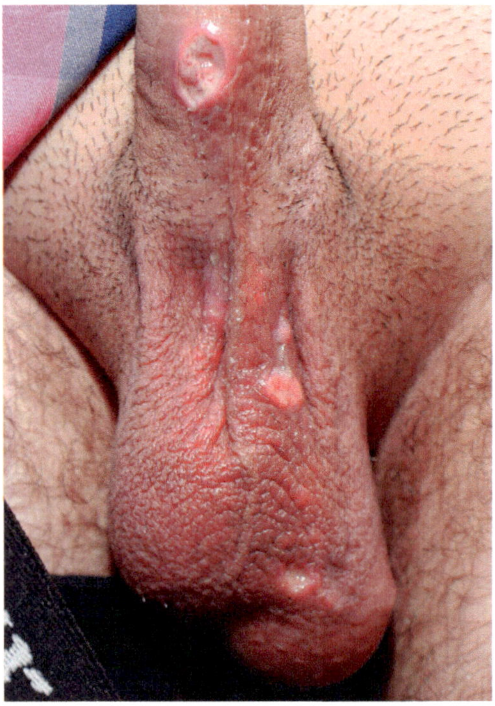

Fig. 7.4 In men, the scrotum is the primary location for genital ulcers

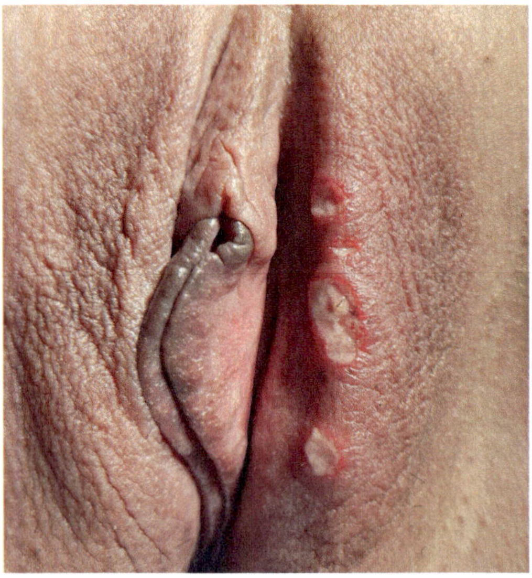

Fig. 7.5 Genital ulcers are most commonly found on labia majora in female patients

active ulcers in the diagnosis of BD. Male patients had a scar formation rate of 89% for large ulcers (>1 cm) and 49% for small ulcers. These rates in female patients were 100% and 40.5%. Ulcers in the labium minus and vestibule can heal without scarring [27]. Additionally, GUs can result in severe pain, dyspareunia, and significant challenges with urination and physical activity. Deep and large ulcers in the vagina can lead to bladder, urethral, or rectal fistulae. Occasionally, tissue loss is a consequence of vulvar ulcerations. The inguinal fold and perianal region can also be affected in both males and females [6, 13].

GUs are the second most common symptom, following OU. These clinical features are crucial for diagnosing due to their high specificity. In the formulation of the International Study Group (ISG) criteria, GUs are measured as the most specific symptom of BD (95%) [28]. In various populations, GUs have been reported as the second most common symptom following OU, with rates ranging from 4.9% to 29.2% [3, 8, 10, 22, 24, 25].

7.4 Cutaneous Lesions

Erythema nodosum (EN)-like lesions can be observed in roughly 1/3 of patients (15 78%), particularly among females (70%) [29]. The main clinical features of these conditions include painful, red, hot subcutaneous nodules, commonly observed in the lower limbs, specifically the pretibial region (Fig. 7.6). Additionally, they can occasionally be found in the gluteal region, upper extremities, face, and neck. EN-like lesions do not ulcerate and typically undergo healing within a period of 2–4 weeks, causing post-inflammatory hyperpigmentation in pigmented patients. Typically, they are accompanied by systemic symptoms including fever, malaise, and arthralgia [1, 6, 15].

Papulopustular lesions (PPL), appearing as folliculitis or acne-like sterile pustules on an erythematous base (Fig. 7.7), are the most frequent cutaneous manifestation. Papules initially appear and subsequently transform into pustules within a span of 24–48 h. Their prevalence is highest on the trunk, lower extremities, and face [30]. Differentiating PPL from acne vulgaris or folliculitis is crucial in patients diagnosed with BD in

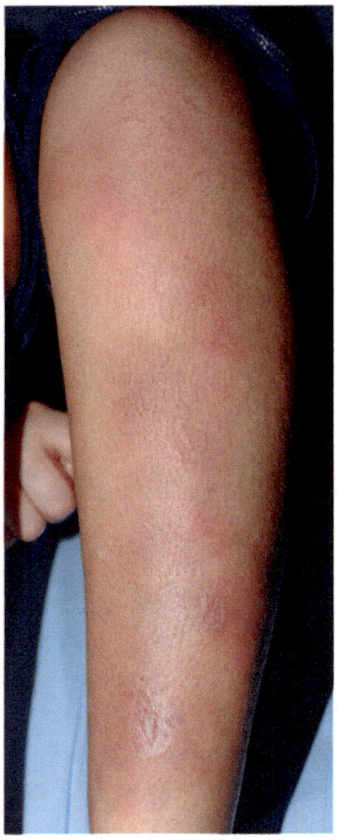

Fig. 7.6 Erythema nodosum-like lesions typically manifest as painful, red, and hot subcutaneous nodules located in the pretibial region

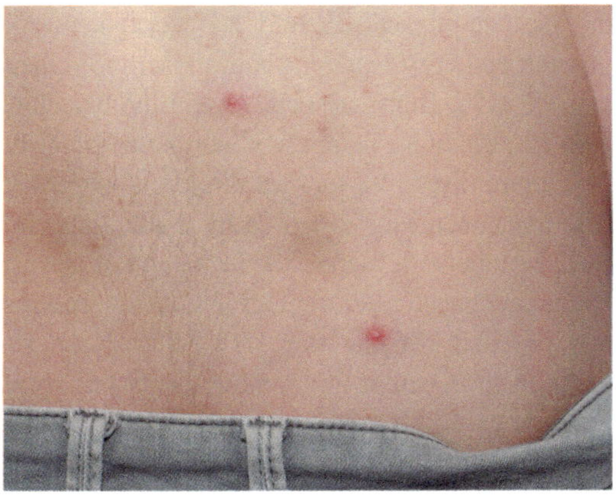

Fig. 7.7 Papulopustular lesions manifest as pustules on an erythematous base, resembling folliculitis or acne

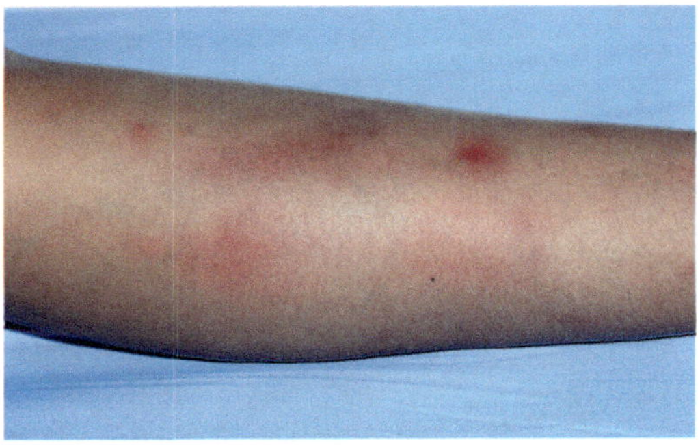

Fig. 7.8 Superficial thrombophlebitis is characterized by painful, erythematous, subcutaneous nodules along a vein

the presence of PPL. In this scenario, our recommendation is to conduct a biopsy on nonfollicular PPL found in nonseborrheic areas of the trunk and extremities, verifying the presence of vascular reaction or vasculitis histopathologically [31]. Patients with skin pathergy reaction (SPR) positivity and arthritis tend to have a higher incidence of PPL [30, 32].

Superficial thrombophlebitis (ST); is observed in 10–20% of BD patients, with a higher prevalence in males. The most common venous involvement of the disease is ST of the lower legs [1, 6]. ST lesions are characterized by painful, erythematous nodules located subcutaneously. These nodules exhibit a linear distribution that follows the vein trace (Fig. 7.8). Palpation can reveal a string-like stiffness caused by thrombosis and sclerosis [6]. ST has prognostic significance due to its potential association with other vascular conditions such as deep vein thrombosis and dural sinus thrombosis [33].

Other Cutaneous Lesions Extragenital ulcer (ExU) is a rare (3%) yet distinctive cutaneous finding of the condition, characterized by deep-seated, punched-out ulcers with erythematous and edematous edges, and a yellow necrotic base. The axilla, thigh (Fig. 7.9), breast, neck, inguinal region, and between the toes are frequent sites of occurrence [34]. ExU shows a recurrent course and is associated with scar formation [1]. Sweet syndrome-like lesions have been documented in 4% of cases [35]. They are identified by painful red nodules/plaques on the face, neck, and limbs, along with fever and leukocytosis. Sweet's syndrome and BD share clinical and histological similarities. Differential diagnosis can be challenging. Leg ulcers, often found between the ankle and knee, are ulcers that involve the reticular dermis and deeper tissues (Fig. 7.10). They

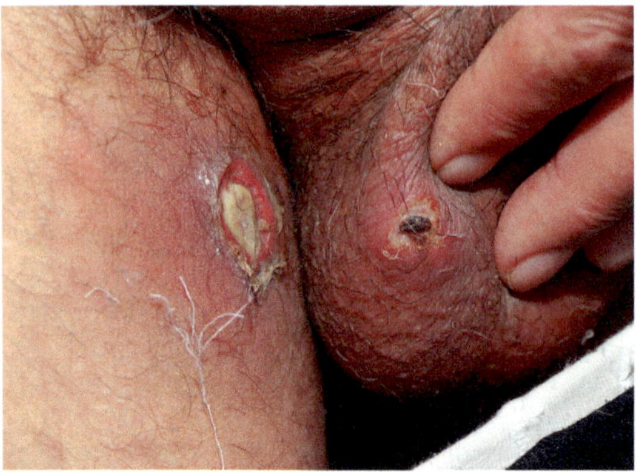

Fig. 7.9 Extragenital ulcer: deep, punched-out ulcers with erythematous edges and yellow necrotic base

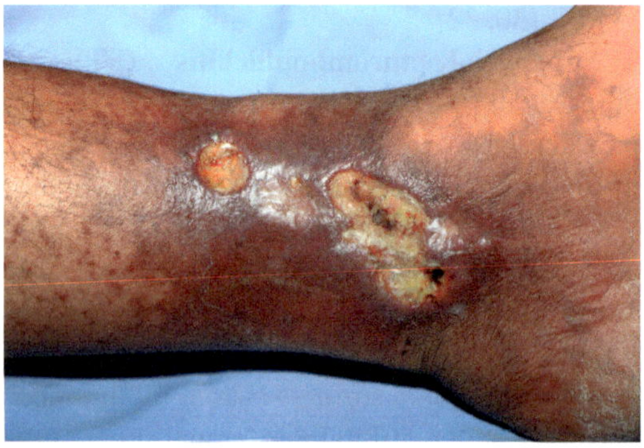

Fig. 7.10 Leg ulcers usually develop between the ankle and knee, involving deeper tissues

have a recurring and treatment-resistant course. Leg ulcers have been found to be associated with deep vein thrombosis [36, 37]. On rare occasions, various cutaneous vasculitic lesions have been documented, including pyoderma gangrenosum-like lesions, palpable purpura, necrotizing bullous vasculitis, pernio-like lesions, polyarteritis nodosa-like lesions, and acral purpuric papulonodular lesions [38–44].

7.5 Skin Pathergy Reaction

Skin pathergy reaction refers to an elevated nonspecific skin hyperreactivity subsequent to needle puncture. The forearm flexor face is punctured

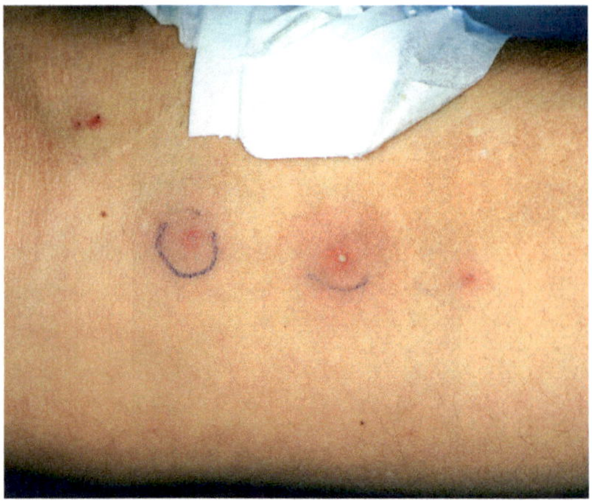

Fig. 7.11 The presence of an erythematous papule or pustule at the needle-prick site, appearing 48 h later, indicates skin pathergy reaction positivity

with a 20G syringe needle at three separate points, inserted intradermally at a 45-degree angle. The presence of an erythematous papule or pustule at the needle-prick site, appearing 48 h after the application, defines the SPR positivity (Fig. 7.11) [1, 6]. Among males, the positivity is more pronounced. Various factors, such as the physical properties of the needles, the number of pricks, and disease-related factors like having an active disease, can impact SPR [45]. It is worth mentioning that pathergy reactions can impact more than just the skin. BD is associated with an exaggerated inflammatory response when tissue integrity is compromised. Various examples of pathergy reactions occurring at different tissue sites are well documented, such as the formation of thrombus or aneurysm after angiographic interventions and vascular surgery [46, 47], ST induced by venipuncture, ocular inflammation resulting from intraocular corticosteroid injections [48], and the occurrence of anastomotic ulcers following surgical treatment of intestinal ulcers [49].

7.6 Differential Diagnosis

Given the absence of a diagnostic laboratory marker for BD, diagnosis relies on clinical manifestations. The diagnostic criteria for BD typically encompass various mucocutaneous manifestations, including OUs, GUs, cutaneous lesions, and SPR positivity. The ISG criteria are widely accepted and commonly used by experts in this field for diagnosis. The diagnosis of BD is made in the presence of any two of recurrent GUs, typical ocular involvement, typical cutaneous lesions, or positive SPR in addition to recurrent OUs [28]. The International Criteria for Behcet's Disease (ICBD) is a newly established and extensively employed set of diagnostic criteria in this particular field. OUs, GUs, and ocular involvement are assigned 2 points, while skin lesions, neurological manifestations, vascular manifestations, and positive SPR are assigned 1 point each. A diagnosis of BD is given to those who score four and above [50]. The Japanese Diagnostic Criteria are commonly used in Far Eastern countries. Mucocutaneous symptoms are included in three out of the four major criteria (OUs, GUs, cutaneous lesions, and ocular involvement) [51].

Diseases with recurrent ulcers in the oral mucosa and/or genitalia are primarily considered in the differential diagnosis, as recurrent OUs and GUs are the most common and characteristic symptoms of the disease. For this particular section of the book chapter, I intend to delve into the differential diagnosis by presenting a genuine case report.

Case 1

A 22-year-old female was referred to our clinic with recurrent OUs for 4 years and GUs for 6 months (Fig. 7.12a, b). Apart from that, her physical examination was normal. The results of the routine laboratory search were within normal limits, ruling out any underlying possible diseases.

While this combination strongly suggests the possibility of BD, it is important to recognize that other conditions may have similar presentations. Because of our patient's complaints, we focused on diseases that present with recurrent OUs and GUs. We considered the conditions summarized in Table 7.1 in the differential diagnosis. However, in daily practice, diseases such as herpes simplex virus (HSV) infection, fixed drug eruption, some cases of erythema multiforme and finally complex aphthosis are often confused with BD. It is therefore important to begin with a brief summary of these conditions.

HSV infection is responsible for the formation of clusters of itchy vesicles that quickly turn into erosions on any mucocutaneous area, including the oral mucosa and genitalia (Fig. 7.13a, b). It is important to note that especially non-dermatologists may misdiagnose HSV infection as BD, particularly when both the oral mucosa and genitalia are affected. In cases of HSV infection, recurrences in the same location are common. However, the patient did not report any

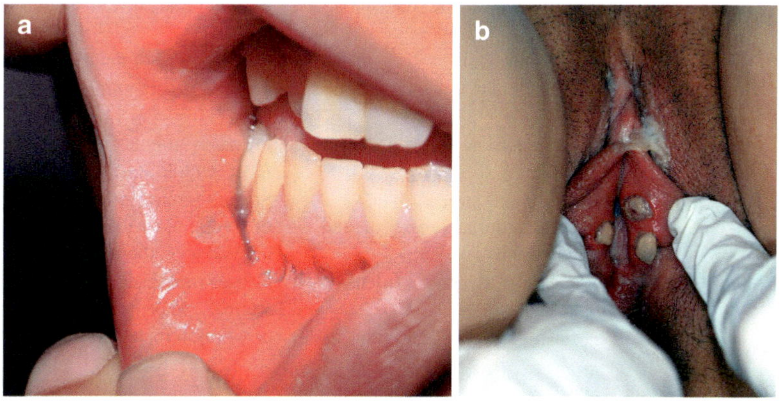

Fig. 7.12 (**a**) Aphthous oral ulcer located on the mucosa of the lower lip. (**b**) Multiple genital ulcers on the labium minus

Table 7.1 Differential diagnosis for mucocutaneous manifestations

Manifestation	Differential diagnosis	Features that distinguish it from BD
Recurrent OU and/or GU	Herpes simplex	Cluster of small, shallow ulcers, recurrence in the same localization and the presence of multinucleated acantholytic cells in Tzanck smear and/or *HSV-PCR positivity*
	Bullous fixed drug eruption	Each intake of the causative drug results in recurring erosions at the same "fixed" site, with a nummular erythematous base, and leaving a residual post-inflammatory pigmentation
	Erythema multiforme	Target lesions found mainly on acral and periorificial areas
	Complex aphthosis	No mucocutaneous symptoms, except for OU and GU, or organ involvement.
	Sweet's syndrome	Painful red plaques with a vesicle-like appearance; diverse overlapping extracutaneous manifestations from BD (e.g. asymmetric polyarthralgia, conjunctivitis and episcleritis), fever
	MAGIC syndrome	Relapsing polychondritis, as well as OU and GU
	Haploinsufficiency A20 (HA20)	Positive family history and early onset (<10 years) with a variety of symptoms (e.g. OU, GU, fever, gastrointestinal ulcers, skin lesions, autoimmunity, joint involvement)
	Autoimmune bullous diseases (e.g. pemphigus vulgaris)	Blistering diseases affecting the mucous membranes and the skin, erosions
	Erosive lichen planus	Painful erosions in the oral mucosa and the genital area with itchy, violaceous (purple), polygonal, flat-topped papules and plaques on the skin
	Hand-foot-mouth disease	Painful vesicles on the hands, feet and diaper area in addition to OU following the vesicles
	Acatalasemia	For childhood cases involving the alveolar region, acatalasemia should be ruled out with a hydrogen peroxide test
	Recurrent aphthous stomatitis	There is no further involvement of mucocutaneous or organ systems.
	Reiter's syndrome	Diverse cutaneous and overlapping extracutaneous manifestations (e.g. keratoderma blennorrhagicum, circinate balanitis, conjunctivitis, urethritis)
	Deficiency of iron, vitamin B12 or folic acid	Laboratory proof of the deficiency and positive response to replacement.
	Inflammatory bowel diseases (Crohn's disease and ulcerative colitis)	GU are extremely rare
	Systemic lupus erythematosus	Irregular and slit-like lesions on the palate with ANA positivity
	Cyclic neutropenia	The presence of neutropenia during attacks
	HIV infection	The lesions are numerous, deep, and cause severe weight loss
	PFAPA syndrome	Primarily affects children under 5; it is the leading cause of fever in children
	Syphilis, chancroid, lymphogranuloma venereum, and HIV infection	Sexually transmitted infections can lead to the development of genital ulcer disease, which can be identified by using clinical and laboratory markers.
	Acute genital ulceration (ulcus vulvae acutum)	Causes rapid painful ulcerations of the vulva or lower vagina, and primarily affects sexually inactive adolescents or young females

(continued)

Table 7.1 (continued)

Manifestation	Differential diagnosis	Features that distinguish it from BD
EN-like lesions	Classical EN	Presents with septal panniculitis, without vasculitis or vascular reaction seen in BD's EN-like lesions.
	Superficial thrombophlebitis	Linear distribution along the vein, hypoechoic pattern on ultrasound (EN-like lesions show hyperechoic pattern)
	Nodular vasculitis	Red-purple nodules primarily found on the posterior or lateral lower limbs can lead to ulceration, atrophy, and scarring
Papulopustular lesions	Acne vulgaris	Presence of polymorphic lesions and comedones, mostly facial location
	Folliculitis	Localisation of follicles and positive culture (e.g., staphylococcus)

BD Behçet disease, *EN* erythema nodosum, *GU* genital ulcer, *HSV* herpes simplex virus, *OU* oral ulcer, *PCR* polymerase chain reaction, *MAGIC syndrome* mouth and genital ulcer with inflamed cartilage syndrome, *PFAPA* periodic fever, aphthous stomatitis, pharyngitis, and cervical adenitis

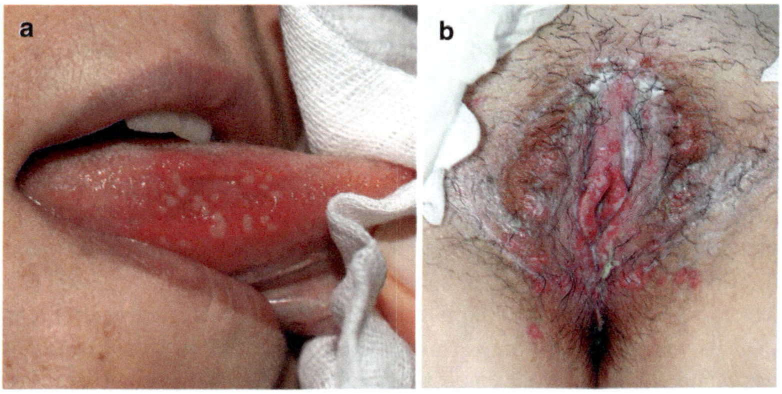

Fig. 7.13 (**a**) Small closely grouped vesicles in the mouth quickly develop into shallow ulcers within a day. (**b**) Multiple shallow ulcers on the external genital organs and mucosal surfaces of the vulva are accompanied by pain and sometimes dysuria

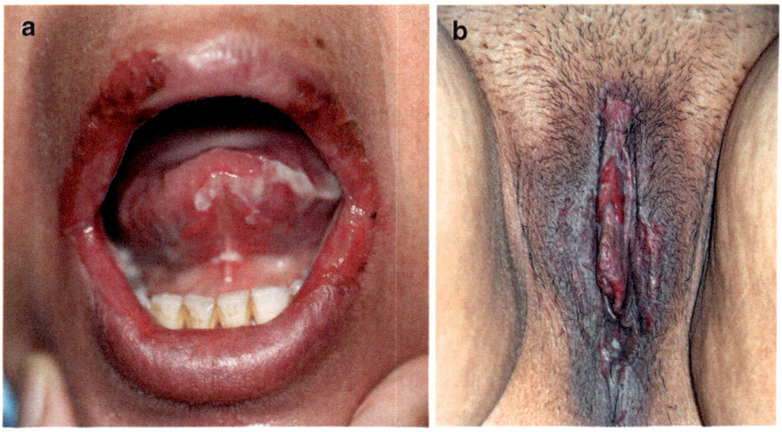

Fig. 7.14 (**a**) Bullous fixed drug eruption on the lip and oral mucosa can cause ulcers that resemble aphthae. (**b**) Erythematous plaques with bullae at the centre rapidly progress to erosion and subsequently regress with pigmentation within a few days to weeks

recurrence following grouped vesicles in the same anatomical area, and the Tzanc test did not detect multinucleated acantholytic cells. *Bullous fixed drug eruption* is a distinctive eruption characterized by solitary or multiple round or oval-shaped inflamed patches or plaques with a blister. This eruption always reappears in the same area upon reexposure to the offending drug. After the rash disappears, a dark brown patch remains, which can last for several weeks to months (Fig. 7.14a, b). The patient did not have a history of any drug or recurrence in the same anatomical area. Additionally, there was no erosion or residual post-inflammatory pigmentation observed during the clinic visit. *Erythema multiforme* is characterized by tense blisters that arise from the center of a ring or target-like lesion, particularly in the acral and periorificial areas. It may also be associated with oral or genital erosions or ulcers. However, the patient did not have target-like lesions clinically, and there was no history of any medication that could trigger this reaction. *Complex aphthosis* is the term used to describe almost constant multiple (>3) oral aphthous lesions or recurrent oral and genital aphthae without systemic symptoms of BD [52]. The symptoms of the case presented here overlap with the diagnosis of complex aphthosis. As BD usually starts in the oral and genital areas, the likelihood of complex aphthosis being the initial stage of BD is not low, especially in places where the disease is endemic. It is therefore recommended that these patients be followed closely at regular intervals using clinical criteria for progression to BD [1].

Additional conditions that should be given less priority in the differential diagnosis of patients who present with recurrent OU and GU symptoms, similar to our case, are briefly discussed below. *Sweet's syndrome* is distinguished by painful erythematous plaques showing the "illusion of vesicles". There are overlapping extracutaneous manifestations different from BD (e.g., asymmetric polyarthralgia, conjunctivitis, and episcleritis) and fever. OUs and GUs are rare. The *Magic syndrome* is defined by the presence of inflammation in cartilage, such as in the ear, nose, throat, and rib cage, as well as recurrent OUs and GUs. *Haploinsufficiency A20 (HA20)* is a monogenic autoinflammatory disease characterized by a variety of symptoms with early onset (<10 years) and a positive family history. These symptoms include (in order of frequency) OUs and GUs, fever, gastrointestinal ulcers, skin lesions, autoimmunity (such as thyroiditis and lupus) and joint involvement [53]. Occasionally, certain mucocutaneous diseases may manifest as nonaphthous oral and/or genital lesions, similar to bullous fixed drug eruption and erythema multiforme, and may need to be differentiated from BD. Autoimmune bullous diseases, such as *pemphigus vulgaris* (Fig. 7.15) and, less commonly, *mucosal pemphigoid*, *bullous pemphigoid*, can cause erosions and/or scars, particularly on the oral mucosa and sometimes on the genitalia, following vesicles and bullae. Although bullous skin lesions often accompany these diseases, they are rarely limited to the oral mucosa and the genitalia. However, the patient did not have a history of blistering diseases affecting the mucous membranes and skin. Upon examination, no vesicle, bullae or scar were observed, and other potential sites of mucosal involvement, such as the conjunctiva and nasopharynx, appeared normal. *Erosive lichen planus* results in painful erosions, specifically in the oral mucosa and occasionally in the genital area. Typical lichen planus lesions, itchy, violaceous (purple), polygonal, flat-topped papules and plaques, may accompany erosive lichen planus. The patient's dermatological examination did not exhibit the characteristic papulosquamous skin manifestations and/or mucosal lesions seen in erosive lichen planus.

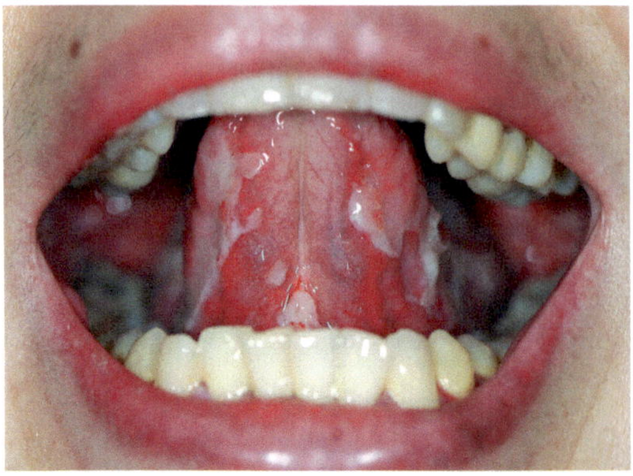

Fig. 7.15 Pemphigus vulgaris typically presents with blisters on the oral mucosa that quickly rupture into painful erosions

Recurrent oral mucosal ulcers should be taken into account as one of the conditions in the differential diagnosis of this case. Conditions like herpes simplex, herpetiform, minor or major forms of RAS, erythema multiforme, fixed drug eruption, hand-foot-mouth disease, and acatalasemia (Takahara's disease) often have a recurring course. We have already mentioned some of these diagnoses above. *Hand–foot–mouth disease* is a viral infection causing painful vesicles on the hands, feet and diaper area in addition to OUs that develop following the vesicles. When dealing with cases that start in childhood and involve the alveolar region, it is important to conduct the hydrogen peroxide test to rule out the possibility of *acatalasemia*, a rare genetic catalase deficiency. This condition can cause an increased incidence of oral ulcers and, in rare cases, gangrene. *RAS* is diagnosed when all these potential causes have been ruled out. The abovementioned MAGIC syndrome, Sweet's syndrome, and BD can all include RAS as a symptom. *Reiter's syndrome*, characterized by a variety of cutaneous and extracutaneous manifestations (e.g., keratoderma blennorrhagicum, circinate balanitis, conjunctivitis, urethritis), can also have an association with RAS. *Anemia* caused by iron, vitamin B12, or folic acid deficiency, as well as *inflammatory bowel diseases* like Crohn's disease and ulcerative colitis, are potential underlying factors for RAS. Oral ulcers are one of the American Rheumatism Association's criteria for the diagnosis of *systemic lupus erythematosus*. Almost half of such lupus erythematosus patients have OUs with irregular and slit-like appearance. Lesions are usually located on the palate (Fig. 7.16) and often heal with scar. The major form of RAS is also called Sutton's disease. It is characterized by well-defined, larger (≥1 cm), deeply punched-out, painful ulcers, which heal with scarring, and may be associated with *cyclic neutropenia* besides the causes mentioned for RAS above. In patients with *HIV infection*, although the incidence of aphthous ulcers is not increased, the lesions are more numerous and deeper, so that they interfere with nourishment and lead to severe weight loss. *PFAPA syndrome*, an autoinflammatory disorder primarily observed in children under the age of 5, may also involve RAS as one of its components. PFAPA, an acronym for periodic fever, aphthous stomatitis, pharyngitis, and cervical adenitis, is the most common cause of periodic fever in childhood. Clinical examination and laboratory tests excluded all of these potential diagnoses in the presented case here.

When considering the differential diagnosis of the patient's GU, it is important to first consider conditions that present with recurrent GUs. Herpes simplex infection is a significant condition that needs to be considered in differential diagnoses. The genital area is a frequent location for both erythema multiforme and fixed drug eruption. Detailed information about all these diseases can be found above. In addition to recurrent GU conditions, if there are rapidly evolving erosions or ulcers without any signs of blistering in both the patient's history and physical examination, it is important to investigate sexually transmitted diseases such as *syphilis* (Fig. 7.17),

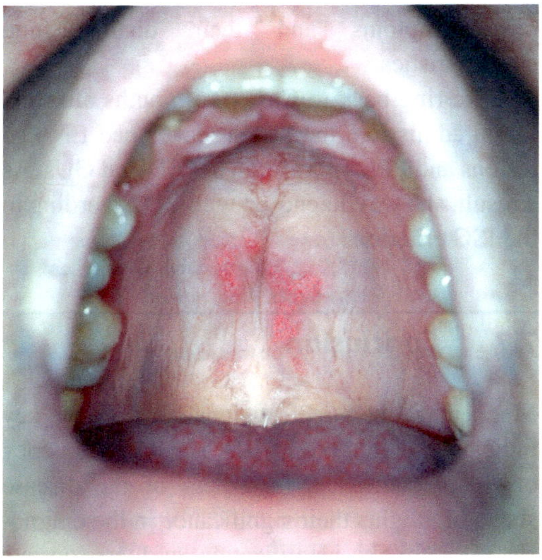

Fig. 7.16 Irregular, painless, erythematous ulcers on the palate are a specific type of ulcer associated with lupus erythematosus

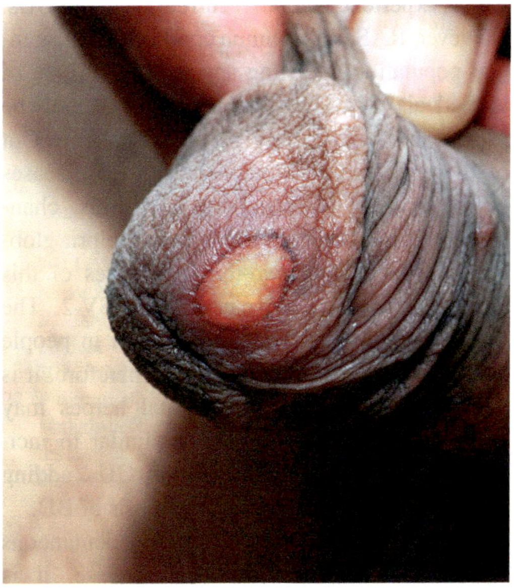

Fig. 7.17 The syphilis chancre begins as a small, painless, red papule on the genital area and quickly develops into a painless ulcer with a well-defined margin and an indurated base

24. El Menyawi MM, Raslan HM, Edrees A. Clinical features of Behcet's disease in Egypt. Rheumatol Int. 2009;29(6):641–6.
25. Zhang Z, He F, Shi Y. Behcet's disease seen in China: analysis of 334 cases. Rheumatol Int. 2013;33(3):645–8.
26. Oh SH, Han EC, Lee JH, Bang D. Comparison of the clinical features of recurrent aphthous stomatitis and Behçet's disease. Clin Exp Dermatol. 2009;34(6):e208–12.
27. Mat MC, Goksugur N, Engin B, Yurdakul S, Yazici H. The frequency of scarring after genital ulcers in Behçet's syndrome: a prospective study. Int J Dermatol. 2006;45(5):554–6.
28. Criteria for diagnosis of Behçet's disease. International study Group for Behçet's disease. Lancet. 1990;335(8697):1078–80.
29. Yazici H, Tüzün Y, Pazarli H, Yurdakul S, Ozyazgan Y, Ozdoğan H, et al. Influence of age of onset and patient's sex on the prevalence and severity of manifestations of Behçet's syndrome. Ann Rheum Dis. 1984;43(6):783–9.
30. Alpsoy E, Aktekin M, Er H, Durusoy C, Yilmaz E. A randomized, controlled and blinded study of papulopustular lesions in Turkish Behçet's patients. Int J Dermatol. 1998;37(11):839–42.
31. Alpsoy E, Uzun S, Akman A, Acar MA, Memişoglu HR, Başaran E. Histological and immunofluorescence findings of non-follicular papulopustular lesions in patients with Behçet's disease. J Eur Acad Dermatol Venereol. 2003;17(5):521–4.
32. Diri E, Mat C, Hamuryudan V, Yurdakul S, Hizli N, Yazici H. Papulopustular skin lesions are seen more frequently in patients with Behçet's syndrome who have arthritis: a controlled and masked study. Ann Rheum Dis. 2001;60(11):1074–6.
33. Tunc R, Saip S, Siva A, Yazici H. Cerebral venous thrombosis is associated with major vessel disease in Behçet's syndrome. Ann Rheum Dis. 2004;63(12):1693–4.
34. Azizlerli G, Ozarmagan G, Ovul C, Sarica R, Mustafa SO. A new kind of skin lesion in Behcet's disease: extragenital ulcerations. Acta Derm Venereol. 1992;72(4):286.
35. Karadoğan SK, Başkan EB, Alkan G, Saricaoğlu H, Tunali S. Generalized Sweet syndrome lesions associated with Behçet disease: a true association or simply co-morbidity? Am J Clin Dermatol. 2009;10(5):331–5.
36. Jung JY, Kim DY, Bang D. Leg ulcers in Behçet's disease. Br J Dermatol. 2008;158(1):178–9.
37. Hatemi G, Christensen R, Bang D, Bodaghi B, Celik AF, Fortune F, et al. 2018 update of the EULAR recommendations for the management of Behçet's syndrome. Ann Rheum Dis. 2018;77(6):808–18.
38. Munro CS, Cox NH. Pyoderma gangrenosum associated with Behçet's syndrome—response to thalidomide. Clin Exp Dermatol. 1988;13(6):408–10.
39. Lee SH, Chung KY, Lee WS, Lee S. Behçet's syndrome associated with bullous necrotizing vasculitis. J Am Acad Dermatol. 1989;21(2 Pt 2):327–30.
40. Cornelis F, Sigal-Nahum M, Gaulier A, Bleichner G, Sigal S. Behçet's disease with severe cutaneous necrotizing vasculitis: response to plasma exchange—report of a case. J Am Acad Dermatol. 1989;21(3 Pt 1):576–9.
41. Ateş A, Karaaslan Y, Aşlar ZO. A case of Behçet's disease associated with necrotizing small vessel vasculitis. Rheumatol Int. 2006;27(1):91–3.
42. Cantini F, Salvarani C, Niccoli L, Senesi C, Truglia MC, Padula A, et al. Behçet's disease with unusual cutaneous lesions. J Rheumatol. 1998;25(12):2469–72.
43. Liao YH, Hsiao GH, Hsiao CH. Behçet's disease with cutaneous changes resembling polyarteritis nodosa. Br J Dermatol. 1999;140(2):368–9.
44. King R, Crowson AN, Murray E, Magro CM. Acral purpuric papulonodular lesions as a manifestation of Behçet's disease. Int J Dermatol. 1995;34(3):190–2.
45. Ergun T. Pathergy phenomenon. Front Med (Lausanne). 2021;8:639404. https://doi.org/10.3389/fmed.2021.639404.
46. Alpagut U, Ugurlucan M, Dayioglu E. Major arterial involvement and review of Behçet's disease. Ann Vasc Surg. 2007;21(2):232–9.
47. Tüzün H, Besirli K, Sayin A, Vural FS, Hamuryudan V, Hizli N, et al. Management of aneurysms in Behçet's syndrome: an analysis of 24 patients. Surgery. 1997;121(2):150–6.
48. Yalcindag FN, Batioglu F. Pathergy-like reaction following intravitreal triamcinolone acetonide injection in a patient with Behçet's disease. Ocul Immunol Inflamm. 2008;16(4):181–3.
49. Choi IJ, Kim JS, Cha SD, Jung HC, Park JG, Song IS, et al. Long-term clinical course and prognostic factors in intestinal Behçet's disease. Dis Colon Rectum. 2000;43(5):692–700.
50. International Team for the Revision of the International Criteria for Behçet's Disease (ITR-ICBD). The international criteria for Behçet's disease (ICBD): a collaborative study of 27 countries on the sensitivity and specificity of the new criteria. J Eur Acad Dermatol Venereol. 2014;28(3):338–47.
51. Mizushima Y. Revised diagnostic criteria for Behçet's disease in 1987. Ryumachi. 1988;28:66–70.
52. Jorizzo JL, Taylor RS, Schmalstieg FC, Solomon AR Jr, Daniels JC, Rudloff HE, et al. Complex aphthosis: a forme fruste of Behçet's syndrome? J Am Acad Dermatol. 1985;13(1):80–4.
53. Elhani I, Riller Q, Boursier G, Hentgen V, Rieux-Laucat F, Georgin-Lavialle S. A20 Haploinsufficiency: a systematic review of 177 cases. J Invest Dermatol. 2023.:S0022-202X(23)03194-9; https://doi.org/10.1016/j.jid.2023.12.007.
54. Patil S, Reddy SN, Maheshwari S, Khandelwal S, Shruthi D, Doni B. Prevalence of recurrent aphthous ulceration in the Indian population. J Clin Exp Dent. 2014;6(1):e36–40.
55. Batteiger TA, Rietmeijer CA. Herpes simplex virus: a practical guide to diagnosis, management, and patient counseling for the primary care clinician. Med Clin North Am. 2024;108(2):311–23.

8 Specificity of Papulopustular Lesions in the Diagnosis of Behçet's Disease

Göknur Kalkan and Ayşe Boyvat

Contents

8.1 Introduction

Behçet's disease (BD) is a chronic multisystemic disease characterized by mucocutaneous lesions and involvement of the ocular, articular, vascular, neurologic, and gastrointestinal systems. There are no distinctive diagnostic laboratory tests, and the diagnosis is based on a thorough review of the patient's medical history, and the identification of typical clinical findings.

Across time, various criteria and classifications have emerged from different groups, aiming to provide greater objectivity in diagnosis. Upon examination of these criteria, a noticeable emphasis is placed on mucocutaneous findings [1–5]. Mucocutaneous lesions are the most commonly observed signs of BD often appearing before the manifestation of systemic involvement. Consequently, identifying mucocutaneous lesions holds immense importance in the disease's early diagnosis and prognosis.

Behçet's disease presents a variety of cutaneous lesions, including erythema nodosum like lesions, papulopustular lesions, extragenital ulcerations, Sweet's syndrome like lesions, pyoderma gangrenosum-like lesions and erythema multiforme-like lesions [6–8]. However, the diagnostic criteria primarily include the most common cutaneous findings—erythema nodosum like lesions and papulopustular lesions—alongside oral aphthous ulceration and genital ulceration.

G. Kalkan (✉)
Department of Dermatology, School of Medicine, Ankara Yıldırım Beyazıt University, Ankara, Türkiye

A. Boyvat
Dermatology and Venereology, Ankara University, Faculty of Medicine, Ankara, Türkiye
e-mail: boyvat@medicine.ankara.edu.tr

E. Alpsoy et al. (eds.), *Behçet's Disease: An Integrated Approach*,
https://doi.org/10.1007/978-3-031-77251-1_8

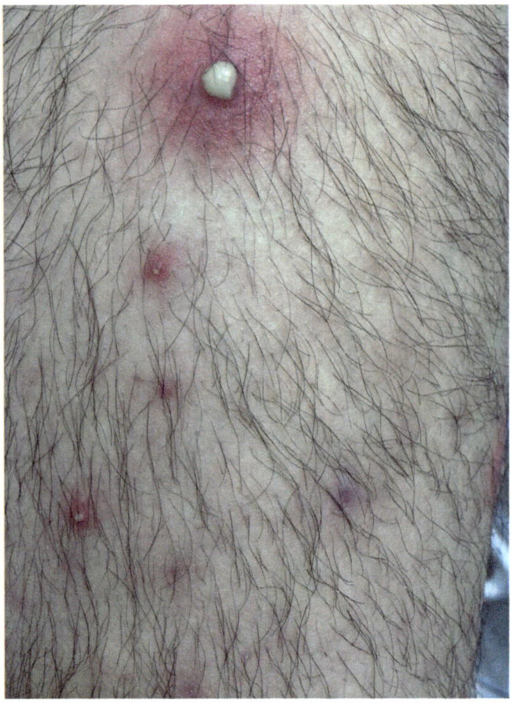

Fig. 8.1 Behçet's disease-associated papulopustular lesions localized on the legs

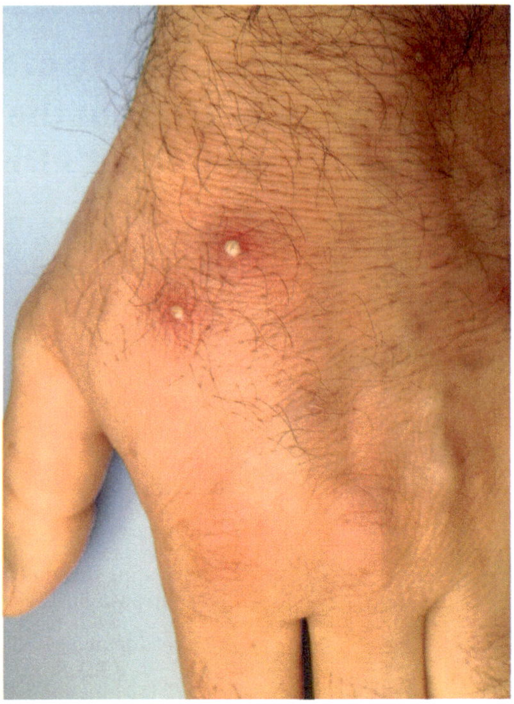

Fig. 8.2 Papulopustular lesions on the hand of a Behçet's disease patient

Papulopustular lesions of BD typically present as erythematous papules or pustules primarily localized on the lower extremities, though they can also manifest on the upper extremities, face, neck, and trunk (Figs. 8.1, 8.2 and 8.3) [6, 7]. These lesions are reported in 40–70% of BD patients with some studies indicating an even higher frequency [9–12]. The International study group (ISG) for BD calculated the sensitivity and specificity of papulopustular lesions as 70% and 76%, respectively [1]. Similarly, in the collaborative study of the "International Criteria for Behçet's Disease" (ICBD) sensitivity and specificity of papulopustular lesions were found as 53% and 92%, respectively [2].

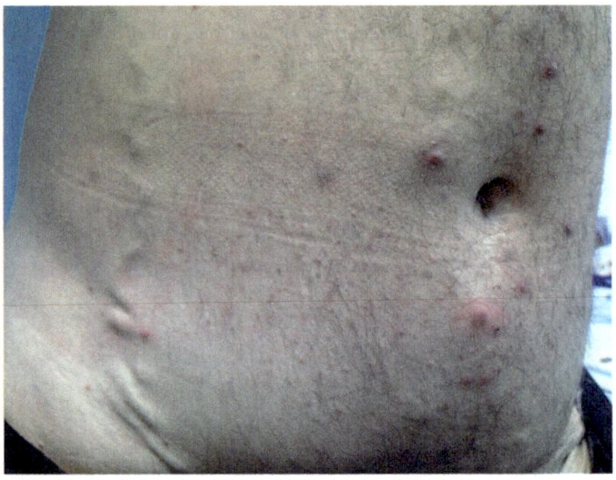

Fig. 8.3 Behçet's disease patient with vena cava inferior syndrome and abdominal papulopustular lesions

8.2 Navigating Diagnostic Challenges: Clinical Similarities of Papulopustular Lesions

While papulopustular lesions are listed in the diagnostic criteria, their diagnostic significance has been a subject of long-standing debate. Despite featuring a typical erythematous base (Fig. 8.4), these lesions pose challenges due to their lack of a distinct clinical appearance, especially when localized on the face and back, making differentiation from acne lesions difficult (Fig. 8.5). Moreover, distinguishing these lesions from the pustules of bacterial folliculitis can also be challenging (Fig. 8.6). This similarity has resulted in various terms like acneiform nodules and pseudo folliculitis being used interchangeably with papulopustular lesions in literature. To avoid confusion, we prefer using "papulopustular lesions" as the singular term. However, "necrotizing folliculitis," another term used in literature to describe papulopustular lesions, should be omitted as papulopustular lesions lack necrosis, do not result in scarring during healing, and frequently do not involve the follicles.

The clinical resemblance of papulopustular lesions to nonspecific follicular lesions raises concerns about their inclusion in the diagnostic criteria. BD typically presents between the ages

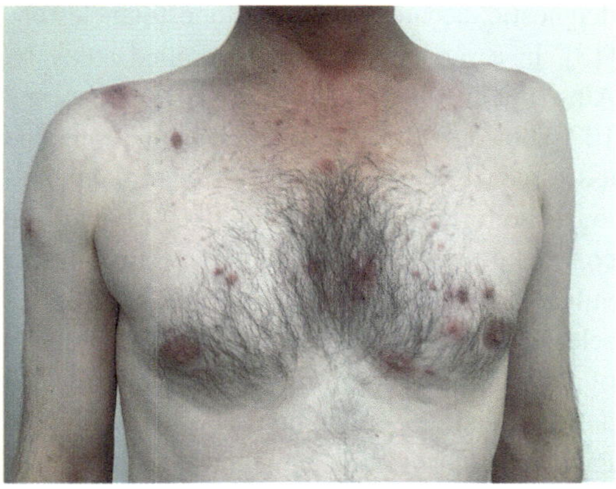

Fig. 8.5 Papulopustular lesions on the chest of a Behçet's disease patient, displaying clinical similarities to acne vulgaris

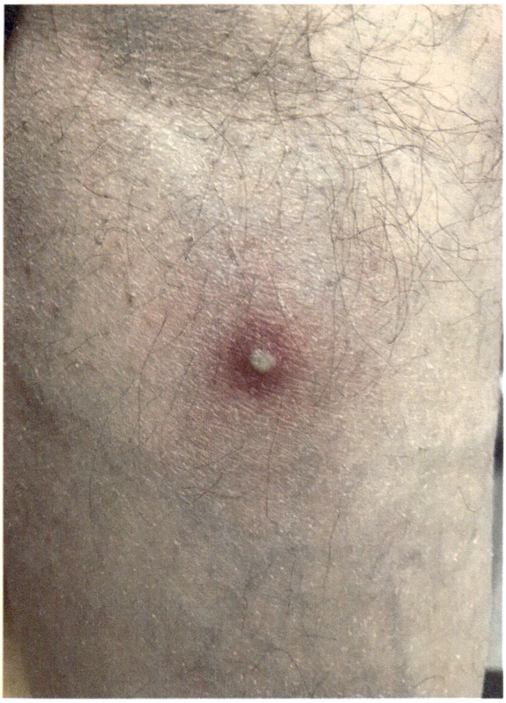

Fig. 8.4 Papulopustular lesion in Behçet's disease characterized by its typical erythematous base

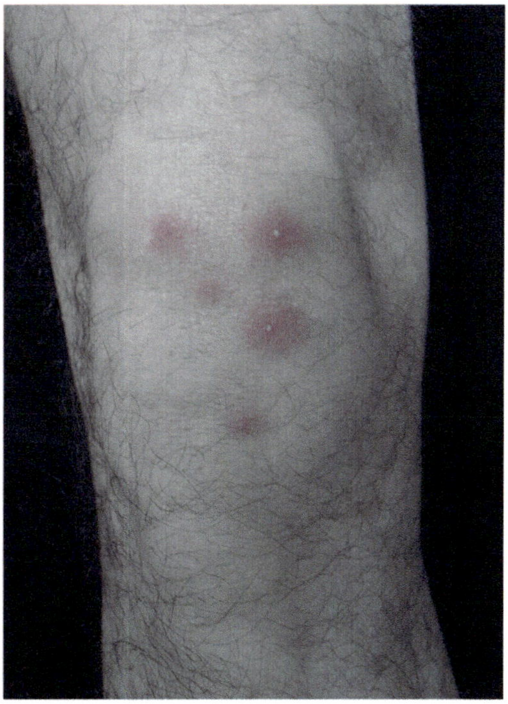

Fig. 8.6 Papulopustular lesions on the legs exhibiting an appearance mimicking bacterial folliculitis

of 20 and 40, and many patients within this age group also exhibit acne vulgaris alongside other nonspecific follicular lesions. Several authors emphasize the challenge in distinguishing between papulopustular lesions of BD and nonspecific lesions. They highlight that including acneiform lesions alongside papulopustular lesions in the diagnostic criteria diminishes the diagnostic accuracy of papulopustular lesions [13]. In a randomized and controlled study by Alpsoy et al. which included 50 BD patients and 100 controls, the authors conducted a blind assessment of papulopustular lesions encompassing acneiform and folliculitis-like lesions. The control group comprised patients with acne vulgaris, and various other dermatologic diseases selected randomly. The study found a frequency of 96% for papulopustular lesions among BD patients and 89% among the control group. Papulopustular lesions exhibited a sensitivity of 96% and a specificity of 11% [10]. This research indicated that while papulopustular lesions of patients with BD exhibit high sensitivity, they lack specificity, particularly when considering lesions resembling acne or follicle-based lesions. Furthermore, the study highlighted the variability of specificity in papulopustular lesions, notably influenced by the composition of the control groups. For instance, if studies conducted by ISG and ICBD had included more patients with dermatologic diseases like acne vulgaris in their control groups, the specificity and diagnostic value of these lesions would likely have been considerably lower.

8.3 Dermatopathological Controversies in the Papulopustular Lesions of BD

As identifying specific papulopustular lesions in BD, which resemble acne and nonspecific follicular lesions, presents a challenge, a persisting question has been whether dermatopathological examination can enhance the specificity of these lesions. Although numerous studies have been conducted thus far in an attempt to address this query, another area of controversy involves the dermatopathologic findings of papulopustular lesions.

Behçet's disease does not possess a specific, definitive histopathologic feature. However, its lesions commonly display histological signs of vasculitis and thrombosis [13–15]. Studies investigating papulopustular lesions have predominantly revealed dermatopathological findings ranging from well-defined leukocytoclastic vasculitis to milder forms of neutrophilic vascular reactions. While acneiform follicle based lesions may appear in BD patients, they are commonly regarded as nonspecific for the disease. Several authors suggest that it is crucial to focus on lesions with perivascular inflammation and advise against including follicular lesions in the diagnostic process [13, 16, 17]. Jorizzo et al. emphasized the necessity of vessel-associated histologic findings in papulopustular lesions to substantiate a diagnosis of BD [13]. They further noted the inability of clinical photographs to reliably predict the histopathological pattern of these lesions. Additionally, other authors also highlighted the significance of biopsy confirmation to identify vessel-related histologic features and to differentiate them from nonspecific follicular lesions [16, 17].

Alpsoy et al. conducted a study on papulopustular lesions in 17 BD patients located on extremities, and the trunk. They excluded follicle-based acneiform lesions and those on the face due to challenges in distinguishing them in such anatomic locations. Biopsies were obtained from both the lesional and approximately 2 cm distant nonlesional skin. Two observers, unaware of the clinical diagnosis, reviewed histological and immunofluorescence findings. The prominent finding was the high incidence of leukocytoclastic vasculitis observed in 11 out of 17 biopsies. Although higher IgM deposition was observed on vessels in the lesional skin as opposed to the nonlesional skin, no discernible correlation emerged between antibody deposition on vessels, types of infiltrating cells, or the clinical manifestations. The authors proposed that selecting nonfollicular lesions located on the trunk or extremities, along with histopathologic examinations improves the specificity of such lesions. They advocated for including only lesions displaying vasculitic changes as fulfilling diagnostic criteria [16].

In another study, Ilknur et al. examined histopathologic features of papulopustular lesions in 18 BD patients, comparing them to a control group of 16 patients (11 with bacterial folliculitis and five with acne vulgaris) [17]. Lymphocytic vasculitis was observed in 27.8% of patients with BD, folliculitis and/or perifolliculitis was observed in 16.7% and perivascular and/or interstitial dermatitis in 55.6%. No instances of vasculitis were detected among patients in the control group. They concluded that only vasculitic changes in histopathologic features of papulopustular lesions could serve as a diagnostic criterion in BD.

Kalkan et al. also conducted a comprehensive study to assess the diagnostic utility of papulopustular lesions in BD [18]. The research, encompassing a larger patient cohort compared to previous studies, aimed to compare histopathological findings of papulopustular lesions in 42 BD patients with those in 21 individuals with acne vulgaris. The results revealed vasculitis, including leukocytoclastic vasculitis (16.7%) and lymphocytic vasculitis (7.1%), in 23.8% of BD patients. Notably, none of the control group specimens exhibited vasculitis. Superficial and/or deep vascular infiltrations and/or interstitial dermatitis were more prevalent than vasculitis, observed in 64.3% of the histopathologic examination of papulopustular lesions of BD patients, aligning with previous studies. Similar vascular infiltrations were noted in the control group, but vasculitis was absent in acne vulgaris patients. The researchers proposed that the identification of vasculitis in the histopathological examination of papulopustular lesions could serve as a valuable diagnostic criterion for BD, distinguishing it from acne vulgaris. This underscores vasculitis as a specific finding in the papulopustular lesions of BD. Discrepancies in vasculitis detection across studies were attributed to factors such as lesion age, disease severity, activity status, and treatment history. Additionally, this study revealed a statistically significant association between vasculitis and male sex, corroborating with the observed severe course of the disease in male BD patients. This finding suggests that papulopustular lesions in males are more likely to be indicative of BD. Nevertheless, to fully elucidate this relationship, further comprehensive studies involving a larger patient cohort and multiple biopsies are required.

However, in other studies, vasculitis or perivascular inflammation was not identified as the dominant histopathologic pattern. Ergun et al. conducted a comparative study analyzing the histopathological aspects of papulopustular lesions in 17 BD patients and six acne vulgaris patients [19]. Biopsies from BD patients exclusively targeted papulopustular lesions localized on the extremities. Follicle-based lesions were also analyzed due to the clinical challenge in distinguishing different clinical patterns. Moreover, the authors noted that diagnostic criteria did not encompass such distinctions for papulopustular lesions. Among the 17 biopsies taken from the papulopustular lesions of BD patients, 15 (88%) exhibited predominantly perifollicular infiltrate, and only two (12%) displayed perivascular infiltrate without leukocytoclastic vasculitis. The authors concluded that both acne vulgaris and papulopustular lesions of BD manifest mainly perifollicular infiltrate, lacking distinctive differences and cannot be distinguished from each other based on histopathological features. According to the researchers, the disease spectrum includes papulopustular lesions characterized by vessel-associated neutrophilic reaction alongside follicle-based lesions. Hence, all papulopustular lesions, encompassing follicular acneiform lesions, ought to be considered indicative of BD. The findings of this study are consistent with those of Chun et al. [20].

Kutlubay et al. conducted a comprehensive evaluation of the clinical and histopathological features of papulopustular lesions in 58 patients with BD, comparing them with 31 acne vulgaris patients [21]. The study revealed that the number of papules, pustules, and comedos were higher on the face of acne vulgaris patients, while BD patients exhibited a higher prevalence of papulopustular lesions on the back and lower extremi-

9 Skin Pathergy Test: How Important Is it for Behcet's Disease?

Zeynep Altan Ferhatoğlu and Zekayi Kutlubay

Contents

9.1 Introduction

The pathergy reaction (PR) is characterized by the hyperreactivity of the skin to minimal trauma [1]. The pathergy test (PT) is a minimally invasive method used to assess this hyperreactivity response of the skin to needle applications [2]. A positive result is indicated by the development of papular lesions or pustules 2 mm or larger, surrounded by erythema at the needle entry sites, after 24–48 h (Figs. 9.1 and 9.2). Notably, bleeding in the relevant area is not considered indicative of a positive result [3]. Although the specific application method may vary among clinics, various studies suggest utilizing 4–6 needle pricks with 20 to 26-gauge needles, at a 45°

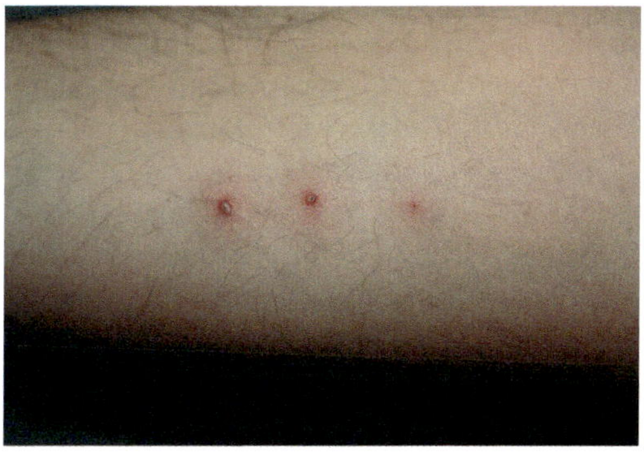

Fig. 9.1 Positive pathergy test (two of three pricks)

Z. Altan Ferhatoğlu (✉) · Z. Kutlubay
Department of Dermatology and Venereology, Istanbul University-Cerrahpaşa, Cerrahpaşa Medical Faculty, Istanbul, Türkiye

E. Alpsoy et al. (eds.), *Behçet's Disease: An Integrated Approach*,
https://doi.org/10.1007/978-3-031-77251-1_9

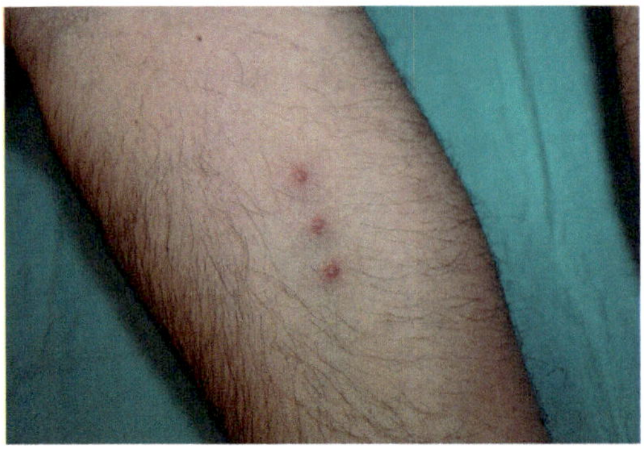

Fig. 9.2 Positive pathergy test (three of three pricks)

angle, on the volar aspect of the forearm [4]. However, the generally accepted approach involves 4–6 perpendicularly or oblique needle pricks with 20-gauge needles, into the hairless skin on the volar aspect of the forearm, targeting the dermis [5]. It is recommended to clean the application area with an antiseptic solution prior to the procedure, preferably alcohol, and to blunt the needle by rubbing it against its plastic cover [6].

The diagnosis of Behçet's disease (BD) is mainly based on clinical criteria, in the absence of a universally accepted pathognomonic test [3]. In addition to the patient's clinical symptoms, PT and human leukocyte antigen (HLA)-B51/5 results can provide valuable diagnostic information. According to the recently developed International Criteria for Behçet's Disease (ICBD), PT is considered optional and its sensitivity and specificity are reported to be 47% and 92%, respectively [3]. In the more commonly used International Study Group for Behcet's Disease (ISG) criteria system, sensitivity and specificity are reported to be 58% and 90%, respectively, and a positive PT is considered having the same diagnostic value as recurrent genital ulcers, eye lesions and other skin findings associated with BD [7]. Davatchi et al. found that sensitivity and accuracy decreased and specificity increased in the absence of PT, in 15 of 16 diagnostic methods, in a large study of 6727 BD patients and 4648 healthy controls [8]. However, PT was not included in the classification and diagnostic criteria for pediatric patients with BD [9]. In a cohort study of 204 children, the sensitivity of the Kone-Paut et al. scoring system was 48%, which was related to the exclusion of PT. Similarly, when PT was added to the classification system as one of the skin lesions or as a stand-alone criterion, the sensitivity increased from 48% to 66.7% and 73%, respectively [10].

It has been suggested that the development of PR provides clues to the etiopathogenesis of BD. For example, the role of an impaired neutrophil response in the pathogenesis of BD was emphasized by the presence of neutrophils in PR. It was emphasized that the term PR is not limited to skin, with examples of patients developing synovitis after arthrocentesis, uveitis after ocular surgery, aneurysms around vascular anastomoses and local ulcer recurrence after bowel resections. Although the PT is considered being specific for BD because it is negative in the control group and in the group of patients with systemic lupus erythematosus, it can also be found to be positive in neutrophilic dermatoses, particularly pyoderma gangrenosum [1].

9.2 History

Pathergy reaction was first described in BD by Blobner in 1937 and demonstrated in 22 BD patients by Katzenellenbogen in 1968 [11, 12]. Haim et al. performed a study in 1976 where they found positive PR in 18 BD patients and also examined the reaction sites histopathologically [13]. Its usefulness in the diagnosis of BD was demonstrated in 1979 in a comparative analysis of 58 patients with BD and a control group of 90 people by Tüzün et al. [14]. In 1981, in a study designed to address uncertainties regarding validation, its clinical usefulness was reinforced by emphasizing that both intra- and inter-observer arithmetic variability values for the assessment of PR positivity were less than one [15]. During the same period, it was reported that PT could be combined with HLA-B5 positivity in the diagnosis of BD, but it might not show parallelism with PT positivity [16]. A report from 1984 on Turkish and British patients showed that PT was positive only in Turkish patients, indicating that there may be racial differences in PR positivity [17]. Yazıcı et al. showed in 1985 that PT positivity was statistically significantly higher in men and that it was not associated with disease activity and PR severity [18]. In the same year, Jorizzo et al. reported a correlation between PT and treatment response with low reproducibility and suggested the use of histopathology and immunopathology of PR lesions instead of clinical assessment for the diagnosis of BD [19]. In 1989, Gilhar et al. observed both clinical and histological positive responses in patients with active BD 24 h after intradermal administration of saline and histamine. They reported that PT is a valuable diagnostic tool for BD, whose clinical findings may overlap with other systemic diseases, and that this method can yield positive results with any intracutaneous injection [20]. In 1990, a publication from Israel reported that PT was positive in 45 out of 46 active BD patients, while it was negative in all patients in the control group of 46 patients with vasculitis-related disease, indicating that it had high sensitivity and specificity [21]. PT was included in the ISG diagnostic criteria in the same year [7].

9.3 Application Methods

The methodology of PT application varies among clinicians and in clinical trials. A survey conducted in Türkiye evaluating PT application methods in practice among dermatologists, highlighted that there was no standardization of PT application due to variations in factors such as injection site, needle type, puncture depth, total number of punctures, puncture site cleaning, injection of saline, needle rotation and evaluation time parameters, among 294 dermatologists participating in the survey [22]. These differences in application methods may potentially have had an impact on the positivity of PT.

PT positivity increases in correlation with the thickness of the needle tip used in the application of the test. A comparative study found 62.5% positivity with 20-gauge needles, but only 35.8% positivity with 26-gauge needles [23]. Similar to needle thickness, the probability of PT positivity increases as the number of needles increases. The observed rates were 13%, 19%, 24%, 28%, 30% and 33% for needle numbers ranging from 1 to 6 in a report investigating the effect of multiple needling on PT positivity [24]. The positivity rate reached 85.7% in another investigation where the number of needles was increased to 16, covering different anatomical regions [25].

The highest positivity rate (81.25%) was found in patients with active BD when PT was administered intradermally with non-disposable/blunt needles in a study of 43 patients with BD from Türkiye compared with a control group. In patients with BD in remission (previously diagnosed and without active symptoms), no positivity was detected with intradermal or intravenous administration of disposable/sharp needles, similar to the control group. In contrast, five out of eleven patients with BD in remission tested positive with intradermal administration of non-disposable/sharp needles. It has been emphasized that disposable sharp needles are inadequate for PT and that PT performed intradermally with blunt non-disposable needles, is more appropriate for the diagnosis of BD and to provide information about the severity of the disease [26].

PT applied intramuscularly has been shown to be more sensitive than classical PT applied intradermally. In addition, multiple punctures have been shown to increase the positivity of intradermal, intravenous and intramuscular applications compared to single punctures [27].

A study investigating the effect of applied body region on PT positivity showed that the most frequent positivity was observed in the forearm flexor, tibial lateral, back scapular and abdominal lumbar regions, respectively [25]. The positivity rates of pathergy testing (PT) applied to the traditional (forearm flexor face), oral, and genital regions were reported as 18.5%, 42.5% and 7.5%, respectively, in a report involving 80 BD patients from Türkiye [28]. On the other hand, in a research report from Iran, the positivity rate of the oral PT described by Sharque et al. was found to be lower (69% vs 47%) than the classical skin PT [29].

The use of argon laser photocoagulation to induce skin PR in patients with BD has shown a positive rate (23%) comparable to that obtained with needling (26%) [30]. Shenavandeh et al. showed that the diagnostic accuracy of using patients' own saliva was statistically significantly higher compared to the dry method and was better correlated with disease activity. However, when compared with patients with recurrent aphthous stomatitis, they found that the sensitivity of the test for BD increased but the specificity declined [31].

PT administered by saline injection did not elicit a positive response in any of the 52 patients with BD, whereas a positive response of 5.8% was observed with needles dipped in the patient's own saliva in a recent report from Europe. An important point in that study is that the application of saliva resulted in an erythema of 15 mm or more in patients with BD, as opposed to patients with axial spondyloarthritis and the control group, without causing induration. This difference was statistically significant (42.3%, 9.6%, and 7.7% respectively) [32]. Elsewhere, it was reported that when the 23-valent polysaccharide pneumococcal vaccine was added to the application site next to a 20-gauge needle puncture site in active-phase BD patients, the sensitivity increased from 6.1% to 80.3% [5].

PT outcomes are thus influenced by many factors, including needle tip thickness, tip sharpness, direction and depth of needle penetration, skin-only or substance injection, number of punctures, and timing of assessments. This variability in factors contributes to differences in positive rates between centers [33].

9.4 Mechanism of the Pathergy Reaction

The pathogenesis of PR has not been clearly elucidated, but it is thought that the cutaneous axon reflex induced by microneedling of the skin, which can also be seen in healthy individuals, and the subsequent release of inflammatory mediators develop more severely in BD patients [4]. Histopathology of positive PT lesions reveals mixed inflammatory cell infiltration, erythrocyte extravasation, leukocytoclastic vasculitis, endothelial swelling and thickening, lymphocytic vasculitis, perivascular cell infiltration, and lymphocytic vascular reaction in the dermis. In the subcutaneous tissue, mixed inflammatory cell infiltration, lymphocyte-rich infiltration, neutrophil-rich infiltration, and lobular panniculitis without vasculitis may be seen [34].

The results of a comparative study with a control group, which aimed to show the distribution of inflammatory cells and measure cytokine levels in areas of skin showing PR positivity, show that BD patients experience marked cell migration to areas of skin trauma. This phenomenon resulted in an exaggerated T helper 1 (Th1) cell response [35]. It is thought that Toll-like receptor-5 expression, which has been shown to be increased in PR-positive BD patients compared with PR-negative patients, may trigger an exaggerated immune response to microbial or injury stimuli in the skin [2]. The identification of the colony-stimulating factor-2 (CSF-2) pathway in a family with extreme pathergy and lesions mimicking BD, may shed light on the pathogenesis of PR [36]. Immunohistochemical studies of biopsies obtained from PR-positive areas have identified E-selectin, P-selectin and CD-105 positivity, suggesting that endothelial proliferation in combination with cellular adhesion molecule interaction may contribute to the development of PT positivity [37]. In conclusion, increased inflammatory mediators and a Th1 cell response to microtrauma have been shown to play a role in the mechanism of PR, with cellular adhesion molecules also contributing.

9.5 Positivity Rates

PR positivity in 84% of BD patients was reported by Tüzün et al. in 1979 [14]. About 20 years later, a study of 2147 BD patients from Türkiye reported a PT-positive rate of 56.8% [38]. In 2000, 43 Israeli patients with BD reported a PT positivity rate of 44.2% [39], while in 2001, a multicenter study from Korea reported a PT positivity rate of 12.7% [40]. A PT positivity rate of 51% was reported in 2006 in a research performed on 519 patients with BD from Tunisia

[41] and a PT positivity rate of 75% was reported from the south-eastern region of Türkiye, where patients were evaluated between 2005 and 2009 [42].

When the positivity rates in country-wide studies were compared by race, the rates reported from Iran, Japan, Korea, and China were 50.8%, 36.8%, 15.4%, and 57.9% respectively [43, 44]. A case series from Thailand reported 33.3% PT positivity [45], and a study from the African continent reported 32% PT positivity in African Americans diagnosed with BD [46].

In Western countries, particularly the UK and United States, the rate of PT positivity has been found to be lower than in countries along the Silk Road [43]. The positivity rate was 15.9% in a cross-sectional study reported from the south-western part of the American continent [47] and the positivity rate was 22.7% in a study from Brazil [48]. The fact that there was no difference in PT positivity between Turks and Germans highlighted that environmental factors other than race and genetics may be possible triggers, in research from Germany in 2012 [49]. In one report from Denmark, PT positivity was found in two out of 26 patients (7.7%), which was similar to the rate of 1 out of 12 patients reported from Sweden [50, 51]. Similar to the rates reported from Scandinavian countries, two patients were found positive for PT in findings including 25 patients with BD from Ireland [52].

When we examine the rates reported around the world in recent literature, it can be seen that there is a decrease in the rate of PT positivity compared to previous years. A positive PT rate of 14.1% was observed in a study published in 2020 that included 489 BD patients from China [53]. A positive PT response was found in 27.1% of patients in another, published in 2021, which collected data over 10 years and included 777 BD patients from the northern region of Türkiye [54]. One report of 514 patients from Iran between 2017 and 2022 reported PT positivity of 20.6% [55], whereas the PT positivity rate was 26.4% in 488 patients from the northwestern region of Türkiye in 2023 [56].

Generally speaking, as a result of the decrease over the years and differences in geographical regions, there are rates varying between 7.7% and 84% in the literature [57].

There may be racial and geographic differences in PT positivity and changes in rates have been observed even in the same regions, over time. The rate of 56.8% reported from Türkiye in 1997 decreased to 37.8% in a multicenter study of 661 patients conducted in Türkiye 10 years later [38, 58]. In research on some 6500 patients with BD reported from Iran, the PT positivity rate was reported as 52.5%. A striking finding of the latter was that while the PT positivity rate was 71.8% in the first 1000 patients in the Iranian registry system over a 20-year period, it decreased to 33.9% between 5000 and 6000 patients [59]. A more comprehensive study with a healthy control group reported from Tehran reported that the sensitivity of PT decreased from 64.2% to 35.8% and the specificity increased from 86.6% to 98.4% over a 35-year period [60].

Based on data reported from around the world, PT test positivity rates have decreased over the years in all countries. In the early stages of discovering the importance of PT positivity in patients with BD, controlled studies in Türkiye reported positivity rates between 72% and 98%. However, after 1986, these rates gradually decreased [26]. Comparing results obtained by Boyvat et al., which included patients between 1998 and 2020, with those from Gürler et al., which included patients between 1976 and 1997, it was reported that the rate of PT positivity decreased from 56.8% to 40.1%. However, there was no statistically significant change in the rates of mucocutaneous involvement (recurrent oral ulcers, genital ulcers, papulopustular lesions, erythema nodosum) or systemic involvement (vascular, neurological, gastrointestinal) [26, 61].

One study compared gross and dermoscopic assessment of PT results and found significant differences between two dermatologists using gross assessment ($p = 0.037$), while this difference between two dermatologists disappeared when using dermoscopic assessment ($p > 0.05$). Therefore, the authors reported that the use of dermoscopy for assessment decreased subjectivity, compared to gross assessment [62]. However, the exact role of dermoscopy in PT and the

3. The international criteria for Behçet's disease (ICBD): a collaborative study of 27 countries on the sensitivity and specificity of the new criteria. J Eur Acad Dermatol Venereol. 2014;28(3):338–47.
4. Scherrer MAR, Rocha VB, Garcia LC. Behçet's disease: review with emphasis on dermatological aspects. An Bras Dermatol. 2017;92(4):452–64.
5. Deniz R, Emrence Z, Yalçınkaya Y, Artım Esen B, İnanç M, Öcal ML, et al. Improved sensitivity of the skin pathergy test with polysaccharide pneumococcal vaccine antigens in the diagnosis of Behçet disease. Rheumatology (Oxford). 2023;62(5):1903–9.
6. Ergun T. Pathergy phenomenon. Front Med. 2021;8:639404.
7. Criteria for diagnosis of Behçet's disease. International Study Group for Behçet's Disease. Lancet (London, England). 1990;335(8697):1078–80.
8. Davatchi F, Sadeghi Abdollahi B, Chams-Davatchi C, Shahram F, Ghodsi Z, Nadji A, et al. Impact of the positive pathergy test on the performance of classification/diagnosis criteria for Behcet's disease. Mod Rheumatol. 2013;23(1):125–32.
9. Koné-Paut I, Shahram F, Darce-Bello M, Cantarini L, Cimaz R, Gattorno M, et al. Consensus classification criteria for paediatric Behçet's disease from a prospective observational cohort: PEDBD. Ann Rheum Dis. 2016;75(6):958–64.
10. Shahram F, Nadji A, Akhlaghi M, Faezi ST, Chams-Davatchi C, Shams H, et al. Paediatric Behçet's disease in Iran: report of 204 cases. Clin Exp Rheumatol. 2018;36(6 Suppl 115):135–40.
11. Blobner F. Zur rezidivierenden hypopyoniritis. Zeitschrift für Augenheilkunde. 1937;91(3–4): 129–39.
12. Kutlubay Z, Tüzün Y, Wolf R. The pathergy test as a diagnostic tool. Skinmed. 2017;15(2):97–104.
13. Haim S, Sobel JD, Friedman-Birnbaum R, Lichtig C. Histohogical and direct immunofluorescence study of cutaneous hyperreactivity in Behçet's disease. Br J Dermatol. 1976;95(6):631–6.
14. Tüzün Y, Yazici H, Pazarli H, Yalçin B, Yurdakul S, Müftüoğlu A. The usefulness of the nonspecific skin hyperreactivity (the pathergy test) in Behçet's disease in Türkiye. Acta Derm Venereol. 1979;59(1):77–9.
15. Altaç M, Tüzün Y, Yurdakul S, Binyildiz P, Yazici H. The validity of the pathergy test (non-specific skin hyperreactivity) in Behçet's disease: a double-blind study by independent observers. Acta Derm Venereol. 1982;62(2):158–9.
16. Yazici H, Tuzun Y, Pazarli H, Yalcin B, Yurdakul S, Muftuoglu A. The combined use of HLA-B5 and the pathergy test as diagnostic markers of Behçet's disease in Türkiye. J Rheumatol. 1980;7(2):206–10.
17. Yazici H, Chamberlain MA, Tüzün Y, Yurdakul S, Müftüoglu A. A comparative study of the pathergy reaction among Turkish and British patients with Behçet's disease. Ann Rheum Dis. 1984;43(1):74–5.
18. Yazici H, Tüzün Y, Tanman AB, Yurdakul S, Serdaroglu S, Pazarli H, et al. Male patients with Behçet's syndrome have stronger pathergy reactions. Clin Exp Rheumatol. 1985;3(2):137–41.
19. Jorizzo JL, Solomon AR, Cavallo T. Behçet's syndrome. Immunopathologic and histopathologic assessment of pathergy lesions is useful in diagnosis and follow-up. Arch Pathol Lab Med. 1985;109(8):747–51.
20. Gilhar A, Winterstein G, Turani H, Landau J, Etzioni A. Skin hyperreactivity response (pathergy) in Behçet's disease. J Am Acad Dermatol. 1989;21(3 Pt 1):547–52.
21. Friedman-Birnbaum R, Bergman R, Aizen E. Sensitivity and specificity of pathergy test results in Israeli patients with Behçet's disease. Cutis. 1990;45(4):261–4.
22. Ozden MG, Bek Y, Aydin F, Senturk N, Canturk T, Turanli AY. Different application techniques of pathergy testing among dermatologists. J Eur Acad Dermatol Venereol. 2010;24(10):1240–2.
23. Ozarmagan G, Saylan T, Azizlerli G, Ovül C, Aksungur VL. Re-evaluation of the pathergy test in Behçet's disease. Acta Derm Venereol. 1991;71(1):75–6.
24. Ozdemir M, Bodur S, Engin B, Baysal I. Evaluation of application of multiple needle pricks on the pathergy reaction. Int J Dermatol. 2008;47(4):335–8.
25. Ozdemir M, Balevi S, Deniz F, Mevlitoğlu I. Pathergy reaction in different body areas in Behçet's disease. Clin Exp Dermatol. 2007;32(1):85–7.
26. Akmaz O, Erel A, Gürer MA. Comparison of histopathologic and clinical evaluations of pathergy test in Behçet's disease. Int J Dermatol. 2000;39(2):121–5.
27. Kalay Yildizhan İ, Boyvat A. Diagnostic sensitivity of different applications of Pathergy test for Behçet's disease. Arch Rheumatol. 2020;35(1):29–34.
28. Gül U, Gönül M. Oral and genital pathergy in Behçet's disease. Dermatology (Basel, Switzerland). 2007;215(1):80–1.
29. Sharquie KE, Al-Araji A, Hatem A. Oral pathergy test in Behçet's disease. Br J Dermatol. 2002;146(1):168–9.
30. Sayarlioglu M, Calka O, Cinal A, Sayarlioglu H, Akdeniz N, Topcu N, et al. Comparison of argon laser photocoagulation-induced cutaneous inflammation and skin pathergy test in Behçet's disease. Clin Rheumatol. 2010;29(1):59–63.
31. Shenavandeh S, Sadeghi SMK, Aflaki E. Pathergy test with a 23G needle with and without self-saliva in patients with Behçet's disease, recurrent aphthous stomatitis and control group compared to the 20G test. Rheumatologia. 2021;59(5):302–8.
32. Vitale A, Berlengiero V, Caggiano V, Barneschi S, Mourabi M, Sota J, et al. The diagnostic role of pathergy test in patients with Behçet's disease from the Western Europe. Intern Emerg Med. 2023;18(1):77–83.
33. Davatchi F, Shahram F, Nadji A, Jamshidi AR, Chams C, Chams H, et al. Influence of pathergy test on the accuracy of different diagnosis criteria for Behçet's disease. Adv Exp Med Biol. 2003;528:109–12.

34. Ozluk E, Balta I, Akoguz O, Kalkan G, Astarci M, Akbay G, et al. Histopathologic study of pathergy test in Behçet's disease. Indian J Dermatol. 2014;59(6):630.
35. Melikoglu M, Uysal S, Krueger JG, Kaplan G, Gogus F, Yazici H, et al. Characterization of the divergent wound-healing responses occurring in the pathergy reaction and normal healthy volunteers. J Immunol. (Baltimore, Md : 1950). 2006;177(9):6415–21.
36. Rösler B, Heinhuis B, Wang X, Silvestre R, Joosten LAB, Netea MG, et al. Mimicking Behçet's disease: GM-CSF gain of function mutation in a family suffering from a Behçet's disease-like disorder marked by extreme pathergy. Clin Exp Immunol. 2021;204(2):189–98.
37. Inaloz HS, Evereklioglu C, Unal B, Kirtak N, Eralp A, Inaloz SS. The significance of immunohistochemistry in the skin pathergy reaction of patients with Behçet's syndrome. J Eur Acad Dermatol Venereol. 2004;18(1):56–61.
38. Gürler A, Boyvat A, Türsen U. Clinical manifestations of Behçet's disease: an analysis of 2147 patients. Yonsei Med J. 1997;38(6):423–7.
39. Krause I, Molad Y, Mitrani M, Weinberger A. Pathergy reaction in Behçet's disease: lack of correlation with mucocutaneous manifestations and systemic disease expression. Clin Exp Rheumatol. 2000;18(1):71–4.
40. Bang D, Lee JH, Lee ES, Lee S, Choi JS, Kim YK, et al. Epidemiologic and clinical survey of Behcet's disease in Korea: the first multicenter study. J Korean Med Sci. 2001;16(5):615–8.
41. B'Chir Hamzaoui S, Harmel A, Bouslama K, Abdallah M, Ennafaa M, M'Rad S, et al. Behçet's disease in Tunisia. Clinical study of 519 cases. La Revue de Medecine interne. 2006;27(10):742–50.
42. Sula B, Batmaz I, Ucmak D, Yolbas I, Akdeniz S. Demographical and clinical characteristics of Behcet's disease in Southeastern Türkiye. J Clin Med Res. 2014;6(6):476–81.
43. Davatchi F, Shahram F, Chams-Davatchi C, Shams H, Nadji A, Akhlaghi M, et al. Behcet's disease: from east to west. Clin Rheumatol. 2010;29(8):823–33.
44. Davatchi F, Shahram F, Chams-Davatchi C, Shams H, Abdolahi BS, Nadji A, et al. Behcet's disease in Iran: analysis of 7641 cases. Mod Rheumatol. 2019;29(6):1023–30.
45. Arromdee E, Tanakitivirul M. Epidemiology of Behcet's disease in Thai patients. J Med Assoc Thail. 2006;89(Suppl 5):S182–S6.
46. Ndiaye M, Sow AS, Valiollah A, Diallo M, Diop A, Alaoui RA, et al. Behçet's disease in black skin. A retrospective study of 50 cases in Dakar. J Dermatol Case Rep. 2015;9(4):98–102.
47. Muruganandam M, Rolle NA, Sibbitt WL Jr, Cook GB, Emil NS, Fangtham M, et al. Characteristics of Behcet's disease in the American Southwest. Semin Arthritis Rheum. 2019;49(2):296–302.
48. Oliveira AC, Buosi AL, Dutra LA, de Souza AW. Behçet disease: clinical features and management in a Brazilian tertiary hospital. J Clin Rheumatol Pract Rep Rheum Musculoskelet Dis. 2011;17(8):416–20.
49. Altenburg A, Mahr A, Maldini C, Kneifel CE, Krause L, Kötter I, et al. Epidemiology and clinical aspects of Adamantiades-Behçet disease in Germany. Current data. Der Ophthalmologe: Zeitschrift der Deutschen Ophthalmologischen Gesellschaft. 2012;109(6):531–41.
50. Gyldenløve M, Tvede N, Larsen JL, Jacobsen S, Thyssen JP. Low prevalence of positive skin pathergy testing in Danish patients with Behçet's disease. J Eur Acad Dermatol Venereol. 2014;28(2):259–60.
51. Ek L, Hedfors E. Behçet's disease: a review and a report of 12 cases from Sweden. Acta Derm Venereol. 1993;73(4):251–4.
52. Adeeb F, Stack AG, Fraser AD. New insights into Behçet's disease in Ireland: the Midwest cohort study. Clin Exp Rheumatol. 2018;36(6 Suppl 115):33–9.
53. Li C, Li L, Wu X, Shi J, Liu J, Zhou J, et al. Clinical manifestations of Behçet's disease in a large cohort of Chinese patients: gender- and age-related differences. Clin Rheumatol. 2020;39(11):3449–54.
54. Gürbüz C, Yalçın Kehribar D, Özgen M. Clinical manifestations of Behçet's syndrome: a single-center cohort of 777 patients. Eur J Rheumatol. 2021;8(4):211–6.
55. Parsaei A, Moradi S, Masoumi M, Davatchi F, Najafi A, Kooshki AM, et al. Predictive value of erythrocyte sedimentation rate and C-reactive protein in Behcet's disease activity and manifestations: a cross-sectional study. BMC Rheumatol. 2022;6(1):9.
56. Çakan ZK, Yağız B, Pehlivan Y. Clinical features of Behçet's disease and prediction of the use of biologics in 488 cases: a single tertiary center study. Rheumatol Int. 2023;43(11):2089–97.
57. Alibaz-Oner F, Direskeneli H. Update on the diagnosis of Behçet's disease. Diagnostics, Basel. 2022;13:1.
58. Alpsoy E, Donmez L, Onder M, Gunasti S, Usta A, Karincaoglu Y, et al. Clinical features and natural course of Behçet's disease in 661 cases: a multicentre study. Br J Dermatol. 2007;157(5):901–6.
59. Davatchi F, Shahram F, Chams-Davatchi C, Shams H, Nadji A, Akhlaghi M, et al. Behcet's disease in Iran: analysis of 6500 cases. Int J Rheum Dis. 2010;13(4):367–73.
60. Davatchi F, Chams-Davatchi C, Ghodsi Z, Shahram F, Nadji A, Shams H, et al. Diagnostic value of pathergy test in Behcet's disease according to the change of incidence over the time. Clin Rheumatol. 2011;30(9):1151–5.
61. Boyvat A, Oktem A, Kalay Yildizhan I, Ates A, Yalcindag N, Koksoy C, et al. A comparison of adult and juvenile Behcet patients and a look at clinical trends: retrospective data from a Turkish follow-up cohort study. Dermatology (Basel, Switzerland). 2023;239(6):958–65.
62. Kecici AS, Kutlubay Z, Serdaroglu S, Tuzun Y. Pathergy testing: prospective comparison of der-

matoscopic evaluation and naked eye examination. Intern Emerg Med. 2019;14(5):699–703.
63. Wang LY, Zhao DB, Gu J, Dai SM. Clinical characteristics of Behçet's disease in China. Rheumatol Int. 2010;30(9):1191–6.
64. Balta I, Akbay G, Kalkan G, Eksioglu M. Demographic and clinical features of 521 Turkish patients with Behçet's disease. Int J Dermatol. 2014;53(5):564–9.
65. Bonitsis NG, Luong Nguyen LB, LaValley MP, Papoutsis N, Altenburg A, Kötter I, et al. Gender-specific differences in Adamantiades-Behçet's disease manifestations: an analysis of the German registry and meta-analysis of data from the literature. Rheumatology (Oxford). 2015;54(1):121–33.
66. Alpsoy E, Elpek GO, Yilmaz F, Ciftcioglu MA, Akman A, Uzun S, et al. Androgen receptor levels of oral and genital ulcers and skin pathergy test in patients with Behçet's disease. Dermatology (Basel, Switzerland). 2005;210(1):31–5.
67. Askari A, Al-Aboosi M, Sawalha A. Evaluation of pathergy test in North Jordan. Clin Rheumatol. 2000;19(3):249–51.
68. Chang HK, Cheon KS. The clinical significance of a pathergy reaction in patients with Behcet's disease. J Korean Med Sci. 2002;17(3):371–4.
69. Faezi ST, Chams-Davatchi C, Ghodsi SZ, Shahram F, Nadji A, Akhlaghi M, et al. Genital aphthosis in Behçet's disease: is it associated with less eye involvement? Rheumatol Int. 2014;34(11):1581–7.
70. Faezi ST, Paragomi P, Shahram F, Shams H, Shams-Davatchi C, Ghodsi Z, et al. Clinical features of Behcet's disease in patients without oral aphthosis. Mod Rheumatol. 2014;24(4):637–9.
71. Tomizuka T, Kikuchi H, Okubo M, Asako K, Miyata S, Kono H. Natural history of Behçet's disease focusing on remission of oral ulcers. Mod Rheumatol. 2023;33(3):566–73.
72. Assar S, Sadeghi B, Davatchi F, Ghodsi SZ, Nadji A, Shahram F, et al. The association of pathergy reaction and active clinical presentations of Behçet's disease. Reumatologia. 2017;55(2):79–83.
73. Zhou J, Shi J, Liu J, Sun L, Li L, Li C, et al. The clinical features, risk factors, and outcome of aneurysmal lesions in Behcet's disease. J Immunol Res. 2019;2019:9198506.
74. Sharquie KE, Al-Rawi Z, Hatem A, Al-Araji A. The influence of age of onset and patient's sex on the prevalence of clinical manifestations of Behcet's disease in Iraqi patients. Ann Saudi Med. 2002;22(3–4):239–41.
75. Çirkinoğlu MS, Demir S, Bilginer Y, Özen S. Behçet's disease in children: single-center experience. Turk Pediatri Ars. 2019;54(3):179–84.
76. Tekgöz N, Tekgöz E, Çolak S, Sezer M, Çelikel E, Tekin Z, et al. Age-related differences in the clinical phenotypes of Behçet's disease: the experience of two referral centers. Mod Rheumatol. 2023;34:194.
77. Menashi S, Tribout B, Dosquet C, Le Toumelin P, Piette JC, Wechsler B, et al. Strong association between plasma thrombomodulin and pathergy test in Behçet disease. Ann Rheum Dis. 2008;67(6):892–3.
78. Oral HB, Dilek K, Özçimen AA, Taşkapılıoğlu Ö, Bingöl Ü, Sarandöl A, et al. Interleukin-4 gene polymorphisms confer Behçet's disease in Turkish population. Scand J Immunol. 2011;73(6):594–601.
79. Zarrabi M, Gholijani N, Shenavandeh S, Aflaki E, Amirghofran Z. IL-38 serum levels in patients with Behcet's disease and the relationship with clinical features. Eur Cytokine Netw. 2019;30(3):82–7.
80. Jadideslam G, Kahroba H, Ansarin K, Sakhinia E, Abhar A, Alipour S, et al. Interleukin-17 mRNA expression and serum levels in Behçet's disease. Cytokine. 2020;127:154994.
81. Hamzaoui A, Houman MH, Massouadia M, Ben Salem T, Khanfir MS, Ben Ghorbel I, et al. Contribution of Hla-B51 in the susceptibility and specific clinical features of Behcet's disease in Tunisian patients. Eur J Intern Med. 2012;23(4):347–9.
82. Mizuki Y, Horita N, Horie Y, Takeuchi M, Ishido T, Mizuki R, et al. The influence of HLA-B51 on clinical manifestations among Japanese patients with Behçet's disease: a nationwide survey. Mod Rheumatol. 2020;30(4):708–14.
83. Temiz SA, Balevi S, Oltulu P, Ozer I. Histopathological comparison of pathergy positive and negative areas of newly diagnosed Behçet patients. Int J Clin Pract. 2021;75(12):e14994.
84. Melikoglu M, Fresko I, Mat C, Ozyazgan Y, Gogus F, Yurdakul S, et al. Short-term trial of etanercept in Behçet's disease: a double blind, placebo controlled study. J Rheumatol. 2005;32(1):98–105.
85. Nakamura K, Tsunemi Y, Kaneko F, Alpsoy E. Mucocutaneous manifestations of Behçet's disease. Front Med. 2020;7:613432.

Topical Treatment Approaches of Mucocutaneous Behçet's Disease

10

Osman Köse

Contents

BD is a chronic, relapsing systemic inflammatory vasculitis characterized by oral ulcers, genital ulcers, and various mucocutaneous manifestations (e.g., erythema nodosum, papulopustular lesions, superficial thrombophlebitis), along with other systemic involvement [1–3]. While systemic therapeutic agents are often the primary treatment based on symptom severity, topical treatments play a crucial role, particularly in managing mucocutaneous manifestations such as oral and genital ulcers [4, 5]. This section provides an in-depth review of the current state of knowledge regarding topical treatment for BD.

10.1 Oral Ulcers

Oral ulcers are the most common manifestation of BD, with three clinical presentations: major, minor, and herpetiform ulcers. While oral ulcers can occur anywhere on the oral mucosa, they are most prevalent on the buccal and labial mucosa. Additionally, they can develop on the soft and hard palates, as well as the lateral and ventral aspects of the tongue. The presence of oral ulcers significantly impairs the quality of life due to

O. Köse (✉)
Private Office, Ankara, Türkiye

E. Alpsoy et al. (eds.), *Behçet's Disease: An Integrated Approach*,
https://doi.org/10.1007/978-3-031-77251-1_10

interference with activities such as eating, drinking, and speaking [1, 2, 4]. The aims of treatment in oral ulcers are healing of the existing lesion, relief of pain, and prevention of recurrence. Studies with a high level of evidence are lacking for the majority of treatments used. A considerable proportion of the therapies employed in clinical practice are based on clinical experience. Numerous topical agents have been used for oral ulcers in BD over time, including corticosteroids, sucralfate suspension, pentoxifylline, hyaluronic acid, tacrolimus, and mouthwashes [6, 7]. There are only a few controlled studies on the treatment of OU. The treatments commonly employed in daily practice are agents that are effective in *recurrent aphthous stomatitis* (RAS). Triamcinolone acetonide, sucralfate, and pentoxifylline have demonstrated efficacy in randomized controlled trials for treating oral ulcers in BD [8–10].

10.1.1 Topical Medications

10.1.1.1 Corticosteroids

Corticosteroids are the primary agents for treating oral ulcers in BD. Triamcinolone acetonide (0.1%) was found to be highly effective, especially in the *early stages of oral ulcers* [7]. The application should be done three times a day and continued for 7–10 days. In one comparative-controlled study, the efficacy of triamcinolone acetonide was measured in oral ulcers in BD. It was found that triamcinolone acetonide is more effective than phenytoin syrup for oral ulcers in BD [8]. Topical corticosteroids, alone or in combination with antiseptics, relieve pain and promote healing in oral ulcers.

10.1.1.2 Sucralfate

Sucralfate, as an aluminum salt of sucrose octasulfate, has been widely used for peptic ulcus for a long time. Sucralfate is a treatment modality for oral ulcers. When used as a gargle at a dose of 1 g/5 ml four times a day for 3 months, it not only reduces pain in oral ulcers but also accelerates wound healing and prevents the formation of new oral ulcers [9].

10.1.1.3 Pentoxifylline

Pentoxifylline (PTX) is a methylxanthine derivative that inhibits phosphodiesterase. It has immunomodulatory effects. Pentoxifylline gel (5%) plus colchicine was found to be more effective than colchicine alone in an open-label, randomized clinical trial. Pentoxifylline gel is effective in decreasing the duration and pain of oral ulcers in BD [10].

10.1.1.4 Hyaluronic Acid

Hyaluronic acid (HA), a crucial component of connective tissue, plays a vital role in tissue repair. HA has been used twice a day for 2 weeks. It decreases the healing time and size of developed oral ulcers in BD. The topical application of 0.2% HA gel was found to be effective therapy. It diminished the pain and healing period of ulcers [11].

10.1.1.5 Topical Immunomodulators

Topical immunomodulators such as tacrolimus and pimecrolimus are immunosuppressive medications that work by inhibiting calcineurin, a protein involved in the activation of T cells. By suppressing the immune response, these medications aim to reduce inflammation and prevent further tissue damage. Two of these agents have been used for oral and genital ulcers in BD [12–14]. Topical tacrolimus was used for oral ulcers in BD. Patients used tacrolimus plus colchicine (Group I) or colchicine alone (Group II) in a double-blind placebo-controlled trial. Ulcer Severity Scores (USS) were significantly lower in group I after 3 months of follow-up regarding the number of ulcers, ulcer size, and duration. It was claimed that topical tacrolimus is a safe and effective drug for oral ulcers in BD [12].

10.1.1.6 Topical Antiseptic Mouthwashes

Antiseptic mouthwashes have been widely used for the treatment of oral ulcers in BD. Maintaining a consistent oral hygiene routine and utilizing topical treatments is the most effective strategy for combating dysbiosis, and restoring balance to the oral microbiome, promoting ulcer healing, and alleviating disease symptoms [15]. The efficacy of a new mouthwash formulation for oral ulcers in BD was evaluated. Patients were randomized to use either the Behçet's disease mouthwash (BD MW) (a combination of soluble betamethasone, doxycycline, and nystatin oral suspension dissolved in water), betamethasone mouthwash alone, or no therapeutic mouthwash. Doxycycline shows antimicrobial activity and immunomodulatory effects, while corticosteroids reduce the duration of oral ulcers and prevent scar formation with their anti-inflammatory effects. A new BD mouthwash is effective in treating oral ulcers and improving the quality of life in people with BD. The mouthwash was able to reduce pain and clear ulcers within 10–14 days, and its continued use was recommended until ulcer recurrence ceased. The mouthwash is more effective than betamethasone mouthwash [16].

10.1.1.7 Antiseptics, Antimicrobial and Anti-Inflammatory Agents

Oral ulcers in RAS and BD share similar clinical presentations and symptoms. Therefore, oral antiseptics and antimicrobial solutions used for RAS may also be effective in treating oral ulcers in BD. These agents include chlorhexidine gel, minocycline, tetracycline suspension, triclosan mouth rinse, and diclofenac [17].

Corticosteroids, antiseptics, and anesthetics are the most commonly used treatment options in daily practice, although there are not enough studies with a high level of evidence to evaluate their efficacy.

10.2 Genital Ulcers

Genital ulcers are common symptoms of BD, affecting approximately 70% of patients. These ulcers, in addition to being painful, negatively impact patients' quality of life due to limitations in movement and the risk of scarring [4, 5, 7]. Genital ulcers are reported to be more common in women than in men. In women, they are found on the vulva, labia majora, labia minora, and vaginal mucosa. In men, it primarily affects the scrotum and, less commonly, the glans penis, and shaft. Spontaneous healing of genital ulcers typically occurs within 10–30 days. However, since two-thirds of genital ulcers heal with scar tissue, prompt treatment is crucial to reduce pain, improve quality of life, and minimize scarring. Genital ulcers are often resistant to treatment, highlighting the need for effective therapeutic interventions. Several topical medications have been used to treat genital ulcers in BD [9, 13, 14].

Table 10.1 summarizes the topical agents commonly used for oral ulcers and genital ulcers.

10.2.1 Topical Medications

10.2.1.1 Sucralfate Suspension

Sucralfate suspension was effective for genital ulcers in BD. It was applied topically four times a day for 3 months. Sucralfate reduced the healing time and pain of genital ulcers compared to the pretreatment period [9].

Table 10.1 Efficacy spectrum of agents in oral ulcer and genital ulcer

Topical agents	Efficacy spectrum of sgents
Oral ulcers	
Corticosteroid vs. phenytoin [8]	Pain relief, ulcer size reduction
Sucralfate vs. placebo [9]	Reduce pain, acceralate wound healing
Hyalunaric acide [11]	Decreasing healing time, size of ulcer
Pentoxyfylline + colchicine vs. colchicine [10]	Reduce pain, decreasing duration of ulcer
Tacrolimus + colchicine vs. colchicine [12]	Diminishing pain scores
Mouthwashes (Triorasol) vs. betamethasone [16]	Reduce pain, cleared ulcer
Genital ulcers	
Sucralfate vs. placebo [9]	Reduce healing time and pain relief
Pimecrolimus vs. placebo [13]	Reduce pain, acceralate wound healing
Pimecrolimus + colchicine vs. colchicine [14]	Reduce pain, acceralate wound healing

10.2.1.2 Topical Immunomodulators

Topical immunomodulators are highly effective for genital ulcers in BD. Pimecrolimus has been used for genital ulcers in BD alone or in combination with oral medications. Topical pimecrolimus was compared with a placebo. It was found to reduce pain and accelerate wound healing [13]. In another study, pimecrolimus cream plus colchicine or colchicine alone was used twice a day. Compared to colchicine alone, pimecrolimus cream plus colchicine reduced the pain duration without any significant effect on healing time [14]. While there is some evidence suggesting the potential benefit of topical calcineurin inhibitors in BD, the research on their effectiveness is limited, and more studies may be needed to establish their role in the treatment of this condition. Although there is no placebo-controlled study in the treatment of genital ulcer, topical steroids are one of the treatment options frequently used in clinical practice.

10.3 Laser Treatment

Studies have demonstrated the effectiveness of laser therapy in treating oral ulcers and genital ulcers in BD. Various types of lasers, including diode lasers, CO_2 lasers, Nd:YAG lasers, and non-thermal CO_2 laser therapy, have been employed [18–25]. Laser treatments with diode and CO_2 lasers have been shown to effectively relieve pain and promote wound healing in a short time. Table 10.2 summarizes laser treatment modalities for oral and genital ulcers.

10.3.1 Nd:YAG Laser

Nd:YAG laser therapy has been proven to be effective in a controlled study. Twenty-eight patients were divided into two groups: the aphthous ulcers of patients in group I ($n = 14$) were treated with Nd:YAG laser, while those in group II ($n = 14$) were treated with triamcinolone acetonide. In comparing Nd:YAG laser and triamcinolone acetonide for oral ulcers in BD, Nd:YAG laser therapy is well tolerated by patients and is often preferred over topical corticosteroids. The mean pain score in the Nd:YAG laser group was significantly lower than that of the topical corticosteroid group at 1 week. Nd:YAG laser therapy is associated with a low risk of adverse events. Common side effects include mild discomfort, erythema, and edema, which typically resolve within a few days. Nd:YAG laser therapy has been shown to provide effective pain relief for oral ulcers [18].

10.3.2 CO_2 Laser

A single-arm pilot study reported the effectiveness of CO_2 laser therapy for oral ulcers. This study included 15 patients (ten males and five females) with BD suffering from recurrent oral ulcerations. A 50% improvement in both pain score and QoL scales was observed at the end of therapy [19]. In one case report, Demetriades et al. have declared the effectiveness of CO_2 lasers in reducing oral ulcer size and diminishing pain [20].

Table 10.2 Laser treatment in oral ulcer and genital ulcer

Laser type	Application	Patients (n)	Mean healing time (days)	Evidence
Nd: YAG laser [18]	OU	14	7	Diminish pain score
CO_2 laser [19]	OU	15	3	Reduce oral ulcer size
CO_2 laser [20]	OU	1	3	Diminishing pain
Diode laser [21]	OU	25	3	Reduce oral ulcer size
Diode laser [22]	OU	1	5	Reduce oral ulcer size
Diode laser [23]	OU	1	7	Reduce oral ulcer size
NTCLT [24]	OU	4	4	Relieving pain
NTCLT [25]	GU	1	9	Diminish pain score

OU oral ulcers, *GU* genital ulcers, *NTCLT* non-thermal CO_2 laser therapy

10.3.3 Diode Laser

The efficacy of diode laser therapy compared to topical corticosteroid in the management of oral ulcers of BD. Fifty patients were divided randomly into two parallel groups. The first group received a 980 nm diode laser; the second group received 0.1% triamcinolone acetonide. A comparison of the diode laser and topical triamcinolone acetonide revealed that diode laser was more effective in pain control and reducing oral ulcer activity [21]. Babu et al. declared a case report of spontaneous relief of pain in an oral ulcer 5 days after management with two diode laser sessions. In another case report, Marinho et al. reported complete healing of oral ulcers on the seventh day after being treated with a diode laser. These case reports have documented the effectiveness of diode lasers in reducing the size of oral ulcer and alleviating pain [22, 23].

10.3.4 Non-thermal CO_2 Laser

The CO_2 laser (10,600 nm) has emerged as a promising therapeutic tool for alleviating acute pain associated with oral lesions. Clinical studies have demonstrated the efficacy of CO_2 laser therapy in reducing pain intensity and accelerating the healing of various oral lesions [24, 25]. Operating at a low-level, non-thermal energy output, the CO_2 laser exerts its effect through photobiomodulation, a process that stimulates cellular repair and regeneration mechanisms. This procedure was termed NTCLT (non-thermal CO_2 laser therapy). Non-thermal CO_2 laser treatment is another laser method that has shown significant improvement in lesions without any complications in a series of four cases. This study has shown that NTCLT can effectively relieve pain from oral ulcers in BD [24]. In one case report, Zand et al. declared a case of BD whose painful genital ulcers were irradiated with NTCLT. The pain was relieved immediately, and no visible complications were detected [25]. These studies suggest that both the Nd:YAG laser and the CO_2 laser are highly effective in the treatment of oral ulcers in BD. Nd:YAG laser appears to be more effective than topical corticosteroids, and the CO_2 laser appears to be effective in reducing pain scores. Non-thermal CO_2 laser treatment has provided rapid pain reduction without significant side effects in the treatment of genital ulcers. More research is needed to confirm these findings and to determine the long-term efficacy of Nd:YAG laser and CO_2 laser in the treatment of oral ulcers in BD. Laser therapies are promising treatments that are mostly applied experimentally today. However, their use is limited due to the cost of their application, difficulties, and the lack of a standardized dose and frequency of application.

10.4 Other Skin Manifestations

Various mucocutaneous manifestations (e.g., erythema nodosum, superficial thrombophlebitis, papulopustular lesions), along with other systemic involvement can be observed in BD. Wet dressings such as aluminum acetate 3–5% were found effective in the early stages of erythema nodosum and superficial thrombophlebitis [7]. Bed rest is useful for these patients.

10.5 Conclusions

Topical agents play a crucial role in managing the mucocutaneous manifestations of BD, particularly oral and genital ulcers. The choice of topical treatment depends on the individual patient's needs and preferences. Topical agents' effects are likely confined to the applied area. They are often used as an adjunct to systemic therapy in BD treatment. However, for a specific subset of patients, such as elderly and female patients, topical treatment alone may suffice. On the other hand, laser therapy can be an effective way to manage the symptoms of BD and improve the quality of life for people with this condition.

References

1. Alpsoy E. Behçet's disease: a comprehensive review with a focus on epidemiology, etiology and clinical features, and management of mucocutaneous lesions. J Dermatol. 2016;43:620–32. https://doi.org/10.1111/1346-8138.13381.
2. Leccese P, Alpsoy E. Behçet's disease: an overview of etiopathogenesis. Front Immunol. 2019;10:1067. https://doi.org/10.3389/fimmu.2019.01067.
3. International Study Group for Behcet's Disease. Criteria for diagnosis of Behçet's disease. Lancet. 1990;335:1078–80.
4. Alpsoy E, Donmez L, Onder M, Gunasti S, Usta A, Karincaoglu Y, et al. Clinical features and natural course of Behçet's disease in 661 cases: a multicentre study. Br J Dermatol. 2007;157:901–6. https://doi.org/10.1111/j.1365-2133.2007.08116.x.
5. Alpsoy E, Zouboulis CC, Ehrlich CE. Mucocutaneous lesions of Behçet's disease. Yonsei Med J. 2007;48:573–85. https://doi.org/10.3349/ymj.2007.48.4.573.
6. Köse O. Development of immunopathogenesis strategies to treat Behçet's disease. Pathol Res Int. 2012:261989. https://doi.org/10.1155/2012/261989.
7. Alpsoy E, Leccese P, Emmi G, Ohno S. Treatment of Behçet's disease: an algorithmic multidisciplinary approach. Front Med (Lausanne). 2021;28(8):624795. https://doi.org/10.3389/fmed.2021.624795.
8. Fani MM, Ebrahimi H, Pourshahidi S, Aflaki E, Shafiee SS. Comparing the effect of phenytoin syrup and triamcinolone acetonide ointment on aphthous ulcers in patients with Behcet's syndrome. Iran Red Crescent Med J. 2012;14(2):75–8.
9. Alpsoy E, Er H, Durusoy C, Yilmaz E. The use of sucralfate suspension in the treatment of oral and genital ulcerations of Behçet's disease: a randomized, placebo-controlled and double-blind study. Arch Dermatol. 1999;135:529–32. https://doi.org/10.1001/archderm.135.5.529.
10. Hatemi G, Yurttas B, Kutlubay Z, Cote T, Derkunt SB, Yazızı Y, et al. Pentoxifylline gel for oral ulcers in patients with Behçet's syndrome. Arthritis Rheumatol. 2019;71(suppl10):3077–9.
11. Lee JH, Jung JY, Bang D, D. The efficacy of topical 0.2% hyaluronic acid gel on recurrent oral ulcers: comparison between recurrent aphthous ulcers and the oral ulcers of Behçet's disease. J Eur Acad Dermatol Venereol. 2008;22(5):590–5. https://doi.org/10.1111/j.1468-3083.2007.02564.x.
12. Hassanien M, Moshrif GM, Abuzaid F, Fathalla D, Talaat E. Valuation of the efficacy of topically applied tacrolimus in the treatment of oral ulcers in Behçet's diseases: a double blind placebo-controlled study. Ann Rheum Dis. 2022; https://doi.org/10.1136/annrheumdis-2022-eular.5305.
13. Chams-Davatchi C, Barikbin B, Shahram F, Nadji A, Moghaddassi M, Maryam Yousefi M, et al. Pimecrolimus versus placebo in genital aphthous ulcers of Behcet's disease: a randomized double-blind controlled trial. Int J Rheum Dis. 2010;13:253–8. https://doi.org/10.1111/j.1756-185X.2010.01531.x.
14. Kose O, Dinc A, Simsek I. Randomized trial of pimecrolimus cream plus colchicine tablets versus colchicine tablets in the treatment of genital ulcers in Behçet's disease. Dermatology. 2009;218:140–5. https://doi.org/10.1159/000182257.
15. Mumcu G, Fortune F. Oral health and its aetiological role in Behçet's disease. Front Med (Lausanne). 2021;20(8):613419. https://doi.org/10.3389/fmed.2021.613419.
16. Senusi A, Kang A, Buchanan JAG, Adesanya A, Aloraini G, Stanford M, et al. New mouthwash: an efficacious intervention for oral ulceration associated with Behcet's disease. Br J Oral Maxillofac Surg. 2020;58(8):1034–9. https://doi.org/10.1016/j.bjoms.2020.07.02777.
17. Alpsoy E. Behçet's disease: treatment of mucocutaneous lesions. Clin Exp Rheumatol. 2005;23(4):532–9.
18. Arabacı T, Kara C, Çiçek Y. Relationship between periodontal parameters and Behçet's disease and evaluation of different treatments for oral recurrent aphthous stomatitis. J Periodontal Res. 2009;44(6):718–25. https://doi.org/10.1111/j.1600-0765.2008.01183.
19. Kassem I, Assad SH. Laser management of resistant oral ulcer in a patient with Behçet's disease. Br J Oral Maxillofac. 2013; https://doi.org/10.1016/j.bjoms.2013.05.081.
20. Demetriades N, Hanford H, Laskarides C. General manifestations of Behçet's syndrome and the success of CO2-laser as treatment for oral lesions: a review of the literature and case presentation. J Mass Dent Soc. 2009;58(3):24–7.
21. Nagieb CS, Harhash TA, Fayed HL, Ali S. Evaluation of diode laser versus topical corticosteroid in management of Behcet's disease-associated oral ulcers: a randomized clinical trial. Clin Oral Investig. 2022;6(1):697–704. https://doi.org/10.1007/s00784-021-04047-8.
22. Babu DB, Chavva S, Waghray S, Allam NS, Kondaiah M. Low level laser therapy to reduce recurrent oral ulcers in Behçet's disease. Case Rep Dent. 2016:4283986. https://doi.org/10.1155/2016/4283986.
23. Marinho KCT, Giovani EM. The treatment of oral lesions in Behçet's syndrome: case report. Revista Espanola de Cirugia Oral Maxilofacial. 2016;38(2):101–4. https://doi.org/10.1016/j.maxilo.2014.05.00122.
24. Zand N, Ataie-Fashtami L, Mansouri P, Fateh M, Shirkavand A. Clinical effect of non-thermal CO_2 laser therapy (NTCLT) on pain relief of oral aphthous ulcers of Behçet's disease. J Lasers Med Sci. 2021;7(12):e72. https://doi.org/10.34172/jlms.2021.72.eCollection2021.
25. Zand N, Mansouri P, Rezaee Khiabanloo S, Fateh M, Ataie-Fashtami L, Safaee Naraghi Z, et al. The immediate pain-relieving effects of non-thermal CO_2 laser therapy on genital ulcers of Behcet's disease: a case report. J Lasers Med Sci. 2020;11(1):108–11. https://doi.org/10.15171/jlms.2020.18.

Systemic Treatments for Mucocutaneous Behçet's Disease

11

Nilgün Şentürk and Ayşe Boyvat

Contents

N. Şentürk (✉)
Faculty of Medicine, Department of Dermatology, Ondokuz Mayis University, Samsun, Türkiye

A. Boyvat
Dermatology and Venereology, Ankara University, Faculty of Medicine, Ankara, Türkiye
e-mail: boyvat@medicine.ankara.edu.tr

11.1 Introduction

Patients with resistant mucocutaneous lesions, and/or systemic involvement can be treated with systemic immunosuppressive and/or immunomodulatory agents. Due to the clinical

E. Alpsoy et al. (eds.), *Behçet's Disease: An Integrated Approach*,
https://doi.org/10.1007/978-3-031-77251-1_11

effectiveness of azithromycin in reducing the frequency of folliculitis and in accelerating the healing time of OU [22, 23].

11.4.3 Minocycline

Hypersensitivity to streptococcal antigens acquired after streptococcal infection is thought to play an important role in the appearance of symptoms of BD since the production of pro-inflammatory cytokines increase when stimulated with streptococcal antigen. Minocycline, has been shown to be effective against certain strains of streptococci and reduce the production of pro-inflammatory cytokines and demonstrated efficacy in reducing the frequency of OU, EN-like lesions, and papulopustular lesions [24].

11.4.4 Dapsone

Dapsone has gained attention for its potential in managing the mucocutaneous manifestations of BD. Dapsone exerts its therapeutic effects through anti-inflammatory and immunomodulatory properties, as well as by inhibiting neutrophil chemotaxis and the generation of reactive oxygen species [25]. Its ability to suppress the inflammatory response makes it a suitable candidate for BD, and its ability to modulate both innate and adaptive immune responses contributes to its potential efficacy in treating mucocutaneous lesions.

Several studies have explored the use of dapsone in BD, with a focus on its impact on mucocutaneous lesions. In an open study, a dose of 100 mg/day has proven effective for mucocutaneous lesions [26]. In a double-blind placebo-controlled clinical trial, dapsone demonstrated relevant effects by decreasing the frequency and duration of OU and the number and frequency of GU [27]. However, no data are available regarding the duration of remission over time.

While dapsone is generally well tolerated, it is essential to consider potential side effects such as hematological abnormalities and hypersensitivity reactions. Regular blood count monitoring and addressing any signs of adverse reactions are crucial. Additionally, the risk of hemolysis in individuals with glucose-6-phosphate dehydrogenase deficiency should be taken into consideration. Despite these considerations, its safety profile compares favorably to immunosuppressive agents.

11.5 Thalidomide

Thalidomide has emerged as an alternative option for the management of refractory mucocutaneous lesions of BD. The anti-inflammatory properties of thalidomide stem from its ability to inhibit tumor necrosis factor alpha (TNF-α), a key pro-inflammatory cytokine implicated in BD pathogenesis. By reducing TNF-α levels, thalidomide alleviates inflammatory cascade, and potentially reduces mucocutaneous symptoms. The drug's immunomodulatory effects extend beyond TNF-α inhibition, influencing various immune pathways. Thalidomide also modulates T-cell function, reduces leukocyte chemotaxis, and alters cytokine profiles, collectively contributing to its anti-inflammatory effects in BD. Given the crucial role of aberrant angiogenesis in the pathogenesis, thalidomide's anti-angiogenic properties, mediated by inhibition of vascular endothelial growth factor (VEGF) may also play a crucial role in reducing severity and frequency of these lesions [28, 29].

Clinical studies and case reports have demonstrated the efficacy of thalidomide in treating mucocutaneous lesions. Patients who are unresponsive or intolerant to conventional therapies may be suitable candidates. The efficacy of thalidomide monotherapy in mucocutaneous lesions was demonstrated in a trial with 96 patients, randomly assigned to receive either thalidomide at 300 mg/day, thalidomide at 100 mg/day, or a placebo. Thalidomide significantly decreased the number of oral and genital ulcers and papulopustular lesions, with both doses proving equally effective. Paradoxically, an increase in the number of EN-like lesions were observed. However, the beneficial effect was short lived after withdrawal. Additionally,

7% of the thalidomide-treated patients developed peripheral neuropathy, a condition that is often irreversible.

In two different open-label studies, thalidomide showed promising results at low (50 mg/day) or medium doses (200 mg/day) [30, 31]. Despite these favorable effects, its use is limited by potential serious side effects. Adverse events, including neuropathy and teratogenicity, necessitate careful patient selection, monitoring, and implementation of strict safety measures. The potential risks and benefits must be thoroughly discussed with patients, and appropriate precautions such as contraception in fertile individuals should be implemented.

11.6 Others

Clinical trials have demonstrated the efficacy of rebamipide [32], zinc sulfate [33], and isotretinoin [34] for mucocutaneous lesions. However, these treatment options are currently considered second-line, as the studies on these agents were conducted with a relatively limited number of patients in the past, and recent studies on these agents are not available in the literature. Moreover, more effective new treatments are now available.

11.7 Apremilast

Apremilast, an oral selective small molecule inhibitor of phosphodiesterase 4, operates by inhibiting phosphodiesterase 4, and enhancing cyclic AMP levels. Consequently, it induces a reduction in the levels of proinflammatory cytokines, including TNF α, IL-23, and IFNγ. Simultaneously it increases the levels of anti-inflammatory cytokines, such as IL-10 [35, 36]. After undergoing a Phase 3 randomized clinical trial known as The RELIEF study, apremilast received approval in multiple countries including United States, Japan, and the European Union for refractory OU associated with BD [37]. This trial demonstrated a significant reduction in the number of OU from baseline to week 12, as well as a decrease in the Behçet's Disease Current Activity Form (BDCAF) [38]. The observed positive effects persisted for a duration of up to 64 weeks [39]. The RELIEF study was designed to investigate only the effects of the drug on OU; therefore, no conclusive evidence was found for the effect on other manifestations of BD. During the recent years, real-world data composed of several observational studies and case series, has started to accumulate on the use of apremilast on patients with BD [1, 35–37, 40–42]. The studies which are limited in number, nonrandomized, and mostly small sample sized, indicated a beneficial effect of apremilast on OU, as well as on extra-oral manifestations of BD, and life quality of the patients. Iizuka et al. performed a systematic review and meta-analysis, pooling data from eight studies spanning from 2015 to 2021. Their analysis aimed to assess the clinical efficacy of apremilast in treating mucocutaneous manifestations, and overall disease activity in patients with BD [41]. The study which included 309 patients with BD receiving apremilast found suggestive evidence of the effectiveness of apremilast on GU, skin lesions and articular manifestations of BD in addition to OU at 12 weeks. Additionally, improvement was observed in overall disease activity. Gastrointestinal symptoms such as diarrhea and nausea were the most common adverse effects, and although not reported in phase 2 and phase 3 studies, depression and suicidal ideation was noted in a small number of cases. Long-term prospective studies conducted on a large number of patients are needed to determine the effect of apremilast on systemic involvements of BD.

11.8 Azathioprine

Azathioprine, an immunosuppressive agent, acts as a purine analogue and, by interfering with DNA synthesis, it inhibits the proliferation of rapidly dividing cells, including activated lymphocytes. Its immunosuppressive effects make it a reasonable option for the treatment of autoimmune and inflammatory conditions, such as BD.

In multiple studies, the efficacy of azathioprine has been investigated in BD, particularly for ocular lesions. The effectiveness of azathioprine on mucocutaneous lesions generally relies on ocular studies. Azathioprine has shown its activity by reducing frequency and severity of OU and GU, papulopustular lesions, and other cutaneous manifestations.

In a randomized trial, 73 male patients with BD, with or without ocular involvement were treated with either azathioprine (2.5 mg/kg per day) or placebo, with glucocorticoids available to both groups [43]. Results after 2 years revealed a lower occurrence of oral and genital ulcers among those treated with azathioprine.

In general, a daily dose of 2–3 mg/kg of Azathioprine is used. Treatment typically begins with 50 mg and is then increased gradually up to the target dose, if tolerated. It may take several weeks for clinical effects to appear. The gradual onset of action necessitates a long-term commitment to treatment. For the disease's acute attacks, faster-acting therapeutic agents, such as systemic corticosteroids, can be used as a bridge, and sustained benefits have been observed with continued use.

Adverse effects of azathioprine may include myelosuppression, hepatotoxicity, and an increased risk of infections. Regular monitoring of complete blood count and liver function tests is essential to promptly detect and manage potential complications. A lower dose is indicated in patients with renal insufficiency. Prior to initiating azathioprine, genetic testing for thiopurine methyltransferase is recommended for dose adjustments.

The decision to initiate azathioprine therapy in BD should be individualized, considering factors such as the severity of mucocutaneous lesions, the involvement of other organ systems, and the patient's overall health. Combining azathioprine with other immunosuppressive agents, such as corticosteroids or biologics, may be considered in refractory cases.

11.9 Calcineurin Inhibitors

11.9.1 Cyclosporine-A (CyA)

Due to its immunosuppressive properties, CyA has emerged as a valuable treatment option, offering relief from the debilitating effects of mucocutaneous lesions of BD.

By inhibiting the calcineurin pathway, CyA suppresses the activation of T-lymphocytes, thereby downregulating the production of pro-inflammatory cytokines. This immunomodulatory effect helps reduce the exaggerated inflammatory response seen in BD. Furthermore, cyclosporine has been shown to enhance regulatory T-cell function, promoting immune tolerance and contributing to the overall anti-inflammatory effect.

Although typically used for ocular manifestations, several clinical studies have reported a significant reduction in the frequency and severity of OU, GU, and skin lesions. In a randomized trial, cyclosporine (10 mg/kg/day in divided doses) demonstrated superiority to colchicine in the managing OU, GU, and other skin lesions, with its effect persisting during long-term follow-up [44].

Subsequent studies have confirmed its effectiveness even at lower doses (5 mg/kg/day) and demonstrated its similar efficacy to the combination of corticosteroid and chlorambucil for mucocutaneous lesions [45, 46].

Due to its long-term adverse effects, CyA should be reserved for selected cases, such as those with resistant mucocutaneous lesions and ocular involvement [47]. Common side effects of CyA treatment include hypertension, hypertrichosis, gingival hyperplasia, and elevated creatine levels [48].

While further research is needed to elucidate the long-term safety and efficacy of CyA, current evidence suggests that it is a key player among the therapeutic options for BD.

11.9.2 Mycophenolate Sodium/ Mycophenolate Mofetil

Mycophenolate sodium demonstrated significant improvement in mucocutaneous lesions without causing serious side effects in patients refractory to previous treatments [49]. However, in a study, mycophenolate mofetil was found to be ineffective, leading to discontinuation of the trial due to its lack of efficacy in the first six patients [50].

11.10 Biologic Treatments

11.10.1 Interferon-α (IFN-α)

IFN-α, known for its immunomodulatory properties, has gained attention for managing mucocutaneous lesions in BD. IFN-α modulates the expression of numerous genes involved in antiviral defense, immune regulation, and cell proliferation. Notably, it aims to restore the low natural killer cell activity in BD, among other effects [51].

Multiple clinical trials and observational studies have investigated the efficacy of IFN-α in mucocutaneous lesions. It has demonstrated notable success in diminishing the frequency and severity of oral and genital ulcers, along with other cutaneous manifestations. The immunomodulatory effects of IFN-α contribute to a comprehensive therapeutic response, often enabling a reduction in the use of immunosuppressive medications.

In comparison to placebo, IFN-α2a (6 MU, administered three times a week, for 3 months), demonstrated efficacy in reducing the duration and pain associated with OU, as well as the frequency of GU and papulopustular lesions. Although the mean frequency and duration of EN-like lesions, thrombophlebitis, and articular symptoms also decreased, the difference was not statistically significant [52]. Similar results were observed in seven open labeled studies [53–59]. The highest efficacy is achieved with a treatment duration of at least 2–4 months of treatment.

In a systematic review, Kötter et al. reported that 86% of patients with mucocutaneous findings responded to the treatment, with IFN-α2a providing higher remission rates than IFN-α2b [60]. The treatment dose and duration of response varied significantly among studies. A recommended approach involves an initial high dose of IFN-α2a (nine million units three times per week) for 3 months, followed by a low maintenance dose (three million units, three times per week) [25].

The safety profile of IFN-α is generally favorable, with side effects typically being mild and reversible. Common adverse effects include flu-like symptoms, fatigue, and hematological abnormalities. While serious adverse events are rare, they may encompass depression, autoimmune phenomena, and exacerbation of preexisting autoimmune conditions. Close monitoring for these potential complications is essential during treatment with IFN-α.

The decision to use IFN-α therapy in BD should be based on a careful assessment of disease severity, organ involvement, and the patient's overall health. IFN-α may be particularly beneficial in cases refractory to conventional therapies or for patients unable to tolerate other immunosuppressive agents. Regular monitoring for side effects and periodic assessment of treatment response are crucial components of clinical management.

11.10.2 TNF Alpha Inhibitors

Identification of the role of tumor necrosis factor alpha (TNF-α) in the pathogenesis of BD has led to the increased use of infliximab and adalimumab in its treatment. According to EULAR treatment guidelines, TNF α inhibitors are recommended in severe refractory BD [47]. While TNF-α inhibitors were initially primarily utilized for refractory ocular BD, their application has recently broadened to include all major organ involvements resistant to conventional immunosuppressive therapies [61–66]. However, their use in mucocutaneous BD is limited and specifically reserved for severe cases unresponsive to conventional therapeutic approaches. There is a limited number of studies exploring the effectiveness of TNF-α inhibitors in treating mucocutaneous lesions of BD. A double-blind placebo controlled study assessed the impact of the TNF-α blocker etanercept on the pathergy test, mucocutaneous manifestations, and arthritis in 38 male patients [67]. While the treatment of etanercept 25 mg twice a week showed no effect on the frequency of pathergy positivity, it significantly reduced the occurrence of OU and skin lesions. No significant effect was observed on the number of GU and the count of swollen joints. Nonetheless, a notable limitation of the study was its brief 1-month duration.

In an observational study, nine patients with refractory mucocutaneous BD were treated with adalimumab 40 mg every 2 weeks, all patients responded significantly to adalimumab without developing anti-adalimumab antibodies, even throughout an extended 5-year follow-up period. Improvement was observed in mucocutaneous lesions and joint involvement. Additionally, elevated serum TNF-α levels detected in five patients, decreased with treatment. Within 1 month and during the follow-up period, there was a significant improvement in BDCAF [68].

Our understanding of how mucocutaneous lesions in BD respond to TNF-α inhibitors primarily derive from numerous case reports, small case series and various prospective series in which anti-TNF treatment was used for the treatment of patients with major organ involvements refractory to conventional therapies. In a systematic review, Arida et al. analyzed the published data of 369 patients who had received anti-TNF therapy due to severe disease manifestations, including ocular, gastrointestinal, central nervous system, and vascular involvement [61]. In general infliximab, adalimumab or etanercept treatment resulted in improvement of mucocutaneous manifestations in most patients. The majority of patients received infliximab treatment leading to rapid remission for 91% of OU, 96% for GU, 81% for EN-like lesions, and 77% for other skin lesions. Although improvement of mucocutaneous lesions was noted in 90% of patients, 21% of patients had complete remission while partial response was obtained in 69%.

In a retrospective multicenter study aimed to evaluate long term efficacy and safety of infliximab and adalimumab in BD, data of 124 patients treated with TNF-α inhibitors for severe or refractory ocular and extraocular manifestations was evaluated. In total, 69 (50.7%) showed complete response, while 54 (39.7%) exhibited partial response. A minority, comprising 13 patients (9.6%), did not respond to therapy. This study highlights the effectiveness of TNF-α inhibitors in the treatment of extraocular manifestations of the disease. Improvement was noted in 88% of mucocutaneous lesions. Similar effectiveness and safety profiles were observed between infliximab and adalimumab. Following a median follow-up of 21 months, side effects occurred in 24 (28%) BD patients. The most commonly encountered side effects were bronchopneumonia, herpes virus infections and abscesses [69].

11.10.3 Secukinumab

The IL-17 axis has been demonstrated to play a significant role in the pathogenesis of BD. In a retrospective study, secukinumab exhibited effectiveness in the management of mucocutaneous lesions and articular manifestations in five female patients with BD. Among these patients four also presented with ankylosing spondylitis, while one met the criteria for psoriatic arthritis [70]. The treatment was well tolerated. Despite concerns regarding Secukinumab's efficacy and safety in patients with ocular and gastrointestinal involvement, none of the treated patients experienced an exacerbation of uveitis or gastrointestinal symptoms. In a multicenter observational study by the same group of authors, data from 15 BD patients with active mucosal and articular phenotypes treated with secukinumab were analyzed [71]. These patients were refractory to or unable to tolerate colchicine, disease modifying anti-rheumatic drugs (DMARDs) treatment and at least one TNF α inhibitor. After 6 months, complete or partial response was observed in 86.7% of the patients. The percentage of complete responders steadily increased throughout the follow-up, with the majority maintaining clinical remission; however, relapses were observed after the first year of therapy. Consistent with the findings of the preliminary study, secukinumab at 300 mg/month exhibited superior effectiveness compared to the 150 mg/month dose. Additionally, the study further demonstrated the steroid sparing and DMARD-sparing effects of secukinumab, with no major organ involvement throughout the study period.

Contrary to the reported beneficial effects of secukinumab in mucocutaneous BD, there have been reported cases of individuals developing BD or experiencing lesions mimicking BD during secukinumab treatment [72–75].

11.10.4 Ustekinumab

Ustekinumab's effectiveness in treating the mucocutaneous lesions of BD has been explored in limited case reports and a small number of studies. The rationale behind utilization of ustekinumab in the treatment of the patients stems from the recognition of the crucial involvement of Th1 and Th17 in the pathogenesis, as well as the identification of an association at the IL23R and IL12RB2 loci in genome-wide association studies.

In 2013, Baerveldt et al. reported a 37-year-old female patient diagnosed with BD, psoriasis and hidradenitis suppurativa, who showed successful treatment response to 45 mg ustekinumab. Remarkably, this patient sustained clinical remission throughout a 36-month follow-up period without requiring additional immunosuppressive therapies [76]. Lopalco et al. reported a case involving a 36-year-old female patient with BD, unresponsive to prior treatments including colchicine, methotrexate, azathioprine, cyclosporine, adalimumab, etanercept, and anakinra. However, this patient experienced rapid resolution of orogenital ulcerations and papulopustular lesions upon treatment with 45 mg ustekinumab [77].

In an open prospective pilot study, 14 BD patients with OU resistant to colchicine treatment were administered either ustekinumab 90 mg or 45 mg, adjusted based on individual patient weight. At week 12, 64% of patients met the criteria for a complete response while 21% showed a partial response. Following a median follow-up period of 7 months, ten patients continued their ustekinumab treatment. However, four patients experienced relapses, primarily manifesting as skin lesions, with one case involving gastrointestinal involvement. At week 12, significantly decreased levels of circulating IL-17 and IL-12 were observed under ustekinumab treatment [78]. In 2019, the same research group published the results of their study examining the therapeutic efficacy of ustekinumab in a larger cohort comprising 30 BD patients with OU refractory to conventional therapies. After 12 weeks of treatment, 18 patients (60%) achieved a complete response, while nine patients (30%) exhibited a partial response. Four patients discontinued therapy due to adverse effects: headache in one patient, and exacerbation of BD manifestations in three patients, including scleritis in one, deep venous thrombosis in another, and papulopustular lesions along with arthralgia in a third patient. Of the initial 30 patients, 26 patients continued ustekinumab therapy. By the end of the 12 months follow-up, complete response rate had risen to 88%, partial response rate was 12% with no non-responding patients. The most frequently reported side effect was headache, observed in four patients [79].

11.10.5 IL-1 Inhibitors

IL-1, a cytokine pivotal in innate immunity, has been effectively used in the treatment of autoinflammatory diseases. BD is believed to involve both autoimmune and autoinflammatory mechanisms in its pathogenesis. Given the clinical resemblances between BD and autoinflammatory diseases, coupled with the observation of elevated IL-1 β levels in the serum and synovial fluid of BD patients, the consideration of anti-IL-1 therapy emerged as a potential treatment approach for BD. So far, the primary emphasis in studies exploring anti-IL-1 therapies in BD has been on evaluating their effects on major organ involvements [62, 80–82]. Conversely, there is only a limited number of case reports, and retrospective studies, that specifically investigate mucocutaneous manifestations, revealing contradictory results. A rapid and enduring response to canakinumab was reported in a small series of three patients with refractory mucocutaneous lesions [83]. In a study evaluating the effect of gevokizumab on ocular involvement promising results were obtained; however, mucocutaneous flares did occur in the study [84]. In a study by Grayson et al., the effectiveness of anakinra on mucocutaneous manifestations of BD was investigated in a two-stage adaptive design [85]. Initially, six patients received anakinra at 100 mg/day subcutaneously, with a potential increase to 200 mg daily if oral and genital ulcers persisted after the first month. For patients with ulcers at month 6, the anakinra dose could be further increased to 300 mg daily. However, after 6 months, only two of the six patients achieved complete response, and two patients had partial remission. Consequently, the randomized phase involving 20 patients was not pursued. The study determined that the optimal dose of anakinra was 200 mg daily and increasing it to 300 mg did not enhance efficacy. Despite a reduction in OU, the effect of anakinra was neither complete nor sustained during the 16-month follow-up for patients showing complete or partial response. The limited number of studies and contradictory results underscore the necessity for further comprehensive research on the efficacy of anti-IL-1 therapies on mucocutaneous BD.

In conclusion, ongoing research efforts contribute to the evolution of BD treatment, incorporating both traditional and emerging therapies. As our understanding of the pathogenesis of BD advances, accompanied by the introduction of new therapeutic modalities, we anticipate better management and improved outcomes in BD in the near future.

References

1. Alpsoy E, Bozca BC, Bilgic A. Behçet disease: an update for dermatologists. Am J Clin Dermatol. 2021;22(4):477–502.
2. Leung YY, Yao Hui LL, Kraus VB. Colchicine—update on mechanisms of action and therapeutic uses. Semin Arthritis Rheum. 2015;45(3):341–50.
3. Terkeltaub RA. Colchicine update: 2008. Semin Arthritis Rheum. 2009;38(6):411–9.
4. Taylor J, Glenny AM, Walsh T, Brocklehurst P, Riley P, Gorodkin R, et al. Interventions for the management of oral ulcers in Behçet's disease. Cochrane Database Syst Rev. 2014;2014(9):Cd011018.
5. Davatchi F, Sadeghi Abdollahi B, Tehrani Banihashemi A, Shahram F, Nadji A, Shams H, et al. Colchicine versus placebo in Behçet's disease: randomized, double-blind, controlled crossover trial. Mod Rheumatol. 2009;19(5):542–9.
6. Yurdakul S, Mat C, Tüzün Y, Ozyazgan Y, Hamuryudan V, Uysal O, et al. A double-blind trial of colchicine in Behçet's syndrome. Arthritis Rheum. 2001;44(11):2686–92.
7. Aktulga E, Altaç M, Müftüoglu A, Ozyazgan Y, Pazarli H, Tüzün Y, et al. A double blind study of colchicine in Behçet's disease. Haematologica. 1980;65(3):399–402.
8. Kazokoglu H, Saatçi O, Cuhadaroglu H, Eldem B. Long-term effects of cyclophosphamide and colchicine treatment in Behçet's disease. Ann Ophthalmol. 1991;23(4):148–51.
9. Calgüneri M, Ertenli I, Kiraz S, Erman M, Celik I. Effect of prophylactic benzathine penicillin on mucocutaneous symptoms of Behçet's disease. Dermatology. 1996;192(2):125–8.
10. Colchicine and other drugs for gout. Med Lett Drugs Ther. 2009;51(1326):93–4.
11. COLCRYSTM (colchicine, USP) tablets for oral use. US Food and Drug Administration (FDA) approved product information. [updated November 2012. Available from: https://www.accessdata.fda.gov/drugsatfda_docs/label/2009/022351lbl.pdf.
12. Pakfetrat A, Mansourian A, Momen-Heravi F, Delavarian Z, Momen-Beitollahi J, Khalilzadeh O, et al. Comparison of colchicine versus prednisolone in recurrent aphthous stomatitis: a double-blind randomized clinical trial. Clin Invest Med. 2010;33(3):E189–95.
13. Femiano F, Buonaiuto C, Gombos F, Lanza A, Cirillo N. Pilot study on recurrent aphthous stomatitis (RAS): a randomized placebo-controlled trial for the comparative therapeutic effects of systemic prednisone and systemic montelukast in subjects unresponsive to topical therapy. Oral Surg Oral Med Oral Pathol Oral Radiol Endod. 2010;109(3):402–7.
14. Mat C, Yurdakul S, Uysal S, Gogus F, Ozyazgan Y, Uysal O, et al. A double-blind trial of depot corticosteroids in Behçet's syndrome. Rheumatology (Oxford). 2006;45(3):348–52.
15. Lessof MHJD, Lehner T, Mattock M, Sanders MD. Corticosteroids and azathioprine: their use in Behçet's syndrome. In: Lehner TBC, editor. Behçet's syndrome: clinical and immunological factors. Academic Press; 1979. p. 267–75.
16. Yazici H, Yurdakul S, Hamuryudan V. Behçet's syndrome. Curr Opin Rheumatol. 1999;11(1):53–7.
17. Bozca BC, Alpsoy E. Experimental therapeutic solutions for Behcet's disease. J Exp Pharmacol. 2021;13:127–45.
18. Direskeneli H. Autoimmunity vs autoinflammation in Behcet's disease: do we oversimplify a complex disorder? Rheumatology (Oxford). 2006;45(12):1461–5.
19. Al-Waiz MM, Sharquie KE, MH AQ, Hayani RK. Colchicine and benzathine penicillin in the treatment of Behçet disease: a case comparative study. Dermatol Online J. 2005;11(3):3.
20. Labro MT. Immunological effects of macrolides. Curr Opin Infect Dis. 1998;11(6):681–8.
21. Isogai E, Ohno S, Kotake S, Isogai H, Tsurumizu T, Fujii N, et al. Chemiluminescence of neutrophils from patients with Behçet's disease and its correlation with an increased proportion of uncommon serotypes of Streptococcus sanguis in the oral flora. Arch Oral Biol. 1990;35(1):43–8.

22. Mumcu G, Ergun T, Elbir Y, Eksioglu-Demiralp E, Yavuz S, Atalay T, et al. Clinical and immunological effects of azithromycin in Behçet's disease. J Oral Pathol Med. 2005;34(1):13–6.
23. Mumcu G, Inanç N, Özdemir FT, Tulunay A, Ekşioğlu-Demiralp E, Ergun T, et al. Effects of azithromycin on intracellular cytokine responses and mucocutaneous manifestations in Behçet's disease. Int J Dermatol. 2013;52(12):1561–6.
24. Kaneko F, Oyama N, Nishibu A. Streptococcal infection in the pathogenesis of Behçet's disease and clinical effects of minocycline on the disease symptoms. Yonsei Med J. 1997;38(6):444–54.
25. Lin P, Liang G. Behçet disease: recommendation for clinical management of mucocutaneous lesions. J Clin Rheumatol. 2006;12(6):282–6.
26. Sharquie KE. Suppression of Behçet's disease with dapsone. Br J Dermatol. 1984;110(4):493–4.
27. Sharquie KE, Najim RA, Abu-Raghif AR. Dapsone in Behçet's disease: a double-blind, placebo-controlled, cross-over study. J Dermatol. 2002;29(5):267–79.
28. Direskeneli H, Ergun T, Yavuz S, Hamuryudan V, Eksioglu-Demiralp E. Thalidomide has both anti-inflammatory and regulatory effects in Behcet's disease. Clin Rheumatol. 2008;27(3):373–5.
29. Hamuryudan V, Mat C, Saip S, Ozyazgan Y, Siva A, Yurdakul S, et al. Thalidomide in the treatment of the mucocutaneous lesions of the Behçet syndrome. A randomized, double-blind, placebo-controlled trial. Ann Intern Med. 1998;128(6):443–50.
30. de Wazières B, Gil H, Magy N, Berthier S, Vuitton DA, Dupond JL. Treatment of recurrent ulceration with low doses of thalidomide. Pilot study in 17 patients. Rev Med Interne. 1999;20(7): 567–70.
31. Gardner-Medwin JM, Smith NJ, Powell RJ. Clinical experience with thalidomide in the management of severe oral and genital ulceration in conditions such as Behçet's disease: use of neurophysiological studies to detect thalidomide neuropathy. Ann Rheum Dis. 1994;53(12):828–32.
32. Matsuda T, Ohno S, Hirohata S, Miyanaga Y, Ujihara H, Inaba G, et al. Efficacy of rebamipide as adjunctive therapy in the treatment of recurrent oral aphthous ulcers in patients with Behçet's disease: a randomised, double-blind, placebo-controlled study. Drugs R D. 2003;4(1):19–28.
33. Sharquie KE, Najim RA, Al-Dori WS, Al-Hayani RK. Oral zinc sulfate in the treatment of Behcet's disease: a double blind cross-over study. J Dermatol. 2006;33(8):541–6.
34. Sharquie KE, Helmi RM, Noiami AA, Al-Hayani RK, Kadhom MA. The therapeutic role of isotretinoin in the management of Behçet's disease: a single-blinded, controlled therapeutic study. J Drugs Dermatol. 2013;12(4):e68–73.
35. Vieira M, Buffier S, Vautier M, Le Joncour A, Jamilloux Y, Gerfaud-Valentin M, et al. Apremilast in refractory Behcet's syndrome: a multicenter observational study. Front Immunol. 2020;11:626792.
36. Takeno M, Dobashi H, Tanaka Y, Kono H, Sugii S, Kishimoto M, et al. Apremilast in a Japanese subgroup with Behcet's syndrome: results from a phase 3, randomised, double-blind, placebo-controlled study. Mod Rheumatol. 2022;32(2):413–21.
37. Hatemi G, Mahr A, Takeno M, Kim D, Melikoglu M, Cheng S, et al. Impact of apremilast on quality of life in Behcet's syndrome: analysis of the phase 3 RELIEF study. RMD Open. 2022;8:2.
38. Hatemi G, Mahr A, Ishigatsubo Y, Song YW, Takeno M, Kim D, et al. Trial of apremilast for oral ulcers in Behcet's syndrome. N Engl J Med. 2019;381(20):1918–28.
39. Hatemi G, Mahr A, Takeno M, Kim DY, Saadoun D, Direskeneli H, et al. Apremilast for oral ulcers associated with active Behcet's syndrome over 68 weeks: long-term results from a phase 3 randomised clinical trial. Clin Exp Rheumatol. 2021;39(Suppl 132(5)):80–7.
40. Ozdede A, Hatemi G. An evaluation of apremilast for the treatment of adult patients with oral ulcers associated with Behcet's syndrome. Expert Opin Pharmacother. 2021;22(12):1533–7.
41. Iizuka Y, Takase-Minegishi K, Hirahara L, Kirino Y, Soejima Y, Namkoong HO, et al. Beneficial effects of apremilast on genital ulcers, skin lesions, and arthritis in patients with Behcet's disease: a systematic review and meta-analysis. Mod Rheumatol. 2022;32(6):1153–62.
42. Azuma N, Matsui K. Effectiveness of apremilast against Behcet's disease-associated mucocutaneous and joint involvement confirmed through switching from adalimumab. Clin Exp Rheumatol. 2022;40(8):1605–6.
43. Yazici H, Pazarli H, Barnes CG, Tüzün Y, Ozyazgan Y, Silman A, et al. A controlled trial of azathioprine in Behçet's syndrome. N Engl J Med. 1990;322(5):281–5.
44. Masuda K, Nakajima A, Urayama A, Nakae K, Kogure M, Inaba G. Double-masked trial of cyclosporin versus colchicine and long-term open study of cyclosporin in Behçet's disease. Lancet. 1989;1(8647):1093–6.
45. Avci O, Gürler N, Güneş AT. Efficacy of cyclosporine on mucocutaneous manifestations of Behçet's disease. J Am Acad Dermatol. 1997;36(5 Pt 1):796–7.
46. BenEzra D, Cohen E, Chajek T, Friedman G, Pizanti S, de Courten C, et al. Evaluation of conventional therapy versus cyclosporine A in Behçet's syndrome. Transplant Proc. 1988;20(3 Suppl 4):136–43.
47. Hatemi G, Christensen R, Bang D, Bodaghi B, Celik AF, Fortune F, et al. 2018 update of the EULAR recommendations for the management of Behçet's syndrome. Ann Rheum Dis. 2018;77(6):808–18.
48. Sajjadi H, Soheilian M, Ahmadieh H, Hassanein K, Parvin M, Azarmina M, et al. Low dose cyclosporin-A therapy in Behçet's disease. J Ocul Pharmacol. 1994;10(3):553–60.
49. Köse O, Simşek I, Pay S. Mycophenolate sodium in the treatment of mucocutaneous Behcet's diseases. Int J Dermatol. 2011;50(7):895–6.

50. Adler YD, Mansmann U, Zouboulis CC. Mycophenolate mofetil is ineffective in the treatment of mucocutaneous Adamantiades-Behçet's disease. Dermatology. 2001;203(4):322–4.
51. Chung RT, Gale M Jr, Polyak SJ, Lemon SM, Liang TJ, Hoofnagle JH. Mechanisms of action of interferon and ribavirin in chronic hepatitis C: summary of a workshop. Hepatology. 2008;47(1):306–20.
52. Alpsoy E, Durusoy C, Yilmaz E, Ozgurel Y, Ermis O, Yazar S, et al. Interferon alfa-2a in the treatment of Behçet disease: a randomized placebo-controlled and double-blind study. Arch Dermatol. 2002;138(4):467–71.
53. Boyvat A, Sişman-Solak C, Gürler A. Long-term effects of interferon alpha 2A treatment in Behçet's disease. Dermatology. 2000;201(1):40–3.
54. O'Duffy JD, Calamia K, Cohen S, Goronzy JJ, Herman D, Jorizzo J, et al. Interferon-alpha treatment of Behçet's disease. J Rheumatol. 1998;25(10):1938–44.
55. Georgiou S, Monastirli A, Pasmatzi E, Gartaganis S, Goerz G, Tsambaos D. Efficacy and safety of systemic recombinant interferon-alpha in Behçet's disease. J Intern Med. 1998;243(5):367–72.
56. Azizlerli G, Sarica R, Köse A, Ovül C, Kavala M, Kayabali M, et al. Interferon alfa-2a in the treatment of Behçet's disease. Dermatology. 1996;192(3):239–41.
57. Alpsoy E, Yilmaz E, Başaran E. Interferon therapy for Behçet's disease. J Am Acad Dermatol. 1994;31(4):617–9.
58. Hamuryudan V, Moral F, Yurdakul S, Mat C, Tüzün Y, Ozyazgan Y, et al. Systemic interferon alpha 2b treatment in Behçet's syndrome. J Rheumatol. 1994;21(6):1098–100.
59. Zouboulis CC, Orfanos CE. Treatment of Adamantiades-Behçet disease with systemic interferon alfa. Arch Dermatol. 1998;134(8):1010–6.
60. Kötter I, Günaydin I, Zierhut M, Stübiger N. The use of interferon alpha in Behçet disease: review of the literature. Semin Arthritis Rheum. 2004;33(5):320–35.
61. Arida A, Fragiadaki K, Giavri E, Sfikakis PP. Anti-TNF agents for Behcet's disease: analysis of published data on 369 patients. Semin Arthritis Rheum. 2011;41(1):61–70.
62. Alibaz-Oner F, Sawalha AH, Direskeneli H. Management of Behcet's disease. Curr Opin Rheumatol. 2018;30(3):238–42.
63. Aksoy A, Yazici A, Omma A, Cefle A, Onen F, Tasdemir U, et al. Efficacy of TNFalpha inhibitors for refractory vascular Behcet's disease: a multicenter observational study of 27 patients and a review of the literature. Int J Rheum Dis. 2020;23(2):256–61.
64. Zou J, Ji DN, Cai JF, Guan JL, Bao ZJ. Long-term outcomes and predictors of sustained response in patients with intestinal Behcet's disease treated with infliximab. Dig Dis Sci. 2017;62(2):441–7.
65. Hibi T, Hirohata S, Kikuchi H, Tateishi U, Sato N, Ozaki K, et al. Infliximab therapy for intestinal, neurological, and vascular involvement in Behcet disease: efficacy, safety, and pharmacokinetics in a multi-center, prospective, open-label, single-arm phase 3 study. Medicine (Baltimore). 2016;95(24):e3863.
66. Calvo-Rio V, Blanco R, Beltran E, Sanchez-Burson J, Mesquida M, Adan A, et al. Anti-TNF-alpha therapy in patients with refractory uveitis due to Behcet's disease: a 1-year follow-up study of 124 patients. Rheumatology (Oxford). 2014;53(12):2223–31.
67. Melikoglu M, Fresko I, Mat C, Ozyazgan Y, Gogus F, Yurdakul S, et al. Short-term trial of etanercept in Behcet's disease: a double blind, placebo controlled study. J Rheumatol. 2005;32(1):98–105.
68. Verboom DM, van der Houwen TB, Kappen JH, van Daele PLA, Dik WA, Schreurs MWJ, et al. Adalimumab provides long-lasting clinical improvement in refractory mucocutaneous Behcet's disease without formation of antidrug antibodies. Clin Exp Rheumatol. 2019;37(Suppl 121(6)):43–7.
69. Vallet H, Riviere S, Sanna A, Deroux A, Moulis G, Addimanda O, et al. Efficacy of anti-TNF alpha in severe and/or refractory Behcet's disease: multicenter study of 124 patients. J Autoimmun. 2015;62:67–74.
70. Di Scala G, Bettiol A, Cojan RD, Finocchi M, Silvestri E, Emmi G. Efficacy of the anti-IL 17 secukinumab in refractory Behcet's syndrome: a preliminary study. J Autoimmun. 2019;97:108–13.
71. Fagni F, Bettiol A, Talarico R, Lopalco G, Silvestri E, Urban ML, et al. Long-term effectiveness and safety of secukinumab for treatment of refractory mucosal and articular Behcet's phenotype: a multicentre study. Ann Rheum Dis. 2020;79(8):1098–104.
72. Dincses E, Yurttas B, Esatoglu SN, Melikoglu M, Hamuryudan V, Seyahi E. Secukinumab induced Behcet's syndrome: a report of two cases. Oxf Med Case Rep. 2019;2019(5):omz041.
73. Barrado-Solis N, Rodrigo-Nicolas B, De la Morena-Barrio I, Perez-Pastor G, Sanchis-Sanchez C, Tomas-Cabedo G, et al. Report of two cases of Behcet's disease developed during treatment with secukinumab. J Eur Acad Dermatol Venereol. 2020;34(10):e587–e9.
74. Calleja Algarra A, Aragon Miguel R, Andres Lencina JJ, Pinilla Martin B, Vico Alonso C, Rodriguez Peralto JL, et al. Behcet's-like disease during secukinumab treatment: new paradoxical reaction? J Dtsch Dermatol Ges. 2021;19(1):116–8.
75. Avci C, Akin G, Akarsu S, Lebe B. Pyoderma gangrenosum and Behcet's-like disease induced by secukinumab: a paradoxical drug reaction. J Dermatolog Treat. 2023;34(1):2235040.
76. Baerveldt EM, Kappen JH, Thio HB, van Laar JA, van Hagen PM, Prens EP. Successful long-term triple disease control by ustekinumab in a patient with Behcet's disease, psoriasis and hidradenitis suppurativa. Ann Rheum Dis. 2013;72(4):626–7.
77. Lopalco G, Fabiani C, Venerito V, Lapadula G, Iannone F, Cantarini L. Ustekinumab efficacy and safety in mucocutaneous multi-refractory Behcet's disease. Clin Exp Rheumatol. 2017;35(Suppl 108(6)):130–1.

78. Mirouse A, Barete S, Monfort JB, Resche-Rigon M, Bouyer AS, Comarmond C, et al. Ustekinumab for Behcet's disease. J Autoimmun. 2017;82:41–6.
79. Mirouse A, Barete S, Desbois AC, Comarmond C, Sene D, Domont F, et al. Long-term outcome of Ustekinumab therapy for Behcet's disease. Arthritis Rheumatol. 2019;71(10):1727–32.
80. Emmi G, Talarico R, Lopalco G, Cimaz R, Cantini F, Viapiana O, et al. Efficacy and safety profile of anti-interleukin-1 treatment in Behcet's disease: a multicenter retrospective study. Clin Rheumatol. 2016;35(5):1281–6.
81. Bettiol A, Silvestri E, Di Scala G, Amedei A, Becatti M, Fiorillo C, et al. The right place of interleukin-1 inhibitors in the treatment of Behcet's syndrome: a systematic review. Rheumatol Int. 2019;39(6):971–90.
82. Cantarini L, Vitale A, Scalini P, Dinarello CA, Rigante D, Franceschini R, et al. Anakinra treatment in drug-resistant Behcet's disease: a case series. Clin Rheumatol. 2015;34(7):1293–301.
83. Vitale A, Rigante D, Caso F, Brizi MG, Galeazzi M, Costa L, et al. Inhibition of interleukin-1 by canakinumab as a successful mono-drug strategy for the treatment of refractory Behcet's disease: a case series. Dermatology. 2014;228(3):211–4.
84. Gul A, Tugal-Tutkun I, Dinarello CA, Reznikov L, Esen BA, Mirza A, et al. Interleukin-1beta-regulating antibody XOMA 052 (gevokizumab) in the treatment of acute exacerbations of resistant uveitis of Behcet's disease: an open-label pilot study. Ann Rheum Dis. 2012;71(4):563–6.
85. Grayson PC, Yazici Y, Merideth M, Sen HN, Davis M, Novakovich E, et al. Treatment of mucocutaneous manifestations in Behcet's disease with anakinra: a pilot open-label study. Arthritis Res Ther. 2017;19(1):69.

12.2 Clinical Features

The mucocutaneous lesions represent the distinctive clinical feature of BD. Their frequent occurrence at the onset or during any phase of the disease highlights the importance of mucocutaneous lesions. Oral ulcers (OU), genital ulcers (GU), and cutaneous lesions, along with ocular and articular involvement, are the most common clinical manifestations [5]. In most cases, the appearance of mucocutaneous lesions precedes the onset of other symptoms. The identification of these symptoms may lead to an earlier diagnosis and treatment, which may result in beneficial outcomes. The presence of painful and recurrent OU and GU is a hallmark of BD. OU, GU, erythema nodosum (EN)-like lesions, papulopustular lesions (PPL), superficial thrombophlebitis (STP), or other less common cutaneous lesions (e.g., extragenital ulcers, Sweet's syndrome-like, and pyoderma gangrenosum-like lesions) can lead to significant pain and/or loss in function [6–8].

Nondeforming arthritis, typically presenting as a monoarticular or oligoarticular pattern, characterizes articular involvement, which is observed in approximately half of the patients. The usual course of the condition is transitory, with episodes lasting from a few days to weeks. Among the joints, the knee is the most frequently affected, followed by the ankle, wrist, and elbow [9, 10].

BD's ocular involvement, which is among the most severe and debilitating complications, is present in roughly half of all patients. The recurrent, explosive inflammatory attacks are characteristic of the condition. Uveitis associated with BD is a potentially sight-threatening condition. The introduction of biologic disease-modifying antirheumatic drugs (DMARDs), particularly anti TNF-alpha agents, has significantly improved visual prognosis. Nowadays, most refractory cases can be treated with an expanding therapeutic armamentarium [11]. Despite the advancements in treatment and improved outcomes over the years, eye complications can still result in the loss of vision. This is frequently a result of patients having limited access to experienced ophthalmologists specialized in BD. Ocular involvement is observed bilaterally in 86% of patients, with a higher frequency and severity in men [12]. The main ocular manifestation of BD is bilateral nongranulomatous panuveitis with retinal vasculitis. Red eyes can be a symptom of episcleritis in some patients. Less common forms of ocular involvement include conjunctival ulcers, scleritis, orbital inflammation, and isolated optic neuritis. Poor visual outcomes can be linked to an increase in the frequency and severity of uveitis attacks, as well as the occurrence of complications like cystoid macular edema and foveal ischemia [12, 13].

Mortality in BD is often caused by the involvement of the vascular system. BD is classified as a variable vessel vasculitis, which can affect veins and arteries of all sizes [14]. Nevertheless, the venous system is the primary affected site, with superficial and deep vein thrombosis being the most common vascular involvements. Additionally, thromboses in the inferior and superior vena cava, dural sinuses, and Budd–Chiari syndrome can be observed and are linked to poor prognosis. Pulmonary artery involvement (pulmonary artery thromboses and/or pulmonary artery aneurysm), albeit uncommon, constitutes the primary cause of death [15].

Neurological involvement is considered one of the most serious complications of the disease because of its severe prognosis. Neurological symptoms, which affect 5–10% of all patients, are more frequently seen in men. The parenchymal and nonparenchymal forms are the two distinct types. The manifestation of neurological involvement can be a single acute attack, relapsing–remitting, or chronic progressive course. Poor prognosis is associated with rapid disease progression, frequent relapse history, and cerebrospinal fluid pleocytosis. The main clinical manifestations in patients with parenchymal involvement may include pyramidal signs, hemiparesis, behavioral changes, and sphincter disturbance. Whereas patients with nonparenchymal involvement may experience raised intracranial pressure due to dural sinus thrombosis [16].

Gastrointestinal involvement is observed in roughly 3–16% of patients, with a higher incidence in Far Eastern countries. Oval, punched-out, volcano-shaped mucosal ulcers are the primary manifestation of this condition, which is typically seen in the ileocecal region but can be present in other areas of the gastrointestinal tract as well. The most prevalent symptoms include abdominal pain, nausea, vomiting, diarrhea, and bleeding. Deep punched-out ulcers are the primary cause of common intestinal complications, including severe bleeding and perforation. The occurrence of intestinal lesions is linked to an unfavorable prognosis [17].

12.3 Treatment

This section of the book aims to provide a detailed overview of the disease treatment. Despite the detailed focus on mucocutaneous symptoms, the algorithmic treatment approach also covers the disease's systemic involvement. Treatment success is subject to multiple variables, including but not limited to the affected organ, severity of involvement, duration of the involvement, and frequency of attacks, as well as the patient's age and gender. Nonetheless, the main goal of treatment should be to rapidly suppress and prevent new inflammatory attacks, particularly during the initial, active stages of BD, to avoid irreversible organ damage. The scope of randomized controlled trials is confined to mucocutaneous, articular, and ocular involvement. Our proposed treatment approach in this chapter uses algorithms based on symptoms. In the treatment recommendations for each organ involvement, "Oxford Levels of Evidence" was used to assess the quality of evidence. Categories of evidence and strength of recommendations were formulated in brackets following each treatment recommendation [18]. Even though the recommendations are mainly derived from controlled studies, significant studies, guidelines, expert reviews and, finally, our own clinical experience is also included [1, 4, 5]. Tables 12.1 and 12.2 summarize the activity spectrum of topical [19–28] and systemic therapeutic agents [29–61] on BD in randomized, controlled studies. The multisystemic nature of the disease requires a harmonious collaboration among relevant medical specialties in the management of patients.

Table 12.1 The principal topical therapeutic agents utilized in randomized, controlled studies for the treatment of Behçet's disease

Therapeutic agent and reference	Dose/duration/patient number	Efficacy spectrum
Interferon alpha vs. placebo [19]	1 × 10^5 U/g thrice a day/24 w/30	Not effective on OU outcomes
Interferon alpha vs. placebo [20]	1000/2000 IU a day/12 w/84	No beneficial effects on OU
Cyclosporin A vs. placebo [21]	70 mg/g of Orabase/8 w/24	No significant difference in efficacy between treatment arms for OU
Sucralfate vs. placebo [22]	4 times a day/3 mo/40	Reduces the frequency, healing time, and pain of OU, as well as the healing time and pain of GU
Pimecrolimus + colchicine vs. colchicine [23]	Twice a day/4 w/38	Pain severity of GU significantly decreased in the pimecrolimus group
Pimecrolimus vs. placebo [24]	Twice a day/4 w/45	GU healed more rapidly in the drug group
Triamcinolone acetonide vs. phenytoin [25]	Thrice a day/1 w/60	Triamcinolone acetonide is more effective than phenytoin on OU
Pentoxifylline + colchicine vs. colchicine [26]	1000 mg/d (four divided doses)/14 d/21	Pentoxifylline group experienced significant decrease in OU duration and pain
Tacrolimus + colchicine vs. colchicine [27]	Twice a day/12 w/20	The use of tacrolimus resulted in significantly better scores for OU severity and VAS
Diode laser vs. triamcinolone acetonide [28]	Two sessions for each lesion (1 min duration) with a resting time of 5 min, 3 w, 50 (25/25)	Diode laser was more effective than triamcinolone acetonide in controlling pain and reducing OU activity

Table 12.2 The principal systemic therapeutic agents utilized in randomized, controlled studies for the treatment of Behçet's disease

Therapeutic agent and reference	Dose/duration/patient number	Efficacy spectrum
Levamisole vs. placebo [29]	3 × 50 mg, 2 days/w; 8 w; 47	Improvement in OU, GU, arthritis, and uveitis outcomes
Colchicine vs. placebo [30–32]	1 mg/d; 9 mo; 28	Decrease in EN-like lesions frequency, and efficacy on arthralgia
	1–2 mg/d; 2 y; 116	Decreased frequency of GU, EN-like lesions and arthritis in women, and the occurrence of arthritis in men
	1 mg/d; 4 mo; 169	Significant improvement both in disease activity index, and OU, GU, EN, and PPL outcomes
Acyclovir vs. placebo [33]	800 mg/d; 12 w; 44	Ineffective in reducing the occurrence and severity of OU and GU or other disease symptoms
CsA vs. conventional treatments (prednisolone, chlorambucil) [34]	5–10 mg/kg/d; 3 y; 40	In ocular disease, CsA was more effective than conventional therapy, while conventional therapy was superior to CsA in controlling OU, GU, and arthritis
CsA vs. colchicine [35]	10 mg/kg/d + 1 mg/d; 4 mo; 96	CsA showed improved efficacy in reducing the severity and frequency of OU, GU, and PPL. It also demonstrated greater efficacy than colchicine in reducing the frequency and severity of ocular attacks
CsA vs. conventional treatments (prednisolone, azathioprine) [36]	5 mg/kg/d; 6 mo; 76	CsA was superior to conventional therapy in multiple symptoms, including OU, GU, cutaneous lesions, STP, articular and neurologic symptoms
Azathioprine vs. placebo [37]	2.5 mg/kg/d; 2 y; 63	Decreased frequency of OU, GU, arthritis, and ocular symptoms; protection the occurrence of new eye disease
Azapropazone vs. placebo [38]	900 mg/d; 3 w; 57	Ineffectiveness in controlling the arthritis
Colchicine vs. colchicine + benzathine penicillin [39]	1–2 mg/d + 1.2 MU/3 w; 2 y; 154	Combined treatment was more effective at reducing the frequency of arthritic episodes, duration of OU and EN, and frequency of GU
Thalidomide vs. placebo [40]	100–300 mg/d; 6 mo; 96	Long-lasting remission of OU, GU, and PPL
CP + corticosteroids vs. corticosteroids [41]	1 g/m²/mo + 0.5 mg/kg; 6 mo; 35	The combination of CP and corticosteroids was more effective for eye disease than corticosteroids alone
IFN-α2a vs. placebo [42]	6 MU/d, 3×/w; 12 w; 50	Significant effectiveness in reducing pain and healing time in OU, and frequency in GU and PPL
Dapsone vs. placebo [43]	100 mg/d; 12 w; 20	Efficacy on the number, healing time and frequency OU, number of GU, and frequency of EN and PPL; reduction in arthritis and epididymitis symptoms
Rebamipide vs. placebo [44]	300 mg/d; 6 mo; 35	Reduction in OU number and pain

(continued)

Table 12.2 (continued)

Therapeutic agent and reference	Dose/duration/patient number	Efficacy spectrum
Etanercept vs. placebo [45]	25 mg/d; 2×/w; 4 w; 40	Decrease in the frequency of OU, nodular skin lesions, and PPL
Zinc sulfate vs. placebo [46]	300 mg/d; 6 mo; 30	A significant efficacy in the clinical manifestations index of mucocutaneous lesions
Zinc gluconate vs. placebo [47]	30 mg/d; 12 wk; *n*: 50 (25/25)	Significant improvement in GU
Corticosteroids vs. placebo [48]	40 mg/every 3 w; 27 w; 41	Reduced frequency of EN-like lesions in women
Daclizumab vs. placebo [49]	1 mg/kg/2 w for 6 weeks; 6 mo; 17	No beneficial outcome compared to placebo
Rituximab vs. cytotoxic combination therapy [50]	Two 1000 mg courses (15-day interval); 6 mo; 20	Rituximab group showed a significant improvement in total adjusted disease activity index
Secukinumab vs. placebo [51]	300 mg/2 w or 300 mg/mo; early termination; 118	Ineffective in uveitis recurrence; positive impact on reducing the use of concomitant immunosuppressive medication
Isotretinoin vs. placebo [52]	20 mg/d; 12 w; 30	Significant decrease in the clinical manifestations index, and OU and skin manifestations outcomes
IFN-α2b (pegylated) vs. glucocorticoids and immunosuppressives [53]	0.3 µg/kg/w; 26 w; 72	Peginterferon-α-2b addition to drug regime resulted in significant corticosteroid dose reduction at 1 year for patients with ocular and systemic involvement
Apremilast vs. placebo [54–56]	30 mg/twice a day; 12 w; 207 (104/103)	Effective in treating OU and its pain
	30 mg/twice a day; 12 w; 111 (55/56)	Significant reduction in the number of OU, and decrease in pain of OU
	30 mg BID, 12 wk, *n*: 39 (19/20)	Reduction in the number of OU and overall disease activity
IFN-α2a vs. CsA [57, 58]	3–9 MU/d-3×/w vs. 3–5 mg/kg; 1 y; 26	The IFN alpha arm had a higher number of patients in remission; the switch from CsA to IFN alpha showed a significant increase
	IFN-α2a (3 MIU/d for 4 weeks, followed by 3 MIU every other day), CsA 200 mg/d, 12 mo, *n*: 26 (44 eyes)	A significantly greater improvement in visual acuity, and more stable remission of intraocular inflammation in IFN-α2a group
Alemtuzumab 60 mg vs. Alemtuzumab 30 mg [59]	At baseline and 6 months or earlier where clinically appropriate; 12 mo; *n*: 23 (ANCA-associated vasculitis = 12; BD = 11)	Remission in two-thirds of patients at 6 months
Nanocurcumin vs. placebo [60]	80 mg/day; 8 wk; *n*: 32 (17/15)	Significant reduction in disease activity in nanocurcumin group
Gevokizumab vs. placebo [61]	60 mg/every 4 wk; 28–420 d; *n*: 83 (40/43)	Gevokizumab did not have a significant effect on the risk of ocular exacerbations

CP, cyclophosphamide; CsA, cyclosporine A; IFN, interferon

12.3.1 Topical Treatment

The use of corticosteroids alone, such as *triamcinolone acetonide* in oral paste (*1B/A*) or *dexamethasone* ointment (*3/D*), for OU, and in combination with antiseptics (e.g., *fusidic acid/betamethasone* (*3/D*)) for GU, has been found to be beneficial, especially when administered in the early stages of these lesions [1, 25]. *Sucralfate* (*1B/A*) has demonstrated its efficacy in ameliorating pain and promoting healing in both OU and GU [22]. *Pentoxifylline* 5% gel (*1B/A*) is found to decrease OU pain and duration [26]. The use of *tacrolimus* (*1B/A*) in OU of BD resulted in significant decreases in VAS and ulcer severity scores among patients [27]. The effectiveness and safety of *pimecrolimus* (*1B/A*) have been demonstrated in GU treatment [23, 24]. Although the availability of *diode laser* (*1B/A*) application in clinical practice is questionable, it was found to be more effective than triamcinolone acetonide in controlling pain and reducing OU activity [28]. Besides bed rest, the use of *wet dressings* (*4/D*) containing aluminum acetate at a concentration of 3–5% is recommended during the early phases of EN-like lesions and STP [62].

In view of the similarity between OU resulting from BD and recurrent aphthous stomatitis (RAS), the remedies recommended for RAS can be implemented for OU of BD. The application of topical antibiotics (e.g., tetracyclines and their derivatives), antimicrobial agents (e.g., chlorhexidine), amlexanox, and triclosan has been found to be beneficial in promoting wound healing and can therefore be recommended as first-line treatments. Hydroxypropyl cellulose, diclofenac, lidocaine, silver nitrate, CO_2 laser, and Nd:YAG laser have been proven to have pain-reducing properties and can be employed as second-line options [1, 62].

The effectiveness of topical treatments is possibly restricted to the application site; thus, considering BD is a systemic inflammatory disease, they should be used together with systemic treatments, not alone. Nevertheless, even in the absence of clinical studies, *topical treatment alone* (*4/D*) may be employed for patients with the following features: (1) patients who have not had a new attack for a long time and have no major organ involvement; (2) patients who are female or elderly without severe organ involvement [5, 63].

12.3.2 Systemic Treatment

12.3.2.1 Mucocutaneous Manifestations

Colchicine (*1B/A*), 0.5 mg × 2–4 /d, can be considered the first-line treatment option for OU, GU, EN-like lesions, and PPL [30–32]. The addition of *benzathine penicillin* (*2A/B*), 1.2 MU/mo, to colchicine has the potential to enhance its efficacy [39]. *Apremilast* (*1B/A*), 30 mg × 2/d, offers another viable option for treating mucocutaneous lesions, with its proven efficacy [54–56]. *Azathioprine* (*1B/A*), 2–2.5 mg/kg/d, is recommended for patients who are not effectively managed by the treatments mentioned above [37]. Patients who are unresponsive to previous treatments can benefit from anti-*tumor necrosis factor* (*TNF*)-*α agents* (*1B/A-3/C*) (etanercept 25 mg × 2/w; adalimumab, 80 mg initial dose, followed by 40 mg every other week starting 1 week after initial dose and infliximab, 5 mg/kg at week 0, 2, and 6 and then at 8- to 12-weekly intervals) [45], *interferon* (*IFN*)-*α* (*1B/A*) (3–12 MU × 3/w) [42] and *cyclosporine A* (*CsA*) (*1B/A*) (5 mg/kg/d) [34–36]. *Ustekinumab* (*2B/B*) (90 mg at inclusion, at week 4, and then once every 12 weeks) can achieve high remission rates for oral and genital ulcers [64]. *Secukinumab* (*3/C*) (150–300 mg at weeks 0, 1, 2, 3, and 4 and monthly after that) [65] may be another effective option in mucocutaneous manifestations. *Thalidomide* (*1B/A*), 100–300 mg/d, and *dapsone* (*1B/A*), 100–150 mg/d, are frequently beneficial [40, 43]. Nevertheless, they must be cautiously administered to certain patients due to possible adverse reactions. Other alternatives include, *levamisole* (*1B/A*) (3 × 50 mg/2 days/week) [29], *rebamipide* (*1B/A*) (300 mg/d) [44], *zinc sulfate* (*1B/A*) (300 mg/d) or *Zinc gluconate* (*1B/A*) (30 mg/d) [46, 47], *isotretinoin* (*1B/A*) (20 mg/d) [52], *methotrexate* (*3/C*) (7.5–20 mg/w) [1], and *pentoxifylline* (*3/C*) (400 mg × 3/d) [1].

Because of the availability of controlled studies, dapsone [43], levamisole [29], zinc sulfate or zinc gluconate [46, 47], and isotretinoin [52] treatments could be considered during the algorithm's early stages. However, there have been no recent publications on most of these treatments. Moreover, recent years have witnessed newer and more effective treatments. The evaluation of rebamipide at earlier stages of the algorithm was not possible because its effect is restricted to OU [44].

In the management of acute and severe mucocutaneous lesions attacks, particularly major OU, GU, EN-like lesions and/or STP, *corticosteroids (prednisolone)* (*3/D*) can be employed with efficacy. The initial dose should be 40–60 mg daily for 2–4 weeks, with subsequent tapering over 4–6 weeks. The treatment, in this case, involves the use of corticosteroids in addition to the previous treatment. A combination with a treatment, such as colchicine, would be the more appropriate choice if the patient is not receiving any systemic treatment [4, 5]. A stepwise, symptom-based, algorithmic approach for mucocutaneous BD management is proposed in Table 12.3.

12.3.2.2 Articular Involvement

To prevent arthritis attacks, *colchicine* (*1B/A*) is often the first-line treatment [31]. The combination of *colchicine and benzathine penicillin* (*2A/B*) may be useful for patients who do not respond to colchicine monotherapy [39]. For patients with recurrent arthritis and/or resistant disease, *azathioprine* (*1B/A*) is a treatment to be considered [37]. More severe cases may necessitate the use of *IFN-α* (*1B/A*) and *anti-TNF-α agents* (*3/C*) [66–70]. *Azapropazone* (*1B/A*) or *intramuscular methylprednisolone acetate* (*1B/A*) did not show promising results in controlled studies, despite the widespread use of these compounds to treat arthritis symptoms [38, 48]. For patients with monoarthritis, *intra-articular corticosteroid injections* (*3/C*) can be employed as an adjunct to systemic therapy. Nonetheless, conclusive evidence has not been derived from randomized clinical trials [1, 71]. Limited data imply that *ustekinumab* (*3/C*), *secukinumab* (*3/C*), and *anti-IL-1 agents* (*3/C*) might be considered as alternative treatment options [65, 72, 73] (Table 12.3).

12.3.2.3 Ocular Involvement

The first step in ocular BD treatment should be to suppress acute inflammation in various parts of the eye, including the anterior uvea, retina, retinal vessels, choroid, and optic disc during the exacerbation stage. Conjunctival ulcers and episcleritis typically have a mild course and only affect the ocular surface. If this is the sole clinical presentation, treatment with topical corticosteroids is usually sufficient to control the condition. For patients experiencing an acute attack limited to the anterior part of the eye, *topical corticosteroid* (*3/C*) eye drops containing dexamethasone are recommended. *Mydriatics* (*3/C*) and/or *cycloplegic eye drops* (*3/C*) are often recommended alongside corticosteroids to manage anterior uveitis. These agents can prevent posterior synechiae and alleviate pain and discomfort caused by ciliary muscle spasms. Some patients may require subconjunctival *corticosteroid injection* (*3/C*). Posterior sub-Tenon corticosteroid injection and *oral corticosteroid* (*3/C*) therapy may be necessary for severe ocular fundus inflammation, in addition to topical treatment above. As with many organ involvements of BD, systemic corticosteroids may be used as a bridge therapy in acute exacerbations of ocular involvement due to their rapid and effective anti-inflammatory activity and until the efficacy of systemic immunosuppressants becomes evident. *Azathioprine* (*1B/A*) and/or *CsA* (*1B/A*) should be added to systemic corticosteroids in unresponsive cases or with posterior segment involvement [1, 12]. Anti-TNF-α agents particularly *adalimumab* and *infliximab* (*2A/B*) or *IFN-α* (*1B/A*) are potentially the strongest treatment options in patients who cannot be controlled by these treatments or in those with acute sight-threatening ocular presentation [11, 12, 18]. However, poorly controlled patients using these agents may experience reduced visual function, in which case other treatments such as *methotrexate*, *mycophenolate mofetil* (*MMF*) and *anti-IL-1 agents* (*3/C*) should be considered [74] (Table 12.3).

nolate mofetil (*3/C*), *anti-IL 6* (*3/C*) or *anti-IL-1 agents* (*3/C*) may be considered as alternative options due to limited scientific evidence [85–88]. The reason is not known, but there seems to be a relationship between CsA and an increased risk of developing parenchymal neurological involvement. Therefore, CsA is not recommended in this clinic [1].

The treatment for venous sinus thrombosis involves high-dose corticosteroids and short-term *anticoagulation* (*3/C*). Immunosuppressive treatment should be considered for those experiencing relapses. Azathioprine, CP, and anti-TNF-α agents are possible treatments. Patient characteristics, disease severity, and organ involvement should guide treatment selection. Patients with relapsing disease or hypercoagulability may benefit from long-term anticoagulation [89, 90] (Table 12.3).

12.3.2.6 Gastrointestinal Involvement

Treatment for gastrointestinal involvement depends on its severity. Mild cases can be initially treated with 5-amino salicylate derivatives such as *sulfasalazine* (*3/C*) and *mesalamine* (*3/C*). However, for unresponsive or severe cases, *azathioprine* (*3/C*) should be considered [71]. In the most severe cases, oral or intravenous high-dose *corticosteroids* (*3/C*) may be necessary [17, 91]. However, there is still uncertainty regarding the benefits and risks of using high-dose corticosteroids [71]. The current evidence is insufficient to recommend regular use of high-dose corticosteroids for gastrointestinal involvement [17, 85]. Poorly controlled enteric manifestations with azathioprine may require *anti-TNF-α agents* (*3/C*) or *thalidomide* (*3/C*). The effectiveness of controlling gastrointestinal symptoms can also be seen in other immunomodulating therapies, such as *methotrexate* (*3/C*) and *MMF* (*3/C*) [91]. Given the limited evidence, these treatments should only be utilized as a last resort for gastrointestinal involvement. *Surgery* (*3/C*) is considered as an absolute indication in cases of perforation and massive gastrointestinal bleeding, while abdominal abscess, fistula, and stricture may also warrant surgical intervention (Table 12.3).

12.4 Conclusion

Regular follow-up and proper management of BD are crucial because of the high occurrence of vital organ involvement. Recent advancements in our understanding of disease pathophysiology have led to the introduction of new therapeutic agents, resulting in substantial improvements in morbidity and mortality rates. Potential future therapies could target the epistatic interactions between HLAB*51 and ERAP1 variants, which disrupt T-cell homeostasis [92]. It is noteworthy that neutrophils from individuals with BD display spontaneous formation of neutrophil extracellular traps (NETosis) when compared to those from healthy individuals [93]. Targeting NETosis in the future could be a potential therapeutic strategy to prevent thrombosis and vascular events related to BD. The multisystemic nature of the disease necessitates collaboration between relevant medical specialties in order to enhance patient outcomes. Disease-specific organizations are required to facilitate collaboration among experienced physicians. Multicenter, large-scale controlled trials are essential to promote optimal patient management, particularly in cases involving organs with high mortality rates, such as the vascular, neurological and gastrointestinal systems, or those causing significant morbidity, such as the eye, articular, and mucocutaneous manifestations. The same approach can be employed for less common occurrences of the disease, including rare mucocutaneous manifestations (e.g., extragenital ulcers, leg ulcers), cardiac involvement, epididymitis. OU and other mucocutaneous manifestations are the most frequent reason for BD patients to present to the outpatient clinic. Additionally, OU activity persists in all age groups and significantly impacts the patient's quality of life. There is still a need for drugs that can provide long-term remission of OU, which may also be a precursor to major organ involvement.

In addition to treatment, it is advisable to consider incorporating certain approaches that can enhance overall well-being. These include adopting a healthy diet and exercise regimen, as well as addressing any psychological issues that may impact patients' quality of life.

References

1. Alpsoy E, Leccese P, Emmi G, et al. Treatment of Behçet's disease: an algorithmic multidisciplinary approach. Front Med (Lausanne). 2021;8:624795.
2. Sallakci N, Bacanli A, Coskun M, Yavuzer U, et al. CTLA-4 gene 49A/G polymorphism in Turkish patients with Behçet's disease. Clin Exp Dermatol. 2005;30:546–50.
3. Mumcu G, Yay M, Aksoy A, et al. Predictive factors for work-day loss in Behçet's syndrome: a multicenter study. Int J Rheum Dis. 2020;23(2):240–6.
4. Alpsoy E. Behçet's disease: a comprehensive review with a focus on epidemiology, etiology and clinical features, and management of mucocutaneous lesions. J Dermatol. 2016;43:620–32.
5. Alpsoy E, Bozca BC, Bilgic A. Behçet disease: an update for dermatologists. Am J Clin Dermatol. 2021;22(4):477–502.
6. Alpsoy E, Zouboulis CC, Ehrlich CE. Mucocutaneous lesions of Behçet's disease. Yonsei Med J. 2007;48:573–85.
7. Alpsoy E, Aktekin M, Er H, et al. A randomized, controlled and blinded study of papulopustular lesions in Turkish Behcet's patients. Int J Dermatol. 1998;37:839–3.
8. Alpsoy E, Donmez L, Onder M, et al. Clinical features and natural course of Behçet's disease in 661 cases: a multicentre study. Br J Dermatol. 2007;157(5):901–6.
9. Dalvi SR, Yildirim R, Yazici Y. Behcet's syndrome. Drugs. 2012;72:2223–41.
10. Diri E, Mat C, Hamuryudan V, et al. Papulopustular skin lesions are seen more frequently in patients with Behçet's syndrome who have arthritis: a controlled and masked study. Ann Rheum Dis. 2001;60:1074–6.
11. Accorinti M, Pesci FR, Pirraglia MP, et al. Ocular Behçet's disease: changing patterns over time, complications and long-term visual prognosis. Ocul Immunol Inflamm. 2017;25(1):29–36.
12. Namba K, Goto H, Kaburaki T, et al. A major review: current aspects of ocular Behçet's disease in Japan. Ocul Immunol Inflamm. 2015;23(Suppl 1):S1–S23.
13. Tugal-Tutkun I. Uveitis in Behçet disease—an update. Curr Opin Rheumatol. 2023;35(1):17–24.
14. Jennette JC, Falk RJ, Bacon PA, et al. 2012 revised International Chapel Hill Consensus Conference nomenclature of vasculitides. Arthritis Rheum. 2013;65:1–11.
15. Emmi G, Bettiol A, Silvestri E, et al. Vascular Behçet's syndrome: an update. Intern Emerg Med. 2019;14(5):645–52.
16. Kalra S, Silman A, Akman-Demir G, et al. Diagnosis and management of neuro-Behçet's disease: international consensus recommendations. J Neurol. 2014;261(9):1662–76.
17. Hisamatsu T, Ueno F, Matsumoto T, et al. The 2nd edition of consensus statements for the diagnosis and management of intestinal Behçet's disease: indication of anti-TNFα monoclonal antibodies. J Gastroenterol. 2014;49:156–62.
18. Oxford Centre for Evidence-based Medicine Levels of Evidence. 2009. http://www.cebm.net/?o=1116.
19. Hamuryudan V, Yurdakul S, Rosenkaimer F, et al. Inefficacy of topical alpha interferon in the treatment of oral ulcers of Behçet's syndrome: a randomized, double blind trial. Br J Rheumatol. 1991;30(5):395–6.
20. Kiliç H, Zeytin HE, Korkmaz C, et al. Low-dose natural human interferon-alpha lozenges in the treatment of Behçet's syndrome. Rheumatology (Oxford). 2009;48(11):1388–91.
21. Ergun T, Gürbüz O, Yurdakul S, et al. Topical cyclosporine-A for treatment of oral ulcers of Behçet's syndrome. Int J Dermatol. 1997;36(9):720.
22. Alpsoy E, Er H, Durusoy C, Yilmaz E. The use of sucralfate suspension in the treatment of oral and genital ulcerations of Behçet's disease: a randomised, placebo-controlled and double-blind study. Arch Dermatol. 1999;135:529–32.
23. Kose O, Dinc A, Simsek I. Randomized trial of pimecrolimus cream plus colchicine tablets versus colchicine tablets in the treatment of genital ulcers in Behçet's disease. Dermatology. 2009;218:140–5.
24. Chams-Davatchi C, Barikbin B, Shahram F, et al. Pimecrolimus versus placebo in genital aphthous ulcers of Behcet's disease: a randomized double-blind controlled trial. Int J Rheum Dis. 2010;13:253–8.
25. Fani MM, Ebrahimi H, Pourshahidi S, et al. Comparing the effect of phenytoin syrup and triamcinolone acetonide ointment on aphthous ulcers in patients with Behcet's syndrome. Iran Red Crescent Med J. 2012;14:75–8.
26. Hatemi G, Yurttas B, Kutlubay Z, et al. Pentoxifylline gel for oral ulcers in patients with Behçet's syndrome [abstract]. Arthritis Rheumatol. 2019;71(Suppl 10).
27. Hassanien M, Moshrif, Galal M, Abuzaid F, Fathalla D, Talaat E. Evaluation of the efficacy of topically applied tacrolimus in the treatment of oral ulcers in Behçet's diseases: a double blind placebo-controlled study. Ann Rheum Dis. 2022. https://doi.org/10.1136/annrheumdis-2022-eular.5305.
28. Nagieb CS, Harhash TA, Fayed HL, et al. Evaluation of diode laser versus topical corticosteroid in management of Behcet's disease-associated oral ulcers: a randomized clinical trial. Clin Oral Investig. 2022;26(1):697–704.
29. Lehner T, Wilton JMA. The therapeutic and immunological effects of levamisole in recurrent oral ulcers and Behçet's syndrome. In: Lehner T, Barnes CB, editors. Behçet's syndrome: clinical and immunological features. New York: Academic Press; 1979. p. 291–305.
30. Aktulga E, Altac M, Muftuoglu A, et al. A double blind study of colchicine in Behcet's disease. Haematologica. 1980;65:399–402.
31. Yurdakul S, Mat C, Tuzun Y, et al. A double-blind trial of colchicine in Behcet's syndrome. Arthritis Rheum. 2001;44:2686–92.

32. Davatchi F, Sadeghi Abdollahi B, et al. Colchicine versus placebo in Behçet's disease: randomized, double-blind, controlled crossover trial. Mod Rheumatol. 2009;19:542–9.
33. Davies UM, Palmer RG, Denman AM. Treatment with acyclovir does not affect orogenital ulcers in Behçet's syndrome: a randomized double-blind trial. Br J Rheumatol. 1988;27(4):300–2.
34. BenEzra D, Cohen E, Chajek T, et al. Evaluation of conventional therapy versus cyclosporine A in Behçet's syndrome. Transplant Proc. 1988;20:136–43.
35. Masuda K, Nakajima A, Urayama A, et al. Double-masked trial of cyclosporin versus colchicine and long-term open study of cyclosporin in Behcet's disease. Lancet. 1989;20:1093–6.
36. Assaad-Khalil SH. Low-dose cyclosporin in Behçet's disease: follow-up controlled study with emphasis on extraocular manifestations and neuro-Behçet's disease. In: O'Duffy JD, Kokmen E, editors. Behçet's disease: basic and clinical aspects. New York: Marcel Dekker; 1991. p. 603–12.
37. Yazici H, Pazarli H, Barnes CG, et al. A controlled trial of azathioprine in Behcet's syndrome. N Engl J Med. 1990;322:281–5.
38. Moral F, Hamuryudan V, Yurdakul S, et al. Ineficacy of azapropazone in the acute arthritis of Behçet's syndrome: a randomized, double blind, placebo controlled study. Clin Exp Rheumatol. 1995;13(4):493–5.
39. Calguneri M, Ertenli I, Kiraz S, et al. Effect of prophylactic benzathine penicillin on mucocutaneous symptoms of Behcet's disease. Dermatology. 1996;192:125–8.
40. Hamuryudan V, Mat C, Saip S, et al. Thalidomide in the treatment of the mucocutaneous lesions of the Behçet syndrome. A randomized, double-blind, placebo-controlled trial. Ann Intern Med. 1998;128:443–50.
41. Davatchi F, Shahram F, Chams H, et al. Pulse cyclophosphamide (PCP) for ocular lesions of Behçet's disease: double blind crossover study. Arthritis Rheum. 1999;42:S320.
42. Alpsoy E, Durusoy C, Yilmaz E, et al. Interferon alpha-2a in the treatment of Behçet disease: a randomized, placebo-controlled and double blind study. Arch Dermatol. 2002;138:467–71.
43. Sharquie KE, Najim RA, Abu-Raghif AR. Dapsone in Behcet's disease: a double-blind, placebo-controlled, cross-over study. J Dermatol. 2002;29:267–79.
44. Matsuda T, Ohno S, Hirohata S, et al. Efficacy of rebamipide as adjunctive therapy in the treatment of recurrent oral aphthous ulcers in patients with Behçet's disease: a randomised, double-blind, placebo-controlled study. Drugs R D. 2003;4:19–28.
45. Melikoglu M, Fresko I, Mat C, et al. Short-term trial of etanercept in Behcet's disease: a double blind, placebo controlled study. J Rheumatol. 2005;32:98–105.
46. Sharquie KE, Najim RA, Al-Dori WS, et al. Oral zinc sulfate in the treatment of Behcet's disease: a double blind cross-over study. J Dermatol. 2006;33:541–6.
47. Faghfouri AH, Baradaran B, Khabbazi A, et al. Regulation of NLRP3 inflammasome by zinc supplementation in Behçet's disease patients: a double-blind, randomized placebo-controlled clinical trial. Int Immunopharmacol. 2022;109:108825.
48. Mat C, Yurdakul S, Ozyazgan Y, et al. A double-blind trial of depot corticosteroids in Behçet's syndrome. Rheumatology (Oxford). 2006;45:348–52.
49. Buggage RR, Levy-Clarke G, Sen HN, et al. A double-masked, randomized study to investigate the safety and efficacy of daclizumab to treat the ocular complications related to Behçet's disease. Ocul Immunol Inflamm. 2007;15:63–70.
50. Davatchi F, Shams H, Rezaipoor M, et al. Rituximab in intractable ocular lesions of Behcet's disease; randomized single-blind control study (pilot study). Int J Rheum Dis. 2010;13:246–52.
51. Dick AD, Tugal-Tutkun I, Foster S, et al. Secukinumab in the treatment of noninfectious uveitis: results of three randomized, controlled clinical trials. Ophthalmology. 2013;120:777–87.
52. Sharquie KE, Helmi RM, Noiami AA, et al. The therapeutic role of isotretinoin in the management of Behçet's disease: a single-blinded, controlled therapeutic study. J Drugs Dermatol. 2013;12:e68–73.
53. Lightman S, Taylor SR, Bunce C, et al. Pegylated interferon-alpha-2b reduces corticosteroid requirement in patients with Behcet's disease with upregulation of circulating regulatory T cells and reduction of Th17. Ann Rheum Dis. 2015;74:1138–44.
54. Hatemi G, Melikoglu M, Tunc R, et al. Apremilast for Behçet's syndrome—a phase 2, placebo-controlled study. N Engl J Med. 2015;372:1510–8.
55. Hatemi G, Mahr A, Ishigatsubo Y, et al. Trial of apremilast for oral ulcers in Behçet's syndrome. N Engl J Med. 2019;381(20):1918–28.
56. Takeno M, Dobashi H, Tanaka Y, et al. Apremilast in a Japanese subgroup with Behçet's syndrome: results from a Phase 3, randomised, double-blind, placebo-controlled study. Mod Rheumatol. 2022;32(2):413–21.
57. Kötter I, Vonthein R, Schoenfisch B, et al. Interferon alpha2a versus cyclosporin A for the treatment of severe ocular Behçet's disease—a prospective, randomized, single blind, national multi center trial (INCYTOB). Ann Rheum Dis. 2016;75(Suppl 2):1091.
58. Qian Y, Qu Y, Gao F, Pei M, Liang A, Xiao J, et al. Comparison of the safety and efficacy of interferon alpha-2a and Cyclosporine-A when combined with glucocorticoid in the treatment of refractory Behçet's uveitis: a randomized controlled prospective study. Front Pharmacol. 2021;12:699903. https://doi.org/10.3389/fphar.2021.699903.

59. Gopaluni S, Smith R, Goymer D, et al. Alemtuzumab for refractory primary systemic vasculitis—a randomised controlled dose ranging clinical trial of efficacy and safety (ALEVIATE). Arthritis Res Ther. 2022;24(1):81.
60. Farzaneh R, Khabbazi A, Soltani-Zangbar MS, et al. Effects of nanocurcumin supplementation on T-helper 17 cells inflammatory response in patients with Behcet's disease: a randomized controlled trial. Immunopharmacol Immunotoxicol. 2022;44(2):206–15.
61. Tugal-Tutkun I, Pavesio C, De Cordoue A, Bernard-Poenaru O, Gül A. Use of gevokizumab in patients with Behçet's disease uveitis: an international, randomized, double-masked, placebo-controlled study and open-label extension study. Ocul Immunol Inflamm. 2018;26(7):1023–33.
62. Alpsoy E. Behçet's disease: treatment of mucocutaneous lesions. Clin Exp Rheumatol. 2005;23:532–9.
63. Bozca BC, Alpsoy E. Experimental therapeutic solutions for Behcet's disease. J Exp Pharmacol. 2021;13:127–45.
64. London J, Régent A, Dion J, Jilet L, Jachiet M, Lidove O, et al. Efficacy and safety of ustekinumab in Behçet disease: results from the prospective phase 2 STELABEC trial. J Am Acad Dermatol. 2022;87(3):681–4.
65. Fagni F, Bettiol A, Talarico R, et al. Long-term effectiveness and safety of secukinumab for treatment of refractory mucosal and articular Behçet's phenotype: a multicentre study. Ann Rheum Dis. 2020;79(8):1098–104.
66. Alpsoy E, Yilmaz E, Başaran E. Interferon therapy for Behçet's disease. J Am Acad Dermatol. 1994;31:617–9.
67. Hamuryudan V, Moral F, Yurdakul S, et al. Systemic interferon alpha 2b treatment in Behçet's syndrome. J Rheumatol. 1994;21:1098–100.
68. Kötter I, Vonthein R, Zierhut M, et al. Differential efficacy of human recombinant interferon-alpha2a on ocular and extraocular manifestations of Behçet disease: results of an open 4-center trial. Semin Arthritis Rheum. 2004;33:311–9.
69. Calguneri M, Ozturk MA, Ertenli I, et al. Effects of interferon alpha treatment on the clinical course of refractory Behçet's disease: an open study. Ann Rheum Dis. 2003;62:492–3.
70. Vallet H, Riviere S, Sanna A, et al. Efficacy of anti-TNF alpha in severe and/or refractory Behçet's disease: multicenter study of 124 patients. J Autoimmun. 2015;62:67–74.
71. Hatemi G, Christensen R, Bang D, et al. 2018 update of the EULAR recommendations for the management of Behçet's syndrome. Ann Rheum Dis. 2018;77:808–18.
72. Emmi G, Talarico R, Lopalco G, et al. Efficacy and safety profile of anti-interleukin-1 treatment in Behçet's disease: a multicenter retrospective study. Clin Rheumatol. 2016;35(5):1281–6.
73. Mirouse A, Barete S, Desbois AC, et al. Long-term outcome of ustekinumab therapy for Behçet's disease. Arthritis Rheumatol. 2019;71(10):1727–32.
74. Fabiani C, Vitale A, Rigante D, et al. The presence of uveitis is associated with a sustained response to the interleukin (IL)-1 inhibitors anakinra and canakinumab in Behçet's disease. Ocul Immunol Inflamm. 2020;28(2):298–304.
75. Emmi G, Becatti M, Bettiol A, et al. Behçet's syndrome as a model of thrombo-inflammation: the role of neutrophils. Front Immunol. 2019;10:1085.
76. Seyahi E, Melikoglu M, Akman C, Hamuryudan V, Ozer H, Hatemi G, et al. Pulmonary artery involvement and associated lung disease in Behcet disease: a series of 47 patients. Medicine (Baltimore). 2012;91(1):35–48.
77. Desbois AC, Biard L, Addimanda O, et al. Efficacy of anti-TNF alpha in severe and refractory major vessel involvement of Behcet's disease: a multicenter observational study of 18 patients. Clin Immunol. 2018;197:54–9.
78. Hamuryudan V, Seyahi E, Ugurlu S, et al. Pulmonary artery involvement in Behçet's syndrome: effects of anti-Tnf treatment. Semin Arthritis Rheum. 2015;45(3):369–73.
79. Seyahi E, Melikoglu M, Akman C, et al. Pulmonary artery involvement and associated lung disease in Behçet disease: a series of 47 patients. Medicine (Baltimore). 2012;91(1):35–48.
80. Voiriot G, Parrot A, Antoine M, et al. Transcatheter embolotherapy of pulmonary artery aneurysms as emergency treatment of hemoptysis in Behcet patients: experience of a referral center and a review of the literature. Intern Emerg Med. 2018;13(4):491–500.
81. Gaudric J, Jayet J, Saadoun D, Couture T, Ferfar Y, Davaine JM, et al. Factors influencing the recurrence of arterial involvement after surgical repair in Behcet disease. J Vasc Surg. 2020;72(5):1761–9.
82. Kikuchi H, Aramaki K, Hirohata S. Effect of infliximab in progressive neuro-Behcet's syndrome. J Neurol Sci. 2008;272(1–2):99–105.
83. Zeydan B, Uygunoglu U, Saip S, et al. Infliximab is a plausible alternative for neurologic complications of Behçet disease. Neurol Neuroimmunol Neuroinflamm. 2016;3(5):e258.
84. Ozguler Y, Leccese P, Christensen R, et al. Management of major organ involvement of Behçet's syndrome: a systematic review for update of the EULAR recommendations. Rheumatology (Oxford). 2018;57(12):2200–12.
85. Monastirli A, Chroni E, Georgiou S, et al. Interferon-α treatment for acute myelitis and intestinal involvement in severe Behçet's disease. QJM. 2010;103:787–90.
86. Shugaiv E, Tuzun E, Mutlu M, et al. Mycophenolate mofetil as a novel immunosuppressant in the treat-

ment of neuro-Behcet's disease with parenchymal involvement: presentation of four cases. Clin Exp Rheumatol. 2011;29(4 Suppl 67):S64–7.
87. Addimanda O, Pipitone N, Pazzola G, et al. Tocilizumab for severe refractory neuro-Behçet: three cases IL-6 blockade in neuro-Behçet. Semin Arthritis Rheum. 2015;44(4):472–5.
88. Cantarini L, Vitale A, Scalini P, et al. Anakinra treatment in drug-resistant Behcet's disease: a case series. Clin Rheumatol. 2015;34:1293–301.
89. Saadoun D, Wechsler B, Resche-Rigon M, et al. Cerebral venous thrombosis in Behcet's disease. Arthritis Rheum. 2009;61(4):518–26.
90. Ferro JM, Canhão P, Stam J, Bousser MG, Barinagarrementeria F, ISCVT Investigators. Prognosis of cerebral vein and dural sinus thrombosis: results of the International Study on Cerebral Vein and Dural Sinus Thrombosis (ISCVT). Stroke. 2004;35(3):664–70.
91. Hisamatsu T, Hayashida M. Treatment and outcomes: medical and surgical treatment for intestinal Behçet's disease. Intest Res. 2017;15(3):318–27.
92. Leccese P, Alpsoy E. Behçet's disease: an overview of etiopathogenesis. Front Immunol. 2019;10:1067. https://doi.org/10.3389/fimmu.2019.01067.
93. Kim D, Nakamura K, Kaneko F, Alpsoy E, Bang D. Mucocutaneous manifestations of Behçet's disease: pathogenesis and management from perspectives of vasculitis. Front Med (Lausanne). 2022;9:987393. https://doi.org/10.3389/fmed.2022.987393.

Eye Disease in Behçet's Disease

13

Ilknur Tugal-Tutkun and Pinar Çakar Özdal

Contents

13.1 Introduction

Ocular involvement is one of the main manifestations of Behçet's disease (BD). Because of the multisystemic nature of BD, reports of clinical cohorts may be from different disciplines, such as dermatology, rheumatology, or ophthalmology, and the data may be biased accordingly. The frequency of ocular involvement is around 30% in large series reported from rheumatology or dermatology clinics in Türkiye and even lower in some other countries [1–6]. On the other hand, reports from multidisciplinary BD centers indicate a higher frequency (38–60%) of ocular involvement in BD [7–10].

13.2 Ocular Findings

Bilateral nongranulomatous panuveitis with retinal vasculitis is the primary type of ocular involvement in BD [11]. More often than not, patients may also present with a red eye due to episcleritis. Other rare types of ocular involvement include conjunctival ulcers, scleritis, myositis, orbital inflammation, and isolated optic neuritis [12–18]. Patients with neurological involvement may also present with neuro-ophthalmic manifestations [19, 20].

Cluster analyses in large BD cohorts have shown that BD patients with uveitis constitute a separate cluster [6, 10, 21]. The incidence of genital ulcer and gastrointestinal involvement is low in the uveitis cluster, whereas there may be an

I. Tugal-Tutkun (✉)
Eye Protection Foundation Bayrampasa Eye Hospital, Istanbul, Türkiye

Department of Ophthalmology, Istanbul University, Istanbul Faculty of Medicine, Istanbul, Türkiye
e-mail: itutkun@istanbul.edu.tr

P. Ç. Özdal
Uveacademy Eye Clinic, Ankara, Türkiye

Department of Ophthalmology, University of Health Sciences, Ankara, Türkiye

E. Alpsoy et al. (eds.), *Behçet's Disease: An Integrated Approach*,
https://doi.org/10.1007/978-3-031-77251-1_13

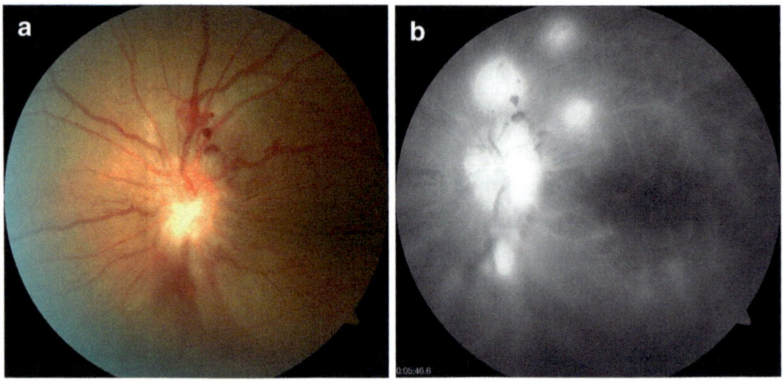

Fig. 13.6 Color fundus photograph (**a**) and FFA image (**b**) of a patient with BD uveitis show neovascularizations around the optic disc and hyperfluorescence due to leakage from new vessels in late phase FFA

pole [29–34]. During clinically quiescent periods between attacks, there are no anterior chamber cells, but there may be cells adherent to the vitreous fibrils, and the fundus exam will reveal only sequelae of past episodes. However, there may be persistent retinal capillaritis that can only be demonstrated by fundus fluorescein angiography (FFA) [31].

Retinal infiltrates, formerly defined as retinitis, were seen in more than 50% of eyes in a large series of BD uveitis [11]. Because of their transient nature, they may be missed if the patient is not seen within a few days after the onset of a uveitis attack. A dense vitreous haze may also hinder fundus visualization, and the infiltrates may resolve by the time fundus details become visible. Rapid resolution of retinal infiltrates in BD uveitis is a significant clue in differentiating from infectious retinal infiltrates or cotton wool spots of various etiology [29]. Large retinal infiltrates are usually associated with retinal hemorrhages, focal serous retinal detachment, and a wider area of retinal edema with indistinct margins. While even large retinal infiltrates resolve without visible retinochoroidal scars, an area of diffuse retinal atrophy may be revealed by optical coherence tomography (OCT) imaging [31].

Occlusive retinal vasculitis is considered a hallmark of ocular involvement in BD. Venular occlusions are mainly seen, which involve small peripheral branches more frequently than main branches of the retinal veins. Central retinal vein occlusion is rare. Branch retinal vein occlusion (BRVO) has been reported in 6–31% of eyes with BD uveitis [11, 30, 35–37]. Retinal arteriolar occlusion may occasionally be an accompanying finding; but an isolated retinal arteriolar occlusion is rare [35, 38, 39]. Occlusive retinal periphlebitis typically presents with diffuse vitritis, fluffy diffuse sheathing of retinal veins and retinal hemorrhages in the involved area. When the blood column is not visible due to the pronounced inflammatory sheathing, it may be described as "frosted branch angiitis" [40]. In BD, BRVO may also develop in the absence of intraocular inflammation [41], especially in patients with vascular BD or dural sinus thrombosis. Retinal nonperfusion caused by occlusive periphlebitis usually results in formation of shunt vessels and vascular rearrangements in BD uveitis, rather than the development of retinal neovascularizations usually seen in noninflammatory BRVO.

Recurrent panuveitis attacks and occlusive retinal vasculitis cause considerable structural damage in the eye resulting in loss of useful vision in patients with long-standing uncontrolled disease. Retinal and optic atrophy as well as macular ischemia and atrophy are irreversible causes of visual impairment [11, 30, 42, 43]. Glaucoma and cataract are mostly due to an excessive use of corticosteroids. Severe macular inflammatory infiltration during a uveitis attack or persistent CME with or without epiretinal membrane or vitreoretinal traction may result in formation of a macular hole and may cause significant visual loss even after closure of the hole spontaneously or surgically [44, 45]. Neovascularization of the optic disc is a serious complication associated with persistent inflammation in 87% and retinal ischemia in 13% of eyes with NVD [46]. Its regression should be achieved with prompt appropriate treatment, because it may cause recurrent intravitreal hemorrhages. In eyes with advanced damage, the fundus picture resembles hereditary retinopathies with diffuse retinal atrophy, pigmentation and optic atrophy. The presence of ghost vessels is a helpful clue in distinguishing end-stage BD uveitis [11].

13.3 Monitoring Behçet's Disease Uveitis

Visual acuity, frequency and severity of uveitis attacks, anterior chamber flare measured by laser flare photometry (LFP), leakage and nonperfusion on FFA, and macular thickness and structural changes on OCT are the routine parameters to be monitored in patients with BD uveitis [31, 47].

Visual acuity varies during the course of the disease, with significant reductions during attacks and improvement after the resolution of acute inflammation. On the other hand, persistent CME may cause long-standing decreased vision. It should be aimed to preserve potential visual acuity, defined as the best level of visual acuity during first remission in the absence of macular edema [11]. Cataract is a reversible cause of decreased vision, and surgical outcome is associated with potential visual acuity.

A subjective and semiquantitative scoring system, Behçet's disease ocular attack score 24 (BOS24), has been developed to monitor severity of uveitis attacks [47, 48]. This scoring system is based on the SUN scoring of anterior chamber cells and vitreous haze [27] and the location of the inflammatory fundus lesions, including peripheral, posterior pole, subfoveal, and optic disc lesions, observed by ophthalmoscopy [47, 48]. A maximum of 24 points are summed from 6 parameters of ocular inflammation for each ocular attack. The sum of BOS24 scores during long-term follow-up has been found to be significantly associated with visual outcome, and the posterior segment lesions had the greatest effect on visual deterioration [49].

Anterior chamber flare due to the protein concentration in the aqueous humor can be noninvasively measured by LFP. Flare levels correlate with the severity of intraocular inflammation [50–52]. There is also a significant correlation between LFP flare and FFA leakage [50, 51, 53]. Importantly, subclinically elevated LFP flare values during remission periods are associated with an increased risk of recurrent uveitis attacks [50].

Fundus fluorescein angiography is the gold standard in monitoring BD uveitis [31, 47]. Both the occlusive and the leaky nature of retinal vasculitis can be demonstrated by FFA. Signs of retinal vasculitis may be detected by FFA in the absence of clinical findings. Hyperfluorescence of the optic disc and retinal capillary leakage in a fern-like pattern are the most frequent FFA findings in BD uveitis [30, 31]. Wide-field FFA is especially useful to reveal retinal vascular/capillary leakage in the peripheral retina [53] (Fig. 13.7). Optic disc staining and/or peripheral leakage can be found even in the absence of overt clinical signs of intraocular inflammation [53, 54]. Using a semiquantitative angiographic scoring system, leakage score has been found to be

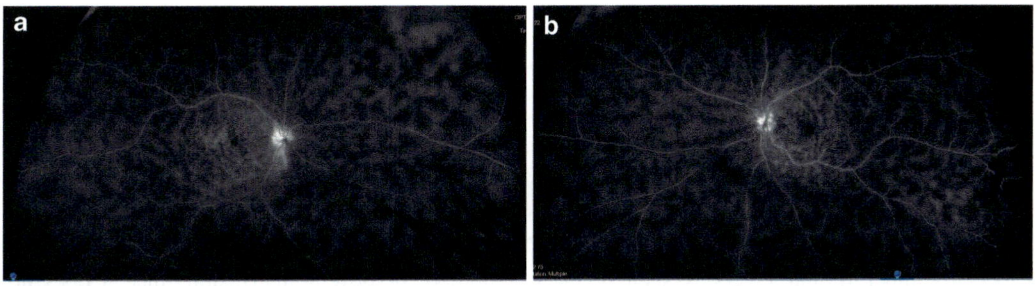

Fig. 13.7 Ultra-wide field FFA shows optic disc staining and diffuse fern-like capillary leakage in both the right (**a**) and the left eye (**b**) of a patient with BD uveitis

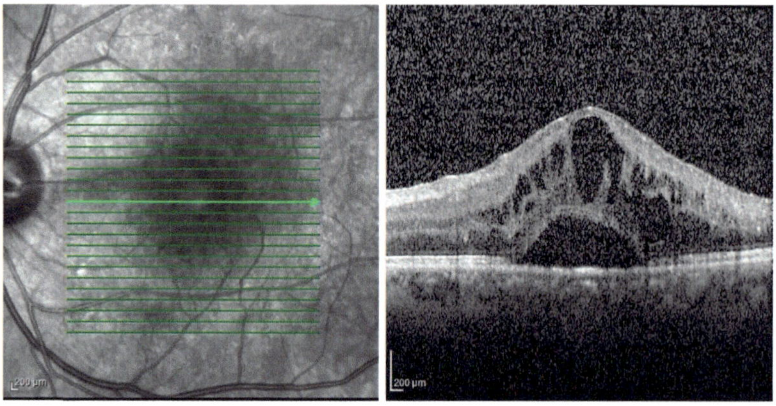

Fig. 13.8 OCT imaging shows cystoid macular edema and serous macular detachment in the left eye of a patient with BD uveitis

lower during quiescence than at times of active inflammation [53, 54]. Of particular importance, persistent leakage during quiescence is associated with an increased risk of relapse [55]. Severe posterior pole leakage is associated with a poor visual prognosis [56].

OCT is routinely used to monitor macular changes, including macular edema (Fig. 13.8), atrophy (Fig. 13.9), epiretinal membrane formation, and development of a macular hole (Fig. 13.10) or scarring. In early stages, before the development of significant macular atrophy, macular thickness correlates with clinical activity, and FFA leakage [57]. At 275 µm cutoff, diagnostic sensitivity and specificity of central foveal thickness for active uveitis were 89% and 72%, respectively, in patients with BD uveitis of less 4-year disease duration [57]. In another study, peripapillary retinal and nerve fiber layer thickness showed a stronger correlation with FFA leakage than the correlation of central macular thickness [58]. The authors of both studies suggested that OCT measurements could be used for noninvasive quantitative monitoring of BD uveitis [57, 58]. Thinning and disruption of the outer retinal layers with increased disease duration and loss of normal foveal contour have been found to be associated with worse visual acuity [59, 60]. OCT also allows documentation of retinal infiltrates and their sequelae at the posterior pole. A hyperreflective retinal thickening with blurring of especially inner retinal layers is seen in OCT scans through retinal infiltrates. The lesion causes shadowing underneath, but there is no choroidal thickening, proving isolated involvement of the retina. After the resolution of the infiltrate, focal atrophy of especially inner retinal layers and elevation of the outer plexiform layer is seen [31, 61]. The location and number of such focal atrophic lesions and retinal nerve fiber layer defects may be monitored by OCT as evidence of prior posterior uveitis attacks [32, 61].

Enhanced depth imaging or swept source OCT can be used to monitor choroidal thickness and vascularity in BD uveitis. While there are conflicting reports of choroidal thickness changes in cross-sectional studies [57, 62–64], progressive choroidal thinning has been reported in longitudinal follow-up studies [65, 66]. Onal et al. reported that there was no significant difference in subfoveal choroidal thickness between eyes with active BD uveitis and healthy controls, but the stroma/vascular lumen ratio of the choroid was higher in active BD uveitis and correlated with FFA leakage [57].

OCT-angiography (OCT-A) is a noninvasive imaging method that has been used to study retinal circulation to the capillary level in patients with BD uveitis. Significantly lower vessel densities of both superficial and deep parafoveal capillary plexus and an enlarged foveal avascular zone have been found in BD patients [67, 68]. Although OCT-A imaging of the fovea will help explain visual loss due to foveal ischemia [69], it should only be used as an adjunct imaging method to show nonperfusion since it does not show capillary leakage as a sign of ongoing inflammation. In a recent study using wide-field

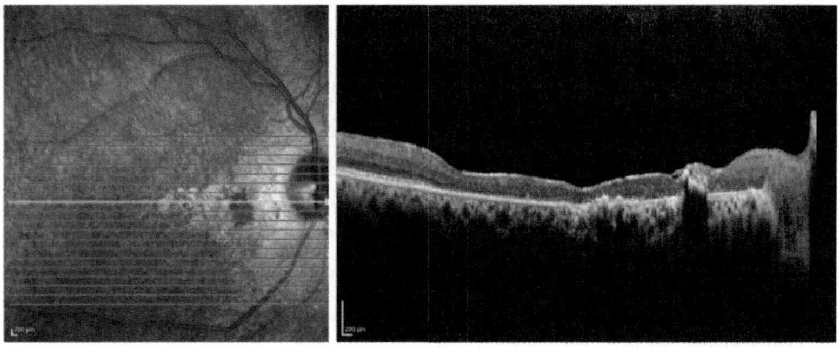

Fig. 13.9 OCT imaging shows diffuse macular thinning and disruption of both inner and outer retinal layers in the right eye of a patient with BD uveitis

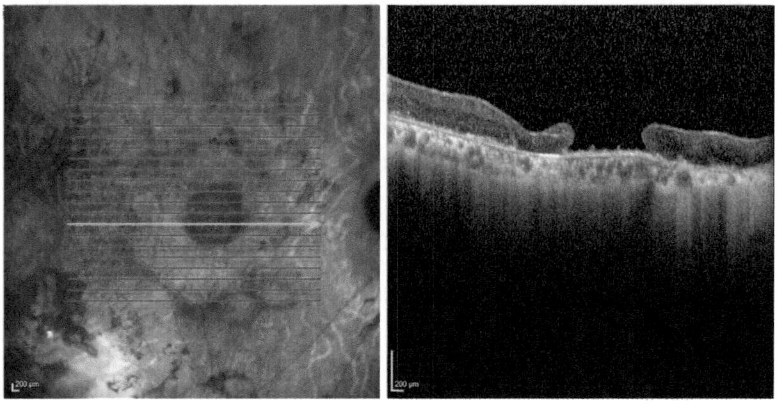

Fig. 13.10 OCT imaging shows a macular hole in the right eye of a patient with BD uveitis

OCT-A, retinal superficial and deep capillary vessel density was found to be reduced especially in the superior and temporal peripheral retina, but the vessel density of choriocapillaris was also found to be lower in all peripheral quadrants of the fundus in BD patients with inactive uveitis [69].

13.4 Treatment of Behçet's Disease Uveitis

BD uveitis is a potentially blinding disease due to cumulative damage caused by recurrent inflammatory attacks. Thus, an immediate and effective inflammation control is crucial to regain the potential visual acuity and prevent irreversible structural damage. However, the treatment should also aim to suppress the chronic subclinical inflammation leading to recurrent attacks, preserve the vision and control the systemic manifestations of the disease [70]. Treatment of BD patients with uveitis requires a multidisciplinary collaboration.

Corticosteroids (CS) are still the most widely used agents for the treatment of acute sight-threatening inflammatory attacks. High dose intravenous methylprednisolone followed by slowly tapered oral prednisolone is the most common way of treating severe posterior segment involvement and associated complications. However, due to its numerous systemic complications, long-term high dose CS therapy and CS monotherapy are no longer accepted in current treatment approaches. Systemic CS should be used concomitantly with immunosuppressives as bridging therapy [33, 71, 72]. Potent topical CS drops should only be used if anterior segment inflammation is present and tapered slowly [70]. Periocular or intravitreal CS injections may be used as an adjunct to systemic treatment in patients with unilateral panuveitis attack, refractory macular edema or in cases where systemic CS cannot be used [33, 71].

Any posterior segment inflammation is an absolute indication for immunosuppressive or biologic treatment [70–72]. European League Against Rheumatism (EULAR) evidence-based recommendations for the treatment of BD uveitis suggest the use of azathioprine (AZA), cyclosporin A (CsA), interferon-alpha (IFN-α), or anti-tumor necrosis factor-alpha (anti-TNF-α) agents in any patient with posterior segment involvement [72]. Conventional immunosuppressive agents combined with CS usually make the first step of treatment. However, in patients presenting with initial or recurrent sight-threatening acute inflammatory attack, biologic agents infliximab (IFX), or IFN-α have been recommended as first-line [72].

AZA and CsA are the only two conventional immunosuppressive agents that have been shown to be effective in randomized controlled trials [73–76]. Their efficacy has also been supported by many clinical studies [77–80]. Despite the availability of many new molecules, AZA and CsA remain to be the mostly used conventional agents, either alone or in combination [33]. Methotrexate, mycophenolate mofetil and tacrolimus however, are not commonly used in BD uveitis. Similarly, alkylating agents still used for some extraocular manifestations of BD, are not preferred for the treatment of ocular involvement due to serious adverse effects such as secondary malignancy and infertility, and the current availability of biologic agents [33, 71].

More potent agents acting rapidly are needed in patients not responding to conventional treatment, having frequent recurrences, and presenting with severe posterior segment involvement and vision loss. Today, the most suitable agents that meet this need are biologics. The introduction of biologic agents has been shown to improve both the visual prognosis and the quality of life of BD patients [81, 82]. Both IFN-α and anti-TNF-α monoclonal antibodies have been widely used for refractory and severe cases of BD uveitis within the last two decades [25].

The efficacy of IFN-α2a has been evaluated in many studies and a partial or complete response of around 90% has been reported in patients with refractory BD uveitis [83–88]. In a recent randomized controlled trial comparing IFN-α with CsA in a small sample size of BD uveitis, better and faster treatment response and complete remission rates, better visual outcome, and more stable remission of intraocular inflammation could be obtained in a 12-month period with IFN-α [89]. Previously published studies showed that the main advantage of IFN-α2a was its ability to induce long-term remission lasting even after drug discontinuation [87, 88]. Unfortunately, IFN-α2a was recently withdrawn from the market. Pegylated interferon IFN-α2a (PEG-IFN-α2a) having slower absorption and longer half-life permitting once-weekly dosing, is still available, at least in some countries. The remission obtained by IFN-α2a could be preserved with the use of PEG-IFN-α2a or PEG-IFN-α2b and the quality of life improved due to fewer injections [90, 91]. However, because the data regarding the use of PEG-IFN-α as induction therapy for BD uveitis are still lacking, the efficacy or the optimum dose for such use is still unknown, needing well designed studies testing its efficacy and tolerability [71].

Anti-TNF-α agents have been reported to be highly effective, associated with efficient inflammation control, reduction in the frequency of uveitis attacks, adequate visual improvement, significant central macular thickness reduction, and significant CS-sparing effect with acceptable safety profile in patients with BD uveitis [92–94]. An expert panel recommended these agents as first-line only for the treatment of BD uveitis [95]. A recent retrospective multicenter study showed that patients with BD uveitis treated with anti-TNF agents had a higher probability of complete response and lower relapse rates compared to those with idiopathic uveitis [96]. These agents are usually combined with a conventional immunosuppressive, mostly an antimetabolite, to prevent anti-chimeric, or anti-human antibody production, which decreases the drug's efficacy leading to secondary failure [95].

Among the anti-TNF-α agents, while there is more experience with IFX and adalimumab (ADA), the experience with golimumab and certolizumab pegol is limited, and etanercept is not a treatment of choice for noninfectious uveitis in general or BD uveitis in particular [71].

IFX has been proven to have a rapid and powerful effect, providing inflammation control within 24 h after a single infusion [97, 98]. It has been reported to be significantly faster in controlling ocular inflammation when compared with intravenous pulse methylprednisolone and intravitreal triamcinolone [97]. It is effective both in reducing the frequency and the severity of inflammatory attacks [48, 82, 99–103]. Most importantly, IFX was also found to be effective in reducing the background retinal vascular and disc leakage in refractory BD uveitis [55, 99–102]. Recently, Yamana et al. reported a continued decrease in ocular attacks and BOS24 even after >5 years of IFX therapy [99]. Previous studies have shown that an earlier initiation of IFX therapy leads to better outcomes [100, 104], and that the drug-free long-term remission can be obtained after a short- or long-term treatment period [105, 106]. Half of the patients who discontinued IFX in remission remained attack free for 12–90 months in Kose et al.'s study [107]. Therefore, an early switch to or an immediate initiation of anti-TNF treatment is crucial in patients presenting with severe posterior segment involvement.

In a meta-analysis comparing IFX and IFN-α2a, rates for sustained remission (71% vs. 44%) and CS cessation (66% vs. 33%) were higher with IFN-α2a, whereas IFX had a more rapid onset of action with higher rate for visual acuity improvement (76% vs. 46%) [108]. Both agents had similar rates for withdrawal due to side effects [108]. In a study comparing IFN-α and IFX therapy in BD uveitis patients resistant to conventional therapy, no difference was reported between the two agents in terms of anti-inflammatory activity or visual acuity improvement, while there were more adverse effects with IFN-α [109].

ADA is the only approved biologic agent for the treatment of noninfectious intermediate, posterior and panuveitis, including BD uveitis [110, 111]. ADA treatment has been reported to be effective and safe for the treatment of BD uveitis including cases with IFX failure [112, 113]. In a retrospective study evaluating treatment-naive BD uveitis patients who were treated with ADA + conventional therapy or conventional therapy alone as first line, significantly better results were reported with ADA regarding relapse rate, FFA scores and CS dependency [114]. In a recent study by Kim et al., ADA treatment led to progressive improvement in ultra-widefield FFA scores after achievement of clinical remission [115]. It has been shown that long-term control of noninfectious uveitis, including BD uveitis could be achieved with ADA even in the absence of concomitant conventional immunosuppressive treatment [116]. A multicenter observational study comparing BD uveitis patients who were treated with either ADA or IFX as first-line biologic agent, demonstrated an improvement in all ocular parameters with both agents after 1 year of therapy, with significantly better outcomes in improvement of visual acuity, anterior chamber inflammation, and vitritis in the ADA group. While inflammation control was more rapid in the IFX group, visual improvement was significantly greater and drug retention rate was higher in the ADA group, even though patients did not receive a loading ADA dose [117]. Thus, even though IFX provides a rapid inflammation control, ADA seems to be more effective in inducing sustained remission.

Intravitreal IFX has been investigated in order to avoid systemic adverse effects. Although it resulted in improvement in all parameters of intraocular inflammation, visual acuity and central macular thickness in the short term, its effect was not as fast as an intravenous infusion of IFX [118, 119]. Furthermore, in an open-label study of monthly intravitreal IFX injections, a high ocular complication rate and failure to control BD uveitis have been reported [120]. Intravitreal ADA administration has also been proposed as a potential adjunctive therapy for controlling breakthrough inflammation in BD patients already on systemic ADA treatment [121]. Off-label intravitreal administration of anti-TNF agents should be considered only as an adjunct to systemic treatment or when systemic treatment is contraindicated or not tolerated [71].

In cases where an adequate response is not achieved with an anti-TNF agent, the dosage and/or the frequency of current anti-TNF agent should first be increased rather than using high dose CS, or switching immediately to another biologic [33, 122]. Encouraging results of weekly administration of ADA have recently been reported in uveitis patients, but not particularly in BD uveitis [122]. If still refractory, a switch between anti-TNF agents should be considered as the second step. Previous studies suggested that when one anti-TNF agent has failed, the second one could be effective [72, 123, 124]. However, when treatment with both anti-TNF agents fails, then an alternative biologic agent should be considered.

Tocilizumab (TCZ) is the most commonly used agent in patients who fail anti-TNF therapy and provides favorable results in BD uveitis patients [125–127]. In five patients treated with monthly infusions of TCZ because of failure of IFN-α and anti-TNF therapy, significant improvements have been reported in visual acuity, LFP values, central macular thickness, and FFA scores [125]. However, the authors stated that a complete resolution of FA leakage could not be obtained in any patient during 5–19 months of treatment period [125]. In another series of 11 patients with refractory BD uveitis, TCZ treatment resulted in rapid and maintained improvement in all ocular parameters and complete remission of intraocular inflammation in eight of them [126]. On the other hand, extraocular manifestations could be controlled in only three patients [126]. TCZ has been reported as an effective therapeutic alternative for major organ involvement in BD, including ocular, neurologic, articular, and peripheral venous involvement, but not for mucocutaneous and intestinal manifestations [126, 127]. Unlike the abovementioned studies, in an observational study of three consecutive Chinese patients with BD uveitis resistant to other biologics and CS, TCZ showed unsatisfactory results [128].

Anakinra and canakinumab which are interleukin-1 antagonists were reported to be successful in treating uveitis in a small Italian cohort of BD patients [129, 130]. In a subsequent report, the authors emphasized that the presence of uveitis in BD patients was associated with a sustained response to IL-1 inhibitors [131]. On the other hand, efficacy of another anti-IL1 agent, gevokizumab, could not be proven in a randomized controlled trial [132].

Although there are reports of successful treatment of noninfectious refractory uveitis with Janus kinase inhibitors (JAKi) [133, 134], experience in BD uveitis is limited, meriting larger prospective controlled trials. Tofacitinib was suggested as an effective alternative treatment in refractory BD uveitis in a recent study by Zou et al. [135]. A favorable clinical response could be obtained in 10 of 13 patients. The drug was well tolerated except for one patient who developed herpes zoster infection [135]. Recently, another JAKi, upadacitinib, has been shown to be effective in two BD patients with chronic ocular inflammation and macular edema resistant to conventional immunosuppressives and ADA. The authors suggested upadacitinib as an important future option in managing recurrent and recalcitrant cases of BD uveitis [136].

“When and how to stop treatment?” is still a question without a definitive answer. Tapering or withdrawal of immunomodulatory treatment should be considered only after a 2-year period of remission. Clinical quiescence of uveitis does not indicate complete remission unless it is associated with no leakage on FFA. Once complete remission is obtained, treatment should be continued for another few years with gradual reduction of the dose of therapeutic agents and/or extending the infusion or injection intervals of biologics with periodic FFA examinations [33].

Currently available therapeutic options improved the management and the visual prognosis of BD uveitis. However, there are still challenges, including the lack of randomized controlled trials, and high cost and off-label use of more effective agents.

References

1. Gürbüz C, Yalçın Kehribar D, Özgen M. Clinical manifestations of Behçet’s syndrome: a single-center cohort of 777 patients. Eur J Rheumatol. 2021;8(4):211–6.
2. Torgutalp M, Eroğlu DŞ, Sezer S, Yayla ME, Karataş G, Özel EM, et al. Patient characteristics in Behçet’s syndrome and their associations with major organ involvement: a single-centre experience of 2118 cases. Scand J Rheumatol. 2022;51(1):50–8.

3. Alpsoy E, Donmez L, Onder M, Gunasti S, Usta A, Karincaoglu Y, et al. Clinical features and natural course of Behçet's disease in 661 cases: a multicentre study. Br J Dermatol. 2007;157(5):901–6.
4. Alharthy F, Almaqati AS, Alsulami S, Ahmad A. Behçet's disease in Saudi Arabia: clinical and demographic characteristics. Cureus. 2023;15(2):e34867.
5. Chang HK, Kim JW. The clinical features of Behcet's disease in Yongdong districts: analysis of a cohort followed from 1997 to 2001. J Korean Med Sci. 2002;17(6):784–9.
6. Oguz E, Bektaş M. Characteristics of patients with Behçet disease from the Van province, Eastern Turkey: definition of disease clusters in a tertiary referral center. J Clin Rheumatol. 2023;29(6):285–90.
7. Tursen U, Gurler A, Boyvat A. Evaluation of clinical findings according to sex in 2313 Turkish patients with Behçet's disease. Int J Dermatol. 2003;42(5):346–51.
8. Davatchi F, Chams-Davatchi C, Shams H, Nadji A, Faezi T, Akhlaghi M, et al. Adult Behcet's disease in Iran: analysis of 6075 patients. Int J Rheum Dis. 2016;19(1):95–103.
9. Kural-Seyahi E, Fresko I, Seyahi N, Ozyazgan Y, Mat C, Hamuryudan V, et al. The long-term mortality and morbidity of Behçet syndrome: a 2-decade outcome survey of 387 patients followed at a dedicated center. Medicine (Baltimore). 2003;82(1):60–76.
10. Soejima Y, Kirino Y, Takeno M, Kurosawa M, Takeuchi M, Yoshimi R, et al. Changes in the proportion of clinical clusters contribute to the phenotypic evolution of Behçet's disease in Japan. Arthritis Res Ther. 2021;23(1):49.
11. Tugal-Tutkun I, Onal S, Altan-Yaycioglu R, Huseyin Altunbas H, Urgancioglu M. Uveitis in Behçet disease: an analysis of 880 patients. Am J Ophthalmol. 2004;138(3):373–80.
12. Jari M, Nasiri S, Ghandehari M. Episcleritis; and posterior uveitis misdiagnosed as orbital cellulitis in a child patient with Behçet's disease. SAGE Open Med Case Rep. 2023;11:2050313X231182237.
13. Parentin F, Lepore L, Rabach I, Pensiero S. Paediatric Behçet's disease presenting with recurrent papillitis and episcleritis: a case report. J Med Case Rep. 2011;5:81.
14. Zamir E, Bodaghi B, Tugal-Tutkun I, See RF, Charlotte F, Wang RC, et al. Conjunctival ulcers in Behçet's disease. Ophthalmology. 2003;110(6):1137–41.
15. Ji YS, Yoon KC. A rare case of peripheral ulcerative keratitis associated with Behçet's disease. Int Ophthalmol. 2014;34(4):979–81.
16. Chang HK, Cho EH. A case of nodular scleritis in association with Behcet's disease. Korean J Intern Med. 2001;16(1):47–9.
17. Dursun D, Akova Y, Yücel E. Myositis and scleritis associated with Behcet's disease: an atypical presentation. Ocul Immunol Inflamm. 2004;12(4):329–32.
18. Kidd DP. Optic neuropathy in Behçet's syndrome. J Neurol. 2013;260:3065–70.
19. Jari M, Mohammadi T, Taheri E. Bilateral retrobulbar optic neuritis as the first manifestation of neuro-Behçet disease. Case Rep Rheumatol. 2020;2020:8834399.
20. Lee WS, Kang MH, Jung WS, Cheon YH, Yoo WH. Homonymous hemianopia in a patient with Behcet's disease. Korean J Intern Med. 2015;30(3):418–9.
21. Seyahi E. Phenotypes in Behçet's syndrome. Intern Emerg Med. 2019;14(5):677–89.
22. Khairallah M, Accorinti M, Muccioli C, Kahloun R, Kempen JH. Epidemiology of Behçet disease. Ocul Immunol Inflamm. 2012;20(5):324–35.
23. Tugal-Tutkun I, Urgancioglu M. Childhood-onset uveitis in Behçet disease:a descriptive study of 36 cases. Am J Ophthalmol. 2003;136(6):1114–9.
24. Koné-Paut I, Darce-Bello M, Shahram F, Gattorno M, Cimaz R, Ozen S, et al. Registries in rheumatological and musculoskeletal conditions. Paediatric Behçet's disease: an international cohort study of 110 patients. One-year follow-up data. Rheumatology (Oxford). 2011;50(1):184–8.
25. Tugal-Tutkun I. Uveitis in Behçet disease—an update. Curr Opin Rheumatol. 2023;35(1):17–24.
26. Ucar-Comlekoglu D, Fox A, Sen HN. Gender differences in Behçet's disease associated uveitis. J Ophthalmol. 2014;2014:820710.
27. Jabs DA, Nussenblatt RB, Rosenbaum JT, Standardization of Uveitis Nomenclature (SUN) Working Group. Standardization of uveitis nomenclature for reporting clinical data. Results of the first international workshop. Am J Ophthalmol. 2005;140(3):509–16.
28. Tugal-Tutkun I, Onal S, Stanford M, Akman M, Twisk JWR, Boers M, et al. An algorithm for the diagnosis of Behçet disease uveitis in adults. Ocul Immunol Inflamm. 2021;29(6):1154–63.
29. Tugal-Tutkun I, Gupta V, Cunningham ET. Differential diagnosis of Behçet uveitis. Ocul Immunol Inflamm. 2013;21(5):337–50.
30. Ozdal PC, Ortaç S, Taşkintuna I, Firat E. Posterior segment involvement in ocular Behçet's disease. Eur J Ophthalmol. 2002;12(5):424–31.
31. Tugal-Tutkun I, Ozdal PC, Oray M, Onal S. Review for diagnostics of the year: multimodal imaging in Behçet uveitis. Ocul Immunol Inflamm. 2017;25(1):7–19.
32. Oray M, Onal S, Bayraktar S, Izgi B, Tugal-Tutkun I. Nonglaucomatous localized retinal nerve fiber layer defects in Behçet uveitis. Am J Ophthalmol. 2015;159(3):475–81.e1.
33. Çakar Özdal P. Behçet's uveitis: current diagnostic and therapeutic approach. Turk J Ophthalmol. 2020;50(3):169–82.
34. Tugal-Tutkun I. Behçet's uveitis. Middle East Afr J Ophthalmol. 2009;16:219–24.
35. Ostrovsky M, Ramon D, Iriqat S, Shteiwi A, Sharon Y, Kramer M, et al. Retinal vascular occlusions in

ocular Behçet disease—a comparative analysis. Acta Ophthalmol. 2023;101:619.
36. Saleh OA, Birnbaum AD, Tessler HH, Goldstein DA. Behçet uveitis in the American midwest. Ocul Immunol Inflamm. 2012;20(1):12–7.
37. Khairallah M, Attia S, Yahia SB, Jenzeri S, Ghrissi R, Jelliti B, et al. Pattern of uveitis in Behçet's disease in a referral center in Tunisia, North Africa. Int Ophthalmol. 2009;29(3):135–41.
38. Yahia SB, Kahloun R, Jelliti B, Khairallah M. Branch retinal artery occlusion associated with Behçet disease. Ocul Immunol Inflamm. 2011;19(4):293–5.
39. Esen E, Sizmaz S, Sariyeva A, Demircan N. Bilateral central retinal artery occlusion in Behçet disease. Ocul Immunol Inflamm. 2015;23(5):416–9.
40. Ferreira BFA, Rodriguez EEC, Prado LLD, Gonçalves CR, Hirata CE, Yamamoto JH. Frosted branch angiitis and cerebral venous sinus thrombosis as an initial onset of neuro-Behçet's disease: a case report and review of the literature. J Med Case Rep. 2017;11(1):104.
41. Ucar D, Mergen B, Gonen B, Ozguler Y, Seyahi E, Hamuryudan V, et al. Investigation of clinical profile of Behçet's syndrome-related versus idiopathic branch retinal vein occlusion. Indian J Ophthalmol. 2020;68(9):1876–80.
42. Kahloun R, Ben Yahia S, Mbarek S, Attia S, Zaouali S, Khairallah M. Macular involvement in patients with Behçet's uveitis. J Ophthalmic Inflamm Infect. 2012;2(3):121–4.
43. Amer R, Alsughayyar W, Almeida D. Pattern and causes of visual loss in Behçet's uveitis: short-term and long-term outcomes. Graefes Arch Clin Exp Ophthalmol. 2017;255(7):1423–32.
44. Alsarhani WK, Saifaldein AA, Abu El-Asrar AM. A novel mechanism of macular holes in patients with Behçet's uveitis. Saudi J Ophthalmol. 2022;36(4):394–6.
45. Uçar D, Atalay E, Özyazgan Y, Özkök A, Yıldırım Y. An exceptional case of full-thickness macular hole closure in a patient with Behçet disease. Ocul Immunol Inflamm. 2014;22(1):79–81.
46. Tugal-Tutkun I, Onal S, Altan-Yaycioglu R, Kir N, Urgancioglu M. Neovascularization of the optic disc in Behçet's disease. Jpn J Ophthalmol. 2006;50(3):256–65.
47. Keino H. Evaluation of disease activity in uveoretinitis associated with Behçet's disease. Immunol Med. 2021;44(2):86–97.
48. Kaburaki T, Namba K, Sonoda KH, Kezuka T, Keino H, Fukuhara T, et al. Behçet's disease ocular attack score 24: evaluation of ocular disease activity before and after initiation of infliximab. Jpn J Ophthalmol. 2014;58(2):120–30.
49. Tanaka R, Murata H, Takamoto M, Ohtomo K, Okinaga K, Yoshida A, et al. Behçet's disease ocular attack score 24 and visual outcome in patients with Behçet's disease. Br J Ophthalmol. 2016;100(7):990–4.
50. Tugal-Tutkun I, Cingü K, Kir N, Yeniad B, Urgancioglu M, Gül A. Use of laser flare-cell photometry to quantify intraocular inflammation in patients with Behçet uveitis. Graefes Arch Clin Exp Ophthalmol. 2008;246(8):1169–77.
51. Yalcindag FN, Bingol Kiziltunc P, Savku E. Evaluation of intraocular inflammation with laser flare photometry in Behçet uveitis. Ocul Immunol Inflamm. 2017;25(1):41–5.
52. Yang P, Fang W, Huang X, Zhou H, Wang L, Jiang B. Alterations of aqueous flare and cells detected by laser flare-cell photometry in patients with Behcet's disease. Int Ophthalmol. 2010;30(5):485–9.
53. Kabaalioglu Guner M, Guner ME, Oray M, Tugal-Tutkun I. Correlation between widefield fundus fluorescein angiography leakage score and anterior chamber flare in Behçet uveitis. Ocul Immunol Inflamm. 2022;32(1):54–61. https://doi.org/10.1080/09273948.2022.2152700.
54. Kang HM, Lee SC. Long-term progression of retinal vasculitis in Behçet patients using a fluorescein angiography scoring system. Graefes Arch Clin Exp Ophthalmol. 2014;252(6):1001–8.
55. Shirahama S, Kaburaki T, Matsuda J, Tanaka R, Nakahara H, Komae K, et al. The relationship between fluorescein angiography leakage after ınfliximab therapy and relapse of ocular ınflammatory attacks in ocular Behçet's disease patients. Ocul Immunol Inflamm. 2020;28(8):1166–70.
56. Keorochana N, Homchampa N, Vongkulsiri S, Choontanom R. Fluorescein angiographic findings and Behcet's disease ocular attack score 24 (BOS24) as prognostic factors for visual outcome in patients with ocular Behcet's disease. Int J Retina Vitreous. 2021;7(1):48.
57. Onal S, Uludag G, Oray M, Mengi E, Herbort CP, Akman M, et al. Quantitative analysis of structural alterations in the choroid of patients with active Behçet uveitis. Retina. 2018;38(4):828–40.
58. Zarei M, Pesarakli H, Yaseri M, Etesali H, Ebrahimiadib N. Peripapillary optical coherence tomography as an alternative to fluorescein angiography for monitoring Behcet's retinal vasculitis. Sci Rep. 2021;11(1):20037.
59. Yalçındağ FN, Temel E, Şekkeli MZ, Kar İ. Macular structural changes and factors affecting final visual acuity in patients with Behçet uveitis. Graefes Arch Clin Exp Ophthalmol. 2021;259(3):715–21.
60. Cheng D, Wang Y, Huang S, Wu Q, Chen Q, Shen M, et al. Macular inner retinal layer thickening and outer retinal layer damage correlate with visual acuity during remission in Behcet's disease. Invest Ophthalmol Vis Sci. 2016;57(13):5470–8.
61. Kido A, Uji A, Morooka S, Kuroda Y, Arichika S, Akagi T, et al. Outer plexiform layer elevations as a marker for prior ocular attacks in patients with Behcet's disease. Invest Ophthalmol Vis Sci. 2018;59(7):2828–32.
62. Coskun E, Gurler B, Pehlivan Y, Kisacik B, Okumus S, Yayuspay R, et al. Enhanced depth imaging opti-

cal coherence tomography findings in Behçet disease. Ocul Immunol Inflamm. 2013;21(6):440–5.
63. Yesilirmak N, Lee W-H, Gur Gungor S, Yaman Pinarci E, Akkoyun I, Yilmaz G. Enhanced depth imaging optical coherence tomography in patients with different phases of Behcet's panuveitis. Can J Ophthalmol. 2017;52(1):48–53.
64. Işık MU, Yalcındag N. Comparison of spectral domain optical coherence tomography (SD OCT) findings with laser flare photometry (LFP) measurements in Behçet's uveitis. Ocul Immunol Inflamm. 2020;28(2):194–9.
65. Ishikawa S, Taguchi M, Muraoka T, Sakurai Y, Kanda T, Takeuchi M. Changes in subfoveal choroidal thickness associated with uveitis activity in patients with Behçet's disease. Br J Ophthalmol. 2014;98(11):1508–13.
66. Park UC, Cho IH, Moon SW, Yu HG. Long-term change of subfoveal choroidal thickness in Behçet's disease patients with posterior uveitis. Ocul Immunol Inflamm. 2018;26(3):397–405.
67. Fan S, Shi X, Chen Z, Li X, Yu S, Li J. Retinal and choroidal microvascular alterations in Behcet's disease without ocular manifestations: a systematic review and meta-analysis. Front Med (Lausanne). 2022;9:911990.
68. Ji KB, Hu Z, Zhang QL, Mei HF, Xing YQ. Retinal microvasculature features in patients with Behcet's disease: a systematic review and meta-analysis. Sci Rep. 2022;12(1):752.
69. Guo S, Liu H, Gao Y, Dai L, Xu J, Yang P. Analysis of vascular changes of fundus in Behcet uveitis by widefield swept source optical coherence tomography angiography and fundus fluorescein angiography. Retina. 2023;43(5):841–50.
70. Zierhut M, Abu El-Asrar AM, Bodaghi B, Tugal-Tutkun I. Therapy of ocular Behçet disease. Ocul Immunol Inflamm. 2014;22(1):64–76.
71. Tugal-Tutkun I, Çakar Özdal P. Behçet's disease uveitis: is there a need for new emerging drugs? Expert Opin Emerg Drugs. 2020;25(4):531–47.
72. Hatemi G, Christensen R, Bang D, Bodaghi B, Celik AF, Fortune F, et al. 2018 update of the EULAR recommendations for the management of Behçet's syndrome. Ann Rheum Dis. 2018;77:808–18.
73. Yazici H, Pazarli H, Barnes CG, Tüzün Y, Ozyazgan Y, Silman A, et al. A controlled trial of azathioprine in Behcet's syndrome. N Engl J Med. 1990;322:281–5.
74. Hamuryudan V, Ozyazgan Y, Hizli N, Mat C, Yurdakul S, Tüzün Y, et al. Azathioprine in Behçet's syndrome: effects on long-term prognosis. Arthritis Rheum. 1997;40:769–74.
75. Masuda K, Urayama A, Kogure M, Nakae K, Kogure M, Inaba G. Double masked trial of cyclosporin versus colchicine and long-term open study of cyclosporin in Behçet'sdisease. Lancet. 1989;1:1093–6.
76. Ozyazgan Y, Yurdakul S, Yazici H, Tüzün B, Işçimen A, Tüzün Y, et al. Low dose cyclosporin a versus pulsed cyclophosphamide in Behçet's syndrome: a single masked trial. Br J Ophthalmol. 1992;76:241–3.
77. Saadoun D, Wechsler B, Terrada C, Hajage D, Le Thi Huong D, Resche-Rigon M, et al. Azathioprine in severe uveitis of Behçet's disease. Arthritis Care Res (Hoboken). 2010;62:1733–8.
78. Díaz-Llopis M, Cervera M, Menezo JL. Cyclosporin a treatment of Behçet's disease: a long-term study. Curr Eye Res. 1990;9(Suppl):17–23.
79. Whitcup SM, Salvo EC Jr, Nussenblatt RB. Combined cyclosporine and corticosteroid therapy for sight-threatening uveitis in Behçet's disease. Am J Ophthalmol. 1994;118:39–45.
80. Özdal PÇ, Ortaç S, Taskıntuna I, Fırat E. Long-term therapy with low dose cyclosporin-A in ocular Behçet's disease. Doc Ophthalmol. 2002;105:301–12.
81. Onal S, Savar F, Akman M, Kazokoğlu H. Vision- and health-related quality of life in patients with Behçet uveitis. Arch Ophthalmol. 2010;128(10):1265–71.
82. Sakai T, Watanabe H, Kuroyanagi K, Akiyama G, Okano K, Kohno H, et al. Health- and vision-related quality of life in patients receiving infliximab therapy for Behcet uveitis. Br J Ophthalmol. 2013;97(3):338–42.
83. Kötter I, Zierhut M, Eckstein AK, Vonthein R, Ness T, Günaydin I, et al. Human recombinant interferon alfa-2a for the treatment of Behçet's disease with sight threatening posterior or panuveitis. Br J Ophthalmol. 2003;87:423–31.
84. Tugal-Tutkun I, Güney-Tefekli E, Urgancioglu M. Results of interferon-alfa therapy in patients with Behçet uveitis. Graefes Arch Clin Exp Ophthalmol. 2006;244:1692–5.
85. Onal S, Kazokoglu H, Koc A, Akman M, Bavbek T, Direskeneli H, et al. Long-term efficacy and safety of low-dose and dose-escalating interferon alfa-2a therapy in refractory Behçet uveitis. Arch Ophthalmol. 2011;129:288–94.
86. Yalçindağ FN, Uzun A. Results of interferon alpha-2a therapy in patients with Behcet's disease. J Ocul Pharmacol Ther. 2012;28:439–43.
87. Deuter CM, Zierhut M, Möhle A, Möhle A, Vonthein R, Stöbiger N, et al. Long-term remission after cessation of interferon-α treatment in patients with severe uveitis due to Behçet's disease. Arthritis Rheum. 2010;62:2796–805.
88. Diwo E, Gueudry J, Saadoun D, Weschler B, LeHoang P, Bodaghi B. Longterm efficacy of interferon in severe uveitis associated with Behçet disease. Ocul Immunol Inflamm. 2017;25:76–84.
89. Qian Y, Qu Y, Gao F, Pei M, Liang A, Xiao J, et al. Comparison of the safety and efficacy of interferon alpha-2a and cyclosporine-A when combined with glucocorticoid in the treatment of refractory Behcet's uveitis: a randomized controlled prospective study. Front Pharmacol. 2021;12:699903.
90. Celiker H, Kazokoglu H, Direskeneli H. Long-term efficacy of pegylated interferon alpha-2b in Behçet's

uveitis: a small case series. Ocul Immunol Inflamm. 2019;27:15–22.
91. Bielefeld P, Devilliers H, Deschasse C, Saadoun D, Sève P, Muselier A, et al. Potential of pegylatedinterferon alpha-2a in Behçet uveitis: a report of five cases. Ocul Immunol Inflamm. 2016;24(5):599–602.
92. Hu Y, Huang Z, Yang S, Chen X, Su W, Liang D. Effectiveness and safety of anti-tumor necrosis factor-alpha agents treatment in Behcets' disease associated uveitis: a systematic review and meta-analysis. Front Pharmacol. 2020;11:941.
93. Zhou X, Shi X, Ren Y, Yan T, Ye Q. Antitumour necrosis factor-alpha agent therapy, compared with conventional therapy, reduces the relapse of uveitis in patients with Behçet's disease: a systematic review of controlled trials. Front Pharmacol. 2022;13:912906.
94. Abolhasani S, Khabbazi A, Hosseini F, Gholizadeh-Ghaleh Aziz S, Alipour S. Effects of anti-TNF biologic drugs on uveitis severity in Behcet patients: systematic review and meta-analysis. Int J Ophthalmol. 2022;15:813–9.
95. Levy-Clarke G, Jabs DA, Read RW, Rosenbaum JT, Vitale A, Van Gelder RN. Expert panel recommendations for the use of anti-tumor necrosis factor biologic agents in patients with ocular inflammatory disorders. Ophthalmology. 2014;12:785–796.e3.
96. Maalouf G, Andrillon A, Leclercq M, Sève P, Bielefeld P, Gueudry J, et al. Lower relapses rate with infliximab versus adalimumab in sight-threatening uveitis: a multicenter study of 330 patients. Am J Ophthalmol. 2022;238:173–80.
97. Markomichelakis N, Delicha E, Masselos S, Fragiadaki K, Kaklamanis P, Sfikakis PP. A single infliximab infusion vs corticosteroids for acute panuveitis attacks in Behcet's disease: a comparative 4-week study. Rheumatology. 2011;50:593–7.
98. Sfikakis PP, Theodossiadis PG, Katsiari CG, Kaklamanis P, Markomichelakis NN. Effect of infliximab on sight-threatening panuveitis in Behçet's disease. Lancet. 2001;358(9278):295–6.
99. Yamana S, Hasegawa E, Takeda A, Yawata N, Sonoda K. Long-term outcomes of infliximab in patients with Behçet's disease-associated uveitis. Int Ophthalmol. 2023;43(3):937–44.
100. Keino H, Watanabe T, Nakayama M, Komagata Y, Fukuoka K, Okada AA. Long-term efficacy of early infliximab-induced remission for refractory uveoretinitis associated with Behçet's disease. Br J Ophthalmol. 2021;105:1525–33.
101. Keino H, Okada AA, Watanabe T, Taki W. Decreased ocular inflammatory attacks and background retinal and disc vascular leakage in patients with Behcet's disease on infliximab therapy. Br J Ophthalmol. 2011;95:1245–50.
102. Keino H, Okada AA, Watanabe T, Taki W. Long-term efficacy of infliximab on background vascular leakage in patients with Behçet's disease. Eye (Lond). 2014;28:1100–6.
103. Takeuchi M, Kezuka T, Sugita S, Keino H, Namba K, Kaburaki T, et al. Evaluation of the long-term efficacy and safety of infliximab treatment for uveitis in Behçet's disease: a multicenter study. Ophthalmology. 2014;121:1877–84.
104. Guzelant G, Ucar D, Esatoglu SN, Hatemi G, Ozyazgan Y, Yurdakul S, et al. Infliximab for uveitis of Behçet's syndrome: a trend for earlier initiation. Clin Exp Rheumatol. 2017;35(Suppl 108):86–9.
105. Sfikakis PP, Arida A, Ladas DS, Markomichelakis N. Induction of ocular Behçet's disease remission after short-term treatment with infliximab: a case series of 11 patients with a follow-up from 4 to 16 years. Clin Exp Rheumatol. 2019;37(Suppl 121):137–41.
106. Sfikakis PP, Arida A, Panopoulos S, Fragiadaki K, Pentazos G, Laskari K, et al. Brief report: drug-free long-term remission in severe Behçet's disease following withdrawal of successful anti-tumor necrosis factor treatment. Arthritis Rheumatol. 2017;69:2380–5.
107. Kose H, Yalcindag N. Clinical follow-up of patients with Behcet uveitis after discontinuation of infliximab therapy. Ocul Immunol Inflamm. 2022;30(1):203–7.
108. Ozguler Y, Leccese P, Christensen R, Esatoglu SN, Bang D, Bodaghi B, et al. Management of major organ involvement of Behçet's syndrome: a systematic review for update of the EULAR recommendations. Rheumatology (Oxford). 2018;57:2200–12.
109. Yalçindag N, Köse HC. Comparison of the treatment results for Behçet uveitis in patients treated with infliximab and interferon. Ocul Immunol Inflamm. 2020;28(2):305–14.
110. Jaffe GJ, Dick AD, Brézin AP, Nguyen QD, Thorne JE, Kestelyn P, et al. Adalimumab in patients with active non-infectious uveitis. N Engl J Med. 2016;375:932–43.
111. Nguyen QD, Merrill PT, Jaffe GJ, Dick AD, Kurup SK, Sheppard J, et al. Adalimumab for prevention of uveitis flare in patients with inactive non-infectious uveitis controlled by corticosteroids (VISUAL II): a multicentre, double-masked, randomised, placebo controlled phase 3 trial. Lancet. 2016;388:1183–92.
112. Interlandi E, Leccese P, Olivieri I, Latanza L. Adalimumab for treatment of severe Behcet's uveitis: a retrospective long-term follow-up study. Clin Exp Rheumatol. 2014;32:S58–62.
113. Fabiani C, Vitale A, Emmi G, Vannozzi L, Lopalco G, Guerriero S, et al. Efficacy and safety of adalimumab in Behçet's disease-related uveitis: a multicenter retrospective observational study. Clin Rheumatol. 2017;36:183–9.
114. Yang S, Huang Z, Hu Y, Zhang J, Liu X, Li H, et al. The efficacy of adalimumab as an initial treatment in patients with Behcet's retinal vasculitis. Front Pharmacol. 2021;12:609148.
115. Kim BH, Park UC, Park SW, Yu HG. Ultra-widefield fluorescein angiography to monitor therapeutic

response to adalimumab in Behcet's uveitis. Ocul Immunol Inflamm. 2022;30(6):1347–53.
116. Bitossi A, Bettiol A, Silvestri E, Di Scala G, Bacherini D, Lopalco G, et al. Adalimumab accounts for long-term control of noninfectious uveitis also in the absence of concomitant DMARD treatment: a multicenter retrospective study. Mediat Inflamm. 2019;2019:1623847.
117. Atienza-Mateo B, Martín-Varillas JL, Calvo-Río V, Demetrio-Pablo R, Beltrán E, Sánchez-Bursón J, et al. Comparative study of infliximab versus adalimumab in refractory uveitis due to Behçet's disease, national multicenter study of 177 cases. Arthritis Rheumatol. 2019;71:2081–9.
118. Markomichelakis N, Delicha E, Masselos S, Sfikakis PP. Intravitreal infliximab for sight-threatening relapsing uveitis in Behcet disease: a pilot study in 15 patients. Am J Ophthalmol. 2012;154(3):534–41.
119. Hamza MME, Macky TA, Sidky MK, Ragab G, Soliman MM. Intravitreal infliximab in refractory uveitis in Behcet's disease: a safety and efficacy clinical study. Retina. 2016;36(12):2399–408.
120. Refaat M, Abdullatif AM, Hamza MM, Macky TA, El-Agha MH, Ragab G, et al. Monthly intravitreal infliximab in Behcet's disease active posterior uveitis: a long-term safety study. Retina. 2021;41:1739–47.
121. Kheir WJ, Mehanna C-J, Abdul Fattah M, Al Ghadban S, El Sabban M, Mansour AM, et al. Intravitreal adalimumab for the control of breakthrough intraocular inflammation. Ocul Immunol Inflamm. 2018;26(8):1206–11.
122. Liberman P, Berkenstock MK, Burkholder BM, Chaon BC, Thorne JE. Escalation to weekly adalimumab for the treatment of ocular inflammation. Ocul Immunol Inflamm. 2021;29:1564–8.
123. Calvo-Río V, Blanco R, Beltrán E, Sánchez-Bursón J, Mesquida M, Adán A, Hernandez MV, et al. Anti-TNF-α therapy in patients with refractory uveitis due to Behçet's disease: a 1-year follow-up study of 124 patients. Rheumatology (Oxford). 2014;53:2223–31.
124. Vallet H, Seve P, Biard L, Baptiste Fraison J, Bielefeld P, Perard L, et al. Infliximab versus adalimumab in the treatment of refractory inflammatory uveitis: a multicenter study from the French Uveitis Network. Arthritis Rheumatol. 2016;68:1522–30.
125. Eser Ozturk H, Oray M, Tugal-Tutkun I. Tocilizumab for the treatment of Behçet uveitis that failed interferon alpha and anti-tumor necrosis factor-alpha therapy. Ocul Immunol Inflamm. 2018;26:1005–14.
126. Atienza-Mateo B, Calvo-Río V, Beltrán E, Martínez-Costa L, Valls-Pascual E, Hernández-Garfella M, et al. Anti-interleukin 6 receptor tocilizumab in refractory uveitis associated with Behçet's disease: multicentre retrospective study. Rheumatology (Oxford). 2018;57(5):856–64.
127. Atienza-Mateo B, Beltrán E, Hernández-Garfella M, Valls Pascual E, Martínez-Costa L, Atanes A, et al. Tocilizumab in Behcet's disease with refractory ocular and/or neurological involvement: response according to different clinical phenotypes. Clin Exp Rheumatol. 2021;39(Suppl 132):37–42.
128. Zhao C, Liu J, Song H, Shi J, Zhang M, Zheng W. Anti-interleukin 6 receptor antibody tocilizumab was not satisfactory for acute attack of Behcet's uveitis in three consecutive patients. Clin Exp Rheumatol. 2022;40(8):1600.
129. Fabiani C, Sota J, Tosi GM, Franceschini R, Frediani B, Galeazzi M, et al. The emerging role of interleukin (IL)-1 in the pathogenesis and treatment of inflammatory and degenerative eye diseases. Clin Rheumatol. 2017;36:2307–18.
130. Fabiani C, Vitale A, Emmi G, Lopalco G, Vannozzi L, Guerriero S, et al. Interleukin (IL)-1 inhibition with anakinra and canakinumab in Behçet's disease related uveitis: a multicenter retrospective observational study. Clin Rheumatol. 2017;36:191–7.
131. Fabiani C, Vitale A, Rigante D, Emmi G, Lopalco G, Di Scala G, et al. The presence of uveitis is associated with a sustained response to the interleukin (IL)-1 inhibitors anakinra and canakinumab in Behçet's disease. Ocul Immunol Inflamm. 2020;28:298–304.
132. Tugal-Tutkun I, Pavesio C, De Cordoue A, Bernard-Poenaru O, Gül A. Use of gevokizumab in patients with Behçet's disease uveitis: an international, randomized, double-masked, placebo-controlled study and open-label extension study. Ocul Immunol Inflamm. 2018;26(7):1023–33.
133. Wen J, Hu H, Chen M, Yang H, Zhao Y, Liu Y. Role of Janus kinase (JAK) inhibitor in autoimmune ocular inflammation: a systematic review. J Immunol Res. 2021;2021:2324400.
134. El-Shabrawi Y, Rath T, Heiligenhaus A. Janus kinase inhibitors: next generation treatment for uveitis. Klin Monatsbl Augenheilkd. 2022;239:695–701.
135. Zou J, Lin CH, Wang Y, Shen Y, Guan JL. Correspondence on 'A pilot study of tofacitinib for refractory Behcet's syndrome'. Ann Rheum Dis. 2023;82(4):e100. https://doi.org/10.1136/annrheumdis-2020-219810.
136. Tao T, He D, Peng X, Huang Z, Su W. Successful remission with upadacitinib in two patients with anti-TNF-refractory macular edema associated with Behçet's uveitis. Ocul Immunol Inflamm. 2023;32(8):1897–900. https://doi.org/10.1080/09273948.2023.2263557.

14 Musculoskeletal Manifestations in Behçet's Syndrome

Mert Öztaş and Gülen Hatemi

Contents

14.1 Introduction

Behçet's syndrome (BS) is a multisystemic, relapsing, variable vessel vasculitis that mainly involves the mucosa, skin, eyes, musculoskeletal, gastrointestinal, and nervous systems. Musculoskeletal involvement is not a sine qua non for BS; nearly one-half of the patients have arthritis and/or arthralgia during their disease course [1]. Arthritis is generally episodic, self-limiting, and nondeforming. Musculoskeletal involvement in BS does not cause life or

M. Öztaş
Division of Rheumatology, Department of Internal Medicine, Istanbul Research and Training Hospital, Istanbul, Türkiye

G. Hatemi (✉)
Division of Rheumatology, Department of Internal Medicine, Istanbul University – Cerrahpaşa, Istanbul, Türkiye

Behçet's Disease Research Center, Istanbul University – Cerrahpaşa, Istanbul, Türkiye

E. Alpsoy et al. (eds.), *Behçet's Disease: An Integrated Approach*,
https://doi.org/10.1007/978-3-031-77251-1_14

organ-threatening complications, but it negatively impacts patients' well-being. Work productivity and daily living activities may be impaired in patients with BS [2]. The treatment of BS-related musculoskeletal involvement is planned according to the severity of the symptoms [3]. This chapter aims to review the epidemiology of the musculoskeletal involvement of BS, immunopathogenesis of BS synovitis, clinical and laboratory findings, synovial morphology and histology, differential diagnosis, and treatment of arthritis in BS patients.

14.2 Epidemiology

The frequency of musculoskeletal manifestations among patients with BS show differences across countries (Fig. 14.1 and Table 14.1, [4–33]. These differences may result from the study setting and definition of musculoskeletal involvement, in addition to real geographic differences. Studies from rheumatology departments may report a higher frequency of musculoskeletal involvement compared with studies from dermatology or ophthalmology departments. Moreover, some studies have included patients with any type of musculoskeletal manifestation or symptom, whereas others included only patients with arthritis episodes confirmed by a physician.

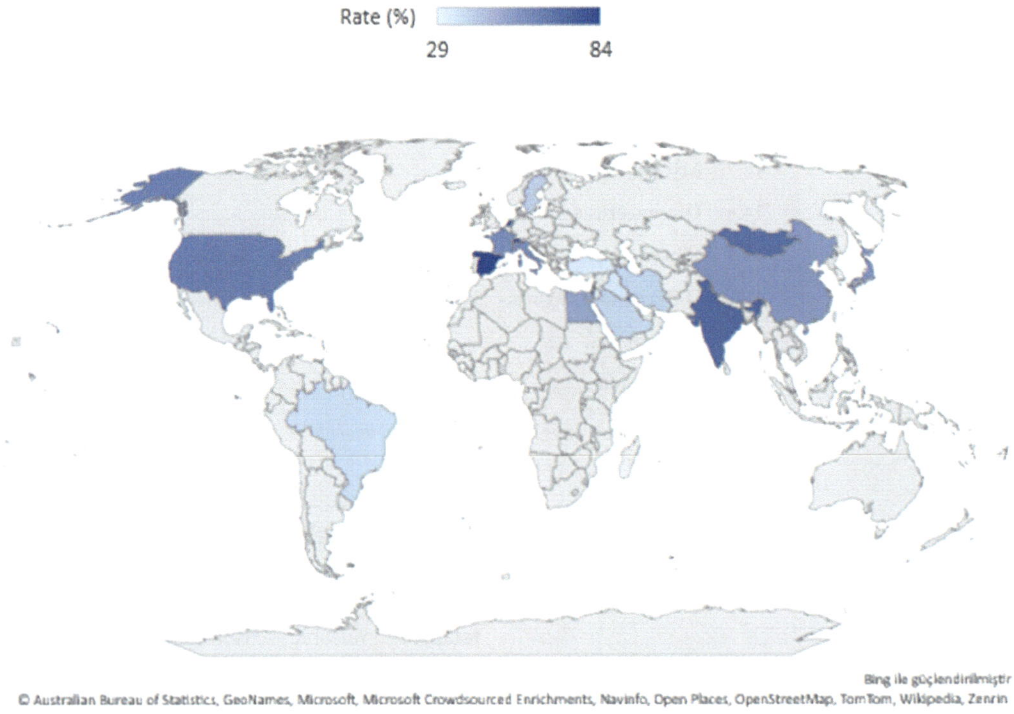

Fig. 14.1 Frequency of musculoskeletal involvement among patients with BS reported from different countries. (Figure created based on the data published by Commonwealth of Australia, licensed under CC-BY 4.0)

Table 14.1 Estimated prevalence of Behçet's syndrome per 100,000 population in each country and frequency of musculoskeletal involvement in each (when more than one study was available for a country, the lowest and highest prevalences were provided in the table)

Country	Author, year	Estimated prevalence per 100,000 population	Frequency of joint involvement	Definition of joint involvement
Brazil	Neves, 2009	–	36	Musculoskeletal complaints
China	Mok, 2002	2,6	54	Arthralgia/arthritis
Egypt	Assaad-Khalil, 1997	7,6	50	Joint involvement
Egypt	Gheita, 2019	3,6	48	Joint involvement
France	Mahr, 2008	7,1	51	Arthropathy
Greece	Vaiopoulos, 2019	–	58	Arthritis
India	Pande, 1995	–	71	Arthritis
Iran	Davatchi, 2010	–	17[a]/24[b]	Arthralgia/arthritis
Iraq	Al-Rawi, 2003	17	33	Arthritis
Ireland	Adeeb, 2018	6,5	40	Arthralgia/arthritis
Israel	Jaber, 2002	120	100	Joint involvement
Israel	Krause, 2007	15,2	70	Joint involvement
Italy	Salvarani, 2007	3,8	50	Arthritis
Italy	Olivieri, 2013	15,9	18	Arthritis
Japan	Nakea, 1993	13,5	57	Joint involvement
Jordan	Madanat, 2017	660	29	Arthritis
Kuwait	Mousa, 1996	2,1	69	Arthritis
Mongolia	Balt, 2020	2,4	68[a]/20[b]	Arthralgia/arthritis
Netherlands	Kappen, 2015	7,6	74[a]/34[b]	Arthralgia/arthritis
Saudi Arabia	Al-Dalaan, 1997	20	37	Arthritis
Scotland	Jankowski, 1992	0,3	93	Arthralgia
Spain	Sanchez Burson, 1998	7,5	30	Joint involvement
Spain	Graña, 2001	5,6	84	Arthritis
Sweden	Ek, 1993	3,5	58	Arthritis
Sweden	Mohammad, 2013	4,9	40	Arthralgia/arthritis
Switzerland	Villiger, 2019	4	77	Arthralgia/arthritis
Türkiye	Azizlerli, 2003	421	32	Arthritis
United Kingdom	Chamberlain, 1977	0,64	63	Arthritis
United States	Calamia, 2009	–	46	Arthritis
United States	Muruganandam, 2019	10,9	71[a]/41[b]	Arthralgia/arthritis

[a] Arthralgia
[b] Arthritis

14.3 Immunopathogenesis

BS is a multifactorial vasculitis where a complex genetic background and environmental factors, especially infections are thought to play a role. Self-limiting, recurrent, and nondeforming arthritis episodes suggest overactivation of the innate immune system. Due to the pathergy phenomenon, arthroscopic investigations are considered risky and there are scarce data on synovial histopathology in the literature. A significant neutrophilic involvement and a striking paucity of plasma cells was disclosed in arthroscopic biopsy samples of BS patients with knee synovitis [1, 34]. Cañete et al. showed a striking difference (13% vs. 4%) between CD15+ neutrophil levels between BS and psoriatic arthritis (PsA) patients in immunochemical analysis [34]. However, no evidence of neutrophilic vasculitis was observed in the same study [34]. Additionally, BS patients had a threefold increased CD3+ T lymphocytes compared to PsA, while no difference in CD4+ and CD8+ T-lymphocyte subsets was observed between the two groups [34]. Further functional studies are needed to clarify the underlying pathogenesis of BS-related arthritis.

14.4 Clinical, Laboratory, and Imaging Findings

Arthritis, arthralgia, and enthesitis, are the typical musculoskeletal manifestations of BS. Recurrent, nonerosive monoarthritis is the most common form of arthritis [1, 35]. On the other hand, oligo- or poly-arthritis were reported as the most common form of arthritis in some cohorts [36, 37]. The knees and ankles are the most frequently involved joints, followed by wrists, elbows, and hands [1, 35] (Fig. 14.2).

The onset of arthritis is generally observed between the third and fourth decades of life in most patients [1, 35, 36]. Elevated acute-phase reactants including an elevated serum C-reactive protein level and erythrocyte sedimentation rate may be observed during arthritis episodes [1, 36]. Arthrocentesis of the affected joints reveals an inflammatory synovial fluid [1, 37]. Anti-nuclear antibody (ANA), anti-cyclic citrullinated peptide (anti-CCP), and rheumatoid factor are almost always negative in BS patients [1, 38]. Arthritis episodes last a few days to a few weeks and resolve in less than 6–8 weeks in the majority of the patients [1, 35]. Although symmetrical polyarthritis is an uncommon type of articular involvement in BS, a small group of BS patients may initially present with symmetric polyarthritis without any additional systemic involvement. This group of patients may be labeled as seronegative rheumatoid arthritis before other BS-related systemic symptoms occur.

In BS-related arthritis, the majority of radiography studies did not disclose erosions or radiographic damage, while few reports described joint destruction [39]. Macroscopic arthroscopic evaluation of morphology (villi or granulous), distribution, vascular changes, and fibrinoid membranes show differences between BS and other rheumatic diseases. A controlled study that compared knee synovitis in BS and PsA patients showed irregular patchy distribution in suprapatellar and intercondylar areas in BS patients while a diffuse involvement in knee synovitis in PsA patients [40]. In the same study, morphologic patterns were quite different. BS patients had a granulous pattern, while PsA patients had villi patterns. In terms of vascular changes, hyperemic synovitis without any other distinctive vascular formation can be observed in BS patients with synovitis. Larger and more prominent fibrinoid membranes were observed in BS synovitis in comparison to PsA patients.

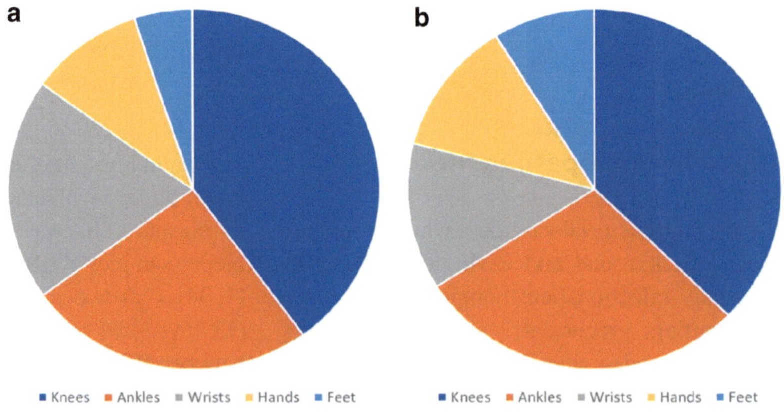

Fig. 14.2 Distribution of the affected joints in two different prospective cohort studies. (**a**) [1], (**b**) [35]

14.5 The Association of Acne, Arthritis, and Enthesitis

The association of acne and arthritis in BS was initially demonstrated in a study that surveyed the frequency of papulopustular lesions among BS patients with arthritis in comparison with BS patients who did not have arthritis, rheumatoid arthritis patients and healthy controls [41]. Both papules and pustules were significantly more common among BS patients with arthritis compared with the control groups. This study suggested that the arthritis in BS may be related to acne-associated arthritis, which is considered to be a form of reactive arthritis, developing through molecular mimicry caused by microorganisms present in acne lesions. This contention was later supported by a study showing that the papulopustular lesions of BS patients were not sterile as previously thought [42]. These lesions were infected with *Staphylococcus aureus* and *Prevotella* spp. bacteria, more commonly than ordinary acne vulgaris lesions. Another study that demonstrated this association was a factor analysis of clinical manifestations among patients with BS. This study identified four distinct clusters and the papulopustular lesion-arthritis cluster was one of the clusters [43]. Years later, another factor analysis study from the same center, this time examining familial patients with BS showed that the same clusters hold true for BS patients who have a first-degree relative with BS [44]. Moreover, the papulopustular lesion-arthritis cluster was observed more frequently among familial BS patients and were shared more commonly by both family members compared to the other three clusters. Enthesopathy was previously reported in few case reports and case series in BS [45, 46]. When enthesopathy was formally studied using musculoskeletal ultrasonography, it was shown that enthesopathy scores were significantly higher among BS patients with acne and arthritis, compared with BS patients without arthritis, rheumatoid arthritis patients, and healthy controls [47]. In order to understand whether the acne-arthritis-enthesopathy in BS patients is associated with sacroiliitis and HLA B27 positivity, the patients included in this study were later studied with sacroiliac X-rays and HLA B27 was tested. No association was observed between this cluster and sacroiliitis or HLA B27 [48].

14.6 Paucity of Sacroiliitis

Some researchers had proposed to classify BS among seronegative spondyloarthropathies (SpA) in the past [49]. This assumption adhered to an increased prevalence of sacroiliitis in BS in previous reports [49, 50]. However, this assumption was falsified for several reasons. When controlled studies that explored the frequency of sacroiliitis in BS were conducted, it was observed that the prevalence of sacroiliitis was not increased in BS compared to controls [51, 52]. Moreover, when HLA B27 was studied among patients with BS, the majority of the studies did not show an association between HLA-B27 and BS, in contrast to what is known for SpA. Finally, venous and arterial involvement, and a variable vessel vasculitis that is thought to underlie different organ manifestations such as retinal vasculitis in eye involvement and venulitis in nervous system involvement are important components of BS that are not present in SpA.

It was suggested that the seemingly increased frequency of sacroiliitis in some studies may be caused by methodological problems [53]. The high inter- and intra-observer variation in the assessment of sacroiliac X-rays, as well as lack of appropriate control groups and blinded reading of X-rays were proposed as possible reasons. Moreover, in a study where sacroiliitis was examined with CT scans in BS patients who seemed to have sacroiliitis on X-rays, it was observed that sacroiliitis was actually not present in 77.5% of those patients [54].

14.7 Myositis

Several case reports and a number of case series have reported the presence of focal myositis in patients with BS [55–59]. The myositis seems to be recurrent, similar to all other manifestations of

BS [60, 61]. The lower extremities were affected in majority of the cases. Creatinine kinase levels were not always elevated. MRI findings included hyperintense signals in the involved muscles and intermuscular fascia on fat-suppressed images, as well as subcutaneous edema [59]. Histopathologic examination suggested vasculitic myositis in the majority of the cases [56–59].

14.8 Osteonecrosis

The frequency of osteonecrosis was reported as 0.22% among patients with BS [62]. Vascular, eye, and nervous system involvement were more common among BS patients with osteonecrosis, suggesting that the underlying cause may be corticosteroid use, similar to the osteonecrosis observed in other diseases. The multifocal nature of osteonecrosis in BS warrants increased awareness for development of the lesion in other sites [63]. The increased association with vascular involvement raises the question whether microangiopathy may also play a role in the pathogenesis of osteonecrosis in BS.

14.9 Fibromyalgia

The prevalence of fibromyalgia was reported to be between 5% and 37% in different cohorts [64–66]. The frequency was generally higher among female patients with BS [64]. No association was found between BS activity and fibromyalgia, while the presence of depression or anxiety was associated with fibromyalgia in BS patients [65]. Moreover, fatigue severity and fatigue impact scores were correlated with fibromyalgia in BS [67].

14.10 Differential Diagnosis

MAGIC (mouth and genital ulcers with inflamed cartilage) syndrome may mimic BS, while chondritis is an unexpected finding in BS [68]. SAPHO syndrome (synovitis, acne, pustulosis, hyperostosis, osteitis) should be considered in patients presenting with acne and arthritis. Hyperostosis and osteitis should be investigated before diagnosing BS. SpA should be considered in the differential diagnosis when the dominant manifestations are arthritis and anterior uveitis. Inflammatory bowel diseases, especially Crohn's disease may be difficult to differentiate from BS, since both conditions can cause arthritis, oral ulcers, nodular lesions, and anterior uveitis in addition to intestinal ulcers [69]. The morphology and distribution of oral manifestations may help the differential diagnosis.

14.11 Treatment

The choice of treatment modalities for BS-related musculoskeletal involvement varies according to the severity and duration of arthritis episodes. Nonsteroidal anti-inflammatory drugs and short-term low-dose glucocorticoids may be used during acute episodes of arthritis with the aim of relieving the pain and shortening the duration of episodes. Immunomodulatory, immunosuppressive, or biologic agents may be required for the prevention of recurrent episodes [3]. Colchicine is usually the first-line treatment modality for preventing arthritis [70]. A moderate dose of prednisolone (up to 15 mg/daily) may be considered for a short duration in patients with recurrent arthritis episodes, whereas in patients with large joint mono-arthritis, intra-articular steroids can be applied [3]. In a randomized controlled trial, benzatin penicillin effectively reduced further arthritis episodes in patients with joint involvement [71]. On the other hand, a randomized controlled study showed that azapropazone was ineffective in controlling arthritis in BS [72]. In patients who continue to have arthritis episodes, azathioprine (2.5 mg/kg/day) may be an alternative or addition to colchicine, confirmed by a randomized controlled study [73]. This may be a reasonable approach before initiating biologic agents. Despite the lack of controlled studies, sulfasalazine and methotrexate may also be tried in such patients. Interferon alpha may be an effective option, if available. Several observational studies revealed that interferon alpha was an effective treatment modality for BS-related arthritides [74, 75]. Among TNF inhibitors (TNFi), only etanercept was studied for BS in a randomized controlled trial [76]. Etanercept showed no superiority to placebo in terms of the mean number of swollen joints and complete response of arthritis at week 4. The possible explanations were the short length of the study and spontaneous remission of the BS arthritides. Several observational studies reported on the successful use of infliximab in different BS manifestations [77, 78]. Adalimumab is another therapeutic option [77]. Ustekinumab showed promising results regarding both mucocutaneous and musculoskeletal involvement of BS in a recent phase 2 trial [79]. An open-label prospective study confirmed positive results with ustekinumab in 16 BS patients with joint involvement [80]. Apremilast is an orally available small-molecule phosphodiesterase four inhibitor. A phase 3 trial had demonstrated the effectiveness of apremilast in BS-related oral ulcers [81]. Although the number of patients with arthritis was small in this study, the proportion of patients with arthritis at week 12 was lower in the apremilast group compared to placebo [82]. An observational study showed favorable results with apremilast for arthralgia and arthritis [83]. No articular involvement was observed in 12 of the 23 BS patients with colchicine and/or DMARDs resistant articular involvement. However, another observational study did not align with the above mentioned study [84]. Only four (25%) of the 16 patients with refractory musculoskeletal involvement had a response to apremilast. A case series showed promising results with secukinumab in BS-related articular manifestations, and long-term efficacy was confirmed by the same group in another study [85, 86]. There are scarce data on tofacitinib in BS-related arthritis. In a small case series, two of the seven BS patients with refractory arthritis improved with tofacitinib [87]. IL-1 may also be tried in treatment-resistant cases. A pilot open-label study showed that four of the six patients had remission with IL-1 receptor antagonist anakinra [88], although the dose had to be increased in the majority of the cases. A number of case reports suggested that anakinra and the anti-IL-1β monoclonal antibody canakinumab, may be effective in refractory patients with joint disease [89, 90].

14.12 Conclusion

Musculoskeletal manifestations may be observed in around one half of patients with BS. Arthritis, arthralgia, and enthesitis are relatively more common forms of musculoskeletal involvement. Myositis and osteonecrosis are rarely seen. Arthritis is usually in the form of a recurrent, mono- or oligo-arthritis that affects the knees, ankles, wrists, or elbows. Although arthritis is usually nondeforming and nonerosive in patients with BS, frequent recurrences may cause difficulty in daily living activities and impair quality of life. Colchicine is usually effective for preventing recurrences and low-dose systemic glucocorticoids or intra-articular injections may be used during acute episodes. Azathioprine, sulfasalazine, and methotrexate may be used in patients who continue to have arthritis episodes despite treatment with colchicine. Biologic agents including interferon alpha and TNFi may be used in refractory cases. Apremilast, ustekinumab, secukinumab, tofacitinib, and IL-1 inhibitors are other promising agents.

Case 1

A 28-year-old woman with a history of mucocutaneous BS presented with a swollen right ankle that had been ongoing for a month. Her chief medical complaint was pain and stiffness in her ankle, which affected her daily living activities. She was diagnosed with BS several years ago with recurrent oral aphthous ulcers, acneiform papulopustular lesions, and a single episode of painful genital ulcer. She had been under colchicine treatment due to recurrent oral aphthous and papulopustular lesions. These complaints had abated after the initiation of colchicine.

On physical examination, she had left ankle arthritis. There were no other tender or swollen joints, and her physical examination was unremarkable otherwise. She had no systemic complaints, such as fever or malaise. Patient's mucocutaneous findings were in remission.

Table 14.2 Laboratory findings of the patient

WBC	11,000/mm^3	ALT	16 IU/L
NEU	5300/mm^3	AST	13 IU/L
LYM	3100/mm^3	CRP	12 g/L
HGB	12 g/dL	ESR	34 mm/h
HCT	36%	CRE	0.5 g/L

WBC, white blood cell count; NEU, neutrophil count; LYM, lymphocyte count; HGB, hemoglobin; HCT, hematocrit; ALT, alanine aminotransferase; AST, aspartate aminotransferase; CRP, C-reactive protein; ESR, erythrocyte sedimentation rate; CRE, serum creatinine

Laboratory tests showed elevated acute-phase reactants and a mildly elevated leukocyte count (Table 14.2).

Intra-articular methylprednisolone acetate injection was performed, but no clinical improvement was observed. Prednisone 15 mg/daily was introduced. After 2 weeks, the patient described improvement in swelling, stiffness, and pain. Prednisone was tapered slowly (2.5 mg per week) and withdrawn at week 6. One month later, the patient presented with arthritis of both ankles. Azathioprine 150 mg/day was added to colchicine, together with prednisiolone 15 mg/day which was tapered and stopped within 1 month. Six months after the initiation of azathioprine the patient was doing well with no further arthritis episodes.

Case 2

A 36-year-old man was referred to our rheumatology outpatient clinic from dermatology with recurrent episodes of right knee pain and swelling that had occured three times during the past year. He reported that his symptoms were aggravated with movement and did not ease with rest. He did not describe any trauma to his knee. Since his childhood, he had suffered from recurring episodes of oral ulcers. Five years ago, after a genital ulcer occurred, he was referred to a dermatology outpatient clinic and was diagnosed with BS with a positive pathergy test and acneiform lesions on his shoulders. The number of oral ulcers and acneiform lesions had significantly decreased with 1 mg daily colchicine. He had no previous complaints about visual, digestive, and neurologic systems.

At the time of his referral to our unit, he stated that his right knee had swollen three times during this year. He described that past episodes had remitted in a week with nonsteroidal antiinflammatory drugs. Between the episodes, he was symptom-free. Even though he restarted the same therapy, his leg pain and swelling were not resolved this time.

The patient described pain during knee flexion and difficulty in walking since the pain in the right knee had started. Physical examination revealed a swollen right knee with effusion. An increased number of new papulopustular eruptions occurred this year while he had few oral ulcers and no new genital ulcers.

Laboratory tests (Table 14.3) disclosed leukocytosis with neutrophilia and elevated acute phase reactants. The remaining blood chemistry was within normal limits. There was no evidence of joint damage on X-ray.

An arthrocentesis was performed, and 60 cc synovial fluid was obtained with a predominance of polymorphonuclear leukocytes with negative microbiological studies indicating inflammatory synovial fluid characteristics. Intra-articular methylprednisolone acetate was administered, and colchicine dose was increased to 1.5 mg/day, but the patient had another episode after 1 month. His physical examination was similar to the first examination. Prednisone 15 mg/daily and azathioprine 150 mg/day were introduced. After 3 weeks, the pain was absent, and the patient described a functional improvement. Prednisolone was tapered slowly (2.5 mg per week) and planned to be withdrawn at week 6. Two months later, the patient suffered from left ankle pain and

Table 14.3 Laboratory findings of the patient

WBC	17,000/mm^3	ALT	22 IU/L
NEU	12,300/mm^3	AST	18 IU/L
LYM	3100/mm^3	CRP	44 g/L
HGB	13 g/dL	ESR	67 mm/h
HCT	37%	CRE	0.9 g/L

WBC, white blood cell count; NEU, neutrophil count; LYM, lymphocyte count; HGB, hemoglobin; HCT, hematocrit; ALT, alanine aminotransferase; AST, aspartate aminotransferase; CRP, C-reactive protein; ESR, erythrocyte sedimentation rate; CRE, serum creatinine

swelling in addition to right knee pain. A mild effusion in his right knee and left ankle arthritis was observed.

Due to the recurrent arthritis episodes, adalimumab 40 mg every 2 weeks was initiated. Colchicine was stopped, and azathioprine was continued. One month later, the patient's musculoskeletal complaints had completely resolved. No effusion was observed in both affected joints. Additionally, the number of acneiform papulopustular eruptions had decreased after adalimumab. At 3 months, acute phase reactants had decreased (CRP: 3 g/L, ESR: 17 mm/h). There were no further arthritis episodes after adalimumab initiation. After a year and a half, the patient was still under adalimumab and azathioprine treatment.

Case 3

A 46-year-old man was referred to our rheumatology outpatient clinic with treatment-resistant left elbow pain, swelling, and stiffness. He complained of elbow stiffness for 2 months. He did not describe any trauma, occupational injury, or hobbies that could be associated with his condition. Six months ago, he was prescribed methotrexate 10 mg/week and prednisolone 5 mg/day in another hospital. He did not have any improvement with this treatment. Before his referral to our clinic, an arthrocentesis was performed, and the synovial fluid analysis showed a white blood count of 10,000/mm^3 with a marked neutrophil ratio (50%). Microbiology results had not revealed any causative microorganisms. No crystal deposits were observed with polarized light microscopy.

A detailed history revealed that the patient had recurrent oral aphthosis since his childhood. He had no additional mucocutaneous complaints. The patient described no previous complaints related to visual, digestive, and nervous systems and no systemic symptoms such as fever or constitutional complaints.

Physical examination verified a swollen left elbow joint with limited extension.

A skin pathergy test was applied, and pustules were observed at 48 h. The patient was diagnosed with BS.

Laboratory tests revealed mild leukocytosis with neutrophilia and elevated acute phase reactants (Table 14.4). The remaining blood chemistry was within normal limits. Autoantibody assays were negative (Table 14.4). Left elbow radiograph did not show any signs of joint destruction (Fig. 14.3).

Due to the severity of symptoms, resistance to methotrexate and corticosteroids, and risk of permanent damage infliximab was initiated (5 mg/kg) without an initial trial of colchicine or other conventional immunosuppressives. After the first infusion, the patient's left elbow pain and swelling decreased. The patient's elbow mobility was significantly improved at the end of three months. Acute phase reactants were also normal (CRP: 1.6 g/L, ESR: 13 mm/h). The patient has still been receiving infliximab (every 8 weeks) with azathioprine for eight months.

Table 14.4 Laboratory findings of the patient

WBC	12,000/mm^3	ALT	31 IU/L
NEU	7000/mm^3	AST	30 IU/L
LYM	3100/mm^3	CRP	23 g/L
HGB	14 g/dL	ESR	44 mm/h
HCT	40%	CRE	1 g/L
RF	7 IU/dL	ANTI-CCP	Negative
ANA	Negative	ANTI-DS DNA	Negative
C3	100 mg/dL	C4	60 mg/dL
Uric acid	6 mg/dL	HLA-B27	Negative

WBC, white blood cell count; NEU, neutrophil count; LYM, lymphocyte count; HGB, hemoglobin; HCT, hematocrit; ALT, alanine aminotransferase; AST, aspartate aminotransferase; CRP, C-reactive protein; ESR, erythrocyte sedimentation rate; CRE, serum creatinine; RF, rheumatoid factor; Anti-CCP, anti-cyclic citrullinated peptide; ANA, antinuclear antibody; Anti-ds DNA, anti-double stranded DNA; C3, complement component 3; C4, complement component 4; HLA-B27, human leukocyte antigen-B27

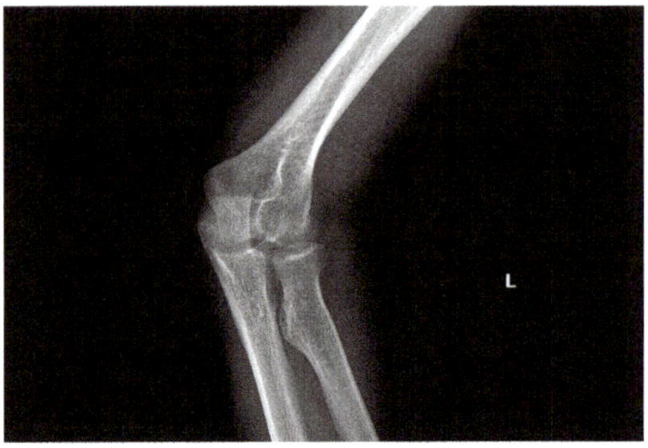

Fig. 14.3 X-ray of the left elbow showing flexion contracture. There was no sign of radiographic joint destruction

References

1. Yurdakul S, Yazici H, Tüzün Y, Pazarli H, Yalçin B, Altaç M, et al. The arthritis of Behçet's disease: a prospective study. Ann Rheum Dis. 1983;42(5):505–15.
2. Mumcu G, Lehimci F, Fidan Ö, Gük H, Alpar U, Ünal AU, et al. The assessment of work productivity and activity impairment in Behçet's disease. Turk J Med Sci. 2017;47(2):535–41.
3. Hatemi G, Christensen R, Bang D, Bodaghi B, Celik AF, Fortune F, et al. 2018 update of the EULAR recommendations for the management of Behçet's syndrome. Ann Rheum Dis. 2018;77(6):808–18.
4. Neves FS, Caldas CAM, Lage LV, Goldenstein-Schainberg C, Gonçalves CR. Faraway from the silk route: demographic and clinical features of Behçet's disease in 106 Brazilian patients. Clin Rheumatol. 2009;28(5):543–6.
5. Mok CC, Cheung TC, Ho CTK, Lee KW, Lau CS, Wong RWS. Behçet's disease in southern Chinese patients. J Rheumatol. 2002;29(8):1689–93.
6. Assaad-Khalil SH, Kamel FA, Ismail EA. Starting a regional registry for patients with Behçet's disease in North West Nile Delta region in Egypt. In: Hamza M, editor. Behçet's disease. Tunis: Pub Adhoua; 1997. p. 173–6.
7. Gheita TA, El-Latif EA, El-Gazzar II, et al. Behçet's disease in Egypt: a multicenter nationwide study on 1526 adult patients and review of the literature. Clin Rheumatol. 2019;38:2565–75.
8. Mahr A, Belarbi L, Wechsler B, Jeanneret D, Dhote R, Fain O, et al. Population-based prevalence study of Behçet's disease: differences by ethnic origin and low variation by age at immigration. Arthritis Rheum. 2008;58(12):3951–9.
9. Vaiopoulos AG, Kapsimali V, Kanakis MA, Vaiopoulos G, Samarkos M, Zouboulis CC, Kaklamanis PG. The frequency of arthritis in Adamantiades-Behçet's disease in Greek patients. J Eur Acad Dermatol Venereol. 2019;33(2):416–20.
10. Pande I, Uppal SS, Kailash S, Kumar A, Malaviya AN. Behçet's disease in India: a clinical, immunological, immunogenetic and outcome study. Br J Rheumatol. 1995;34(9):825–30.
11. Davatchi F, Shahram F, Chams-Davatchi C, Shams H, Nadji A, Akhlaghi M, Faezi T, Ghodsi Z, Larimi R, Ashofteh F, Abdollahi BS. Behcet's disease in Iran: analysis of 6500 cases. Int J Rheum Dis. 2010;13(4):367–73.
12. Al-Rawi ZS, Neda AH. Prevalence of Behçet's disease among Iraqis. Adv Exp Med Biol. 2003;528:37–41.
13. Adeeb F, Stack AG, Fraser AD. New insights into Behçet's disease in Ireland: the Midwest cohort study. Clin Exp Rheumatol. 2018;36(6 Suppl 115):33–9.
14. Jaber L, Milo G, Halpern GJ, et al. Prevalence of Behçet's disease in an Arab community in Israel. Ann Rheum Dis. 2002;61:365–6.
15. Krause I, Yankevich A, Fraser A, Rosner I, Mader R, Zisman D, Boulman N, Rozenbaum M, Weinberger A. Prevalence and clinical aspects of Behçet's disease in the north of Israel. Clin Rheumatol. 2007;26:555–60.

16. Salvarani C, Pipitone N, Catanoso MG, Cimino L, Tumiati B, Macchioni P, et al. Epidemiology and clinical course of Behçet's disease in the Reggio Emilia area of Northern Italy: a seventeen-year population-based study. Arthritis Rheum. 2007;57(1):171–8.
17. Olivieri I, Leccese P, Padula A, Nigro A, Palazzi C, Gilio M, D'Angelo S. High prevalence of Behçet's disease in southern Italy. Clin Exp Rheumatol. 2013;31(3 Suppl 77):28–31.
18. Nakae K, Masaki F, Hashimoto T, Inaba G, Mochizuki M, Sakane T. Recent epidemiological features of Behçet's disease in Japan. In: Wechsler B, Godeau P, editors. Behçet's disease, vol. 14. Amsterdam: Excerpta Medica; 1993. p. 145–51.
19. Madanat WY, Alawneh KM, Smadi MM, Saadeh SS, Omari MM, Bani Hani AB, Yazici H. The prevalence of Behçet's disease in the north of Jordan: a hospital-based epidemiological survey. Clin Exp Rheumatol. 2017;35 Suppl 108(6):51–4.
20. Mousa AR, Marafie AA, Rifai KM, Dajani AI, Mukhtar MM. Behçet's disease in Kuwait, Arabia: a report of 29 cases and a review. Scand J Rheumatol. 1986;15:310–32.
21. Balt J, Jamyanjav B, Jav S, et al. Clinical features of Behcet's disease in Mongolia: a multicenter study. Clin Rheumatol. 2020;39(9):2697–706.
22. Kappen JH, van Dijk EH, Baak-Dijkstra M, van Daele PL, Lam-Tse WK, van Hagen PM, van Laar JA. Behçet's disease, hospital-based prevalence and manifestations in the Rotterdam area. Neth J Med. 2015;73:471–7.
23. Al-Dalaan A, al Balaa S, el Ramahi K, al-Kawi Z, Bohlega S, Bahabri S, et al. Behçet's disease in Saudi Arabia. J Rheumatol. 1994;21:658–61.
24. Jankowski J, Crombie I, Jankowski R. Behçet's syndrome in Scotland. Postgrad Med J. 1992;68:566–70.
25. Sanchez Burson J, Grandal Y, Mendoza M, Montero R, Rejon E, Marenco JL. Clinical characteristics, HLA antigen and mortality in Behçet's syndrome in Spain. In: Olivieri I, Salvarani C, Cantini F, editors. 8th international congress on Behçet's disease: program and abstracts. Milan: Prex; 1998. p. 102.
26. Graña J, Sánchez-Meizoso MO, Galdo F. Epidemiological aspects of Behçet's disease in Galicia. J Rheumatol. 2001;28:2565–6.
27. Ek L, Hedfors E. Behçet's disease: a review and a report of 12 cases from Sweden. Acta Derm Venereol. 1993;73:251–4.
28. Mohammad A, Mandl T, Sturfelt G, Segelmark M. Incidence, prevalence and clinical characteristics of Behcet's disease in southern Sweden. Rheumatology (Oxford). 2013;52(2):304–10.
29. Villiger RA, Stefanski AL, Grobety V, Adler S, Villiger PM. Behçet's syndrome: clinical presentation and prevalence in Switzerland. Swiss Med Wkly. 2019;149:w20072.
30. Azizlerli G, Kose AA, Sarica R, et al. Prevalence of Behçet's disease in Istanbul, Turkey. Int J Dermatol. 2003;42:803–6.
31. Chamberlain MA. Behçet's syndrome in 32 patients in Yorkshire. Ann Rheum Dis. 1977;36:491–9.
32. Calamia KT, Wilson FC, Icen M, Crowson CS, Gabriel SE, Kremers HM. Epidemiology and clinical characteristics of Behçet's disease in the US: a population-based study. Arthritis Rheum. 2009;61(5):600–4.
33. Muruganandam M, Rolle NA, Sibbitt WL Jr, et al. Characteristics of Behçet's disease in the American Southwest. Semin Arthritis Rheum. 2019;49:296–302.
34. Cañete JD, Celis R, Noordenbos T, Moll C, Gómez-Puerta JA, Pizcueta P, et al. Distinct synovial immunopathology in Behçet disease and psoriatic arthritis. Arthritis Res Ther. 2009;11(1):R17.
35. Fatemi A, Shahram F, Akhlaghi M, Smiley A, Nadji A, Davatchi F. Prospective study of articular manifestations in Behçet's disease: five-year report. Int J Rheum Dis. 2017;20(1):97–102.
36. Gur A, Sarac AJ, Burkan YK, Nas K, Cevik R. Arthropathy, quality of life, depression, and anxiety in Behcet's disease: relationship between arthritis and these factors. Clin Rheumatol. 2006;25(4):524–31.
37. Kim HA, Choi KW, Song VW. Arthropathy in Behcet's disease. Scand J Rheumatol. 1997;26(2):125–9.
38. Koca SS, Akbulut H, Dag S, Artas H, Isik A. Anti-cyclic citrullinated peptide antibodies in rheumatoid arthritis and Behçet's disease. Tohoku J Exp Med. 2007;213(4):297–304.
39. Ben Taarit C, Turki S, Ben Maïz H. Les manifestations rhumatologiques de la maladie de Behçet: à propos de 309 cas. Rev Med Interne. 2001;22(11):1049–55.
40. Moll C, Bogas M, Gómez-Puerta JA, Celis R, Vázquez I, Rodríguez F, et al. Macroscopic features of knee synovitis in early untreated Behçet disease and psoriatic arthritis. Clin Rheumatol. 2009;28(9):1053–7.
41. Diri E, Mat C, Hamuryudan V, Yurdakul S, Hizli N, Yazici H. Papulopustular skin lesions are seen more frequently in patients with Behçet's syndrome who have arthritis: a controlled and masked study. Ann Rheum Dis. 2001;60(11):1074–6.
42. Hatemi G, Bahar H, Uysal S, Mat C, Gogus F, Masatlioglu S, Altas K, Yazici H. The pustular skin lesions in Behcet's syndrome are not sterile. Ann Rheum Dis. 2004;63(11):1450–2.
43. Tunc R, Keyman E, Melikoglu M, Fresko I, Yazici H. Target organ associations in Turkish patients with Behçet's disease: a cross sectional study by exploratory factor analysis. J Rheumatol. 2002;29(11):2393–6.
44. Karaca M, Hatemi G, Sut N, Yazici H. The papulopustular lesion/arthritis cluster of Behçet's syndrome also clusters in families. Rheumatology (Oxford). 2012;51(6):1053–60.
45. Takahashi A, Takeda I, Kanno T, Saito N, Kasukawa R. Achilles tendonitis in a patient with Behçet's disease. Mod Rheumatol. 2004;14(6):485–7.
46. Caporn N, Higgs ER, Dieppe PA, Watt I. Arthritis in Behcet's syndrome. Br J Radiol. 1983;56(662):87–91.
47. Hatemi G, Fresko I, Tascilar K, Yazici H. Increased enthesopathy among Behçet's syndrome patients with acne and arthritis: an ultrasonography study. Arthritis Rheum. 2008;58(5):1539–45.

48. Hatemi G, Fresko I, Yurdakul S, Ozdogan H, Yazici H, Altiok E, et al. Reply to letter by Priori et al commenting on whether Behçet's syndrome patients with acne and arthritis comprise a true subset. Arthritis Rheum. 2010;62(1):305–6.
49. Moll JM, Haslock I, Macrae IF, Wright V. Associations between ankylosing spondylitis, psoriatic arthritis, Reiter's disease, the intestinal arthropathies, and Behcet's syndrome. Medicine (Baltimore). 1974;53(5):343–64.
50. Dilsen N, Koniçe M, Övül C. Arthritic patterns in Behçet's disease. Behçet's disease: proceedings of an international symposium on Behçet's disease. Amsterdam: Excerpta Medica; 1979. p. 145–55.
51. Yazici H, Tuzlaci M, Yurdakul S. A controlled survey of sacroiliitis in Behcet's disease. Ann Rheum Dis. 1981;40(6):558–9.
52. Chamberlain MA, Robertson RJ. A controlled study of sacroiliitis in Behçet's disease. Br J Rheumatol. 1993;32(8):693–8.
53. Yazici H, Turunç M, Ozdoğan H, Yurdakul S, Akinci A, Barnes CG. Observer variation in grading sacroiliac radiographs might be a cause of 'sacroiliitis' reported in certain disease states. Ann Rheum Dis. 1987;46(2):139–45.
54. Kotevoglu N, Tasbas I, Bekiroglu N. Computed tomography does not support sacroiliitis as a feature of Behçet disease: a metaanalytic review. J Clin Rheumatol. 2004;10(1):42–5.
55. Motet C, Nubourgh I, Vandergheynst F. Gastrocnemius myositis associated with Behçet's syndrome. Eur J Case Rep Intern Med. 2023;10(5):003828.
56. Gallay L, Hot A, Allenbach Y, Maucort-Boulch D, Comarmond C, Marques C, et al. From the French Behçet's Network. Occurrence of focal myositis during Behçet's disease: the identification of a specific vasculitis-associated focal myopathy. Neuropathol Appl Neurobiol. 2023;49(2):e12900.
57. Conway R, Bergin D, Carey JJ, Coughlan RJ. A case of Behcet's syndrome presenting as focal myositis. Rheumatology (Oxford). 2012;51(6):975.
58. Akansel G, Akgoz Y, Ciftci E, Arslan A, Demirci A. MRI findings of myositis in Behçet disease. Skeletal Radiol. 2004;33(7):426–8.
59. Kim DH, Kim SW, Yeo SM, Kang MS, Yoon YC, Sung DH. Focal vasculitic myositis as a primary manifestation of Behçet's disease: a case series of 10 Korean patients in a locomotive medicine clinic. Rheumatology (Oxford). 2021;60(10):4609–15.
60. Chung SW, Lee JH, Ha YJ, Kang EH, Lee YJ. Recurrent focal myofasciitis of Behçet syndrome mimics infectious myofasciitis: a case report. J Rheum Dis. 2023;30(4):268–71.
61. Ogose T, Tamaki W, Shinahara K, Kaneko M, Wakata Y, Naruse K. A case of recurrent myositis as the main manifestation of Behçet disease. Pediatr Int. 2010;52(2):e101–4.
62. Nejadhosseinian M, Babagoli M, Faezi ST, Haerian H, Shahram F, Alikhani M, Davatchi F. Osteonecrosis as a rare musculoskeletal complication in Behcet's disease—the largest case series with literature review. BMC Rheumatol. 2023;7(1):42.
63. Atas N, Bitik B, Varan O, Babaoglu H, Tufan A, Haznedaroglu S, et al. Clinical characteristics of avascular necrosis in patients with Behçet disease: a case series and literature review. Rheumatol Int. 2019;39(1):153–9.
64. Yavuz S, Fresko I, Hamuryudan V, Yurdakul S, Yazici H. Fibromyalgia in Behçet's syndrome. J Rheumatol. 1998;25(11):2219–20.
65. Haliloglu S, Carlioglu A, Akdeniz D, Karaaslan Y, Kosar A. Fibromyalgia in patients with other rheumatic diseases: prevalence and relationship with disease activity. Rheumatol Int. 2014;34(9):1275–80.
66. Lee SS, Yoon HJ, Chang HK, Park KS. Fibromyalgia in Behçet's disease is associated with anxiety and depression, and not with disease activity. Clin Exp Rheumatol. 2005;23(4 Suppl 38):S15–9.
67. Buyuktas D, Hatemi G, Yuksel-Findikoglu S, Ugurlu S, Yazici H, Yurdakul S. Fatigue is correlated with disease activity but not with the type of organ involvement in Behçet's syndrome: a comparative clinical survey. Clin Exp Rheumatol. 2015;33(6 Suppl 94):S107–12.
68. Luo Y, Bolek EC, Quinn KA, Wells K, Rose E, Sikora K, et al. A prospective observational cohort study and systematic review of 40 patients with mouth and genital ulcers with inflamed cartilage (MAGIC) syndrome. Semin Arthritis Rheum. 2022;52:151924.
69. Hatemi I, Hatemi G, Celik AF, Melikoglu M, Arzuhal N, Mat C, et al. Frequency of pathergy phenomenon and other features of Behçet's syndrome among patients with inflammatory bowel disease. Clin Exp Rheumatol. 2008;26(4 Suppl 50):S91–5.
70. Yurdakul S, Mat C, Tüzün Y, Ozyazgan Y, Hamuryudan V, Uysal O, et al. A double-blind trial of colchicine in Behçet's syndrome. Arthritis Rheum. 2001;44(11):2686–92.
71. Calgüneri M, Ertenli I, Kiraz S, Erman M, Celik I. Effect of prophylactic benzathine penicillin on mucocutaneous symptoms of Behçet's disease. Dermatology. 1996;192(2):125–8.
72. Moral F, Hamuryudan V, Yurdakul S, Yazici H. Inefficacy of azapropazone in the acute arthritis of Behçet's syndrome: a randomized, double blind, placebo controlled study. Clin Exp Rheumatol. 1995;13(4):493–5.
73. Yazici H, Pazarli H, Barnes CG, Tüzün Y, Ozyazgan Y, Silman A, et al. A controlled trial of azathioprine in Behçet's syndrome. N Engl J Med. 1990;322(5):281–5.
74. Hamuryudan V, Moral F, Yurdakul S, Mat C, Tüzün Y, Ozyazgan Y, et al. Systemic interferon alpha 2b treatment in Behçet's syndrome. J Rheumatol. 1994;21(6):1098–100.
75. Kötter I, Vonthein R, Zierhut M, Eckstein AK, Ness T, Günaydin I, et al. Differential efficacy of human recombinant interferon-alpha2a on ocular and extraocular manifestations of Behçet disease: results

of an open 4-center trial. Semin Arthritis Rheum. 2004;33(5):311–9.
76. Melikoglu M, Fresko I, Mat C, Ozyazgan Y, Gogus F, Yurdakul S, et al. Short-term trial of etanercept in Behçet's disease: a double blind, placebo controlled study. J Rheumatol. 2005;32(1):98.
77. Vallet H, Riviere S, Sanna A, Deroux A, Moulis G, Addimanda O, et al. Efficacy of anti-TNF alpha in severe and/or refractory Behçet's disease: multicenter study of 124 patients. J Autoimmun. 2015;62:67–74.
78. Arida A, Fragiadaki K, Giavri E, Sfikakis PP. Anti-TNF agents for Behçet's disease: analysis of published data on 369 patients. Semin Arthritis Rheum. 2011;41(1):61–70.
79. London J, Régent A, Dion J, Jilet L, Jachiet M, Lidove O, et al. Efficacy and safety of ustekinumab in Behçet disease: results from the prospective phase 2 STELABEC trial. J Am Acad Dermatol. 2022;87(3):681–4.
80. Mirouse A, Barete S, Desbois AC, Comarmond C, Sène D, Domont F, et al. Long-term outcome of Ustekinumab therapy for Behçet's disease. Arthritis Rheumatol. 2019;71(10):1727–32.
81. Hatemi G, Mahr A, Ishigatsubo Y, Song YW, Takeno M, Kim D, Melikoğlu M, Cheng S, McCue S, Paris M, Chen M, Yazici Y. Trial of apremilast for oral ulcers in Behçet's syndrome. N Engl J Med. 2019;381(20):1918–28.
82. Hatemi G, Mahr A, Takeno M, Kim D, Melikoglu M, Chen S, et al. Efficacy of apremilast for the treatment of manifestations of Behçet's syndrome other than oral ulcers, including skin lesions and arthritis. ACR 2020 convergence meeting abstracts.
83. Vieira M, Buffier S, Vautier M, Le Joncour A, Jamilloux Y, Gerfaud-Valentin M, et al. Apremilast in refractory Behçet's syndrome: a multicenter observational study. Front Immunol. 2020;11:626792.
84. Atienza-Mateo B, Martín-Varillas JL, Graña J, Espinosa G, Moriano C, Pérez-Sandoval T, et al. Apremilast in refractory orogenital ulcers and other manifestations of Behçet's disease. A national multicentre study of 51 cases in clinical practice. Clin Exp Rheumatol. 2020;38 Suppl 127(5):69–75.
85. Di Scala G, Bettiol A, Cojan RD, Finocchi M, Silvestri E, Emmi G. Efficacy of the anti-IL 17 secukinumab in refractory Behçet's syndrome: a preliminary study. J Autoimmun. 2019;97:108–13.
86. Fagni F, Bettiol A, Talarico R, Lopalco G, Silvestri E, Urban ML, et al. Long-term effectiveness and safety of secukinumab for treatment of refractory mucosal and articular Behçet's phenotype: a multicentre study. Ann Rheum Dis. 2020;79(8):1098–104.
87. Liu J, Hou Y, Sun L, Li C, Li L, Zhao Y, et al. A pilot study of tofacitinib for refractory Behçet's syndrome. Ann Rheum Dis. 2020;79(11):1517–20.
88. Grayson PC, Yazici Y, Merideth M, Sen HN, Davis M, Novakovich E, Joyal E, Goldbach-Mansky R, Sibley CH. Treatment of mucocutaneous manifestations in Behçet's disease with anakinra: a pilot open-label study. Arthritis Res Ther. 2017;19(1):69.
89. Cantarini L, Vitale A, Scalini P, Dinarello CA, Rigante D, Franceschini R, et al. Anakinra treatment in drug-resistant Behcet's disease: a case series. Clin Rheumatol. 2015;34(7):1293–301.
90. Vitale A, Rigante D, Caso F, Brizi MG, Galeazzi M, Costa L, et al. Inhibition of interleukin-1 by canakinumab as a successful mono-drug strategy for the treatment of refractory Behçet's disease: a case series. Dermatology. 2014;228(3):211–4.

Clinical Features and Diagnostic Tools in Vascular and Cardiac Involvement of Behçet's Disease

15

Fatma Alibaz-Oner

Contents

15.1 Introduction

Behçet's disease (BD) is a chronic inflammatory disease characterized by oral and genital ulcers and uveitis. It also involves gastrointestinal, musculoskeletal, neurological systems and major vessels [1]. Vessels of all sizes can be involved both in the arterial and venous system. Therefore, BD is defined as variable vessel vasculitis in Chapel Hill Consensus Conference [2]. Vascular involvement is seen in the range of 15–50% in BD [3]. It is more commonly observed in Middle-Eastern and Northern Africa countries such as Türkiye, Jordan, Israel, Iran, Morocco, and Algeria, and South European countries with immigrant populations, such as France [4] but is quite rare in East Asian countries such as Japan (<10%) [5] and Korea (<5%) [6]. Venous involvement is seen in the rate of 67–84% among all vascular manifestations. Arterial involvement is seen less than 15% in all series. Deep vein thrombosis

F. Alibaz-Oner (✉)
Division of Rheumatology, Department of Internal Medicine, Marmara University School of Medicine Hospital, Istanbul, Türkiye

E. Alpsoy et al. (eds.), *Behçet's Disease: An Integrated Approach*,
https://doi.org/10.1007/978-3-031-77251-1_15

(DVT) in lower extremities is the most frequent type of vascular involvement [7, 8]. Vascular involvement such as pulmonary aneurysm, Budd–Chiari syndrome (BCS) and arterial aneurysm is also the major cause of mortality up to 44% in BD [9]. About 80% of patients with vascular Behçet disease (VBD) are males. A more severe disease course is observed in male BD patients [10, 11]. In about one-fourth of VBD patients, vascular involvement develops before fulfilling International Study Group (ISG) Criteria for BD [12]. In a large cohort from Türkiye, it was reported that the first vascular event develops within 5 years after disease onset. DVT and cerebral sinus thrombosis develop earlier within median 1 year after disease onset, whereas nonpulmonary arterial involvement seems to develop within a median of 5 years during the disease course [7].

15.2 Clinical Features of Vascular and Cardiac Involvement of Behçet's Disease

15.2.1 Deep Vein Thrombosis of Lower Extremities

DVT in the lower extremity is the most frequent manifestation of vascular involvement in BD. It consists of about 70% of all vascular manifestations [8]. Femoral and popliteal veins are the most common involved veins in lower extremities. However, crural, external iliac, and common iliac veins are also involved commonly. Bilateral involvement and less recanalization are more frequent in VBD compared to DVT due to non-BD reasons [13, 14]. Relapses are seen in about one-third of patients during retrospective follow-up studies [7, 8]. However, the relapse rate was found higher (45%) in only a prospective study including 33 patients [15]. Post-thrombotic syndrome (PTS) is the most frequent complication of DVT. It causes different combinations of leg pain, heaviness, swelling, edema, hyperpigmentation, varicose veins, lipodermatosclerosis, and venous ulcers [16]. Venous ulcers are the sign of severe PTS in BD, they should be distinguished from pyoderma gangrenosum and vasculitic ulcers [17]. PTS is observed in up to 64% of BD with DVT, and it causes impaired venous disease-associated QoL [14, 18]. Therefore, prevention of PTS development should also be targeted as well as prevention of relapses in BD (Fig. 15.1).

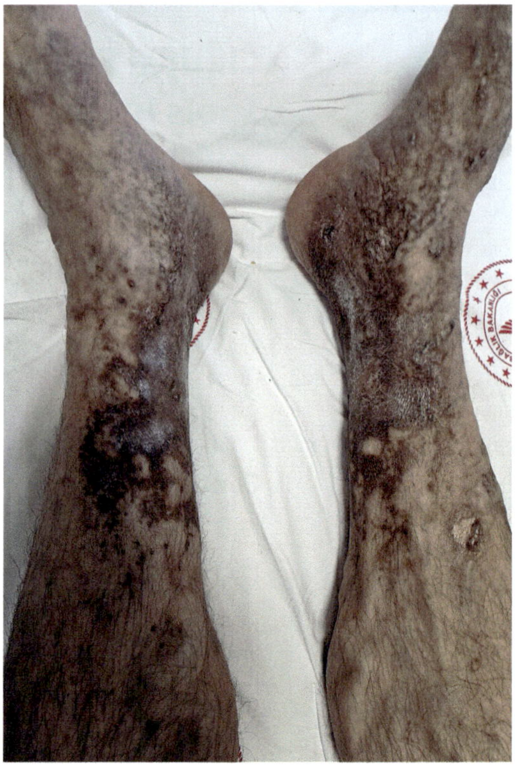

Fig. 15.1 Bilateral post-thrombotic syndrome

15.2.2 Thrombosis of Superior and Inferior Vena Cava

Thrombosis of vena cava (VC) superior and inferior is seen in less than 10% of VBD patients [8]. Cava involvement is commonly associated with other vascular involvement types such as BCS, pulmonary involvement and cerebral sinus thrombosis. When VC superior is involved, patients generally present with VC superior syndrome (VCSS) signs such as swelling and cyanosis of the face, neck and upper extremities. Those patients generally have a benign course due to venous collateral development. When VC inferior is involved, the clinical findings change according to the involved segment. The clinical course is silent if there is no BCS. BCS develops in case of hepatic and suprahepatic segment involvement. On the other hand, infrahepatic involvement is commonly involved with the extension of DVT in the lower extremity. In case of bilateral common femoral vein involvement, vena cava inferior thrombosis is seen in 20% of these patients [19]. Vena cava involvement in BD is generally associated with other vascular involvements such as BCS, pulmonary artery involvement, and cerebral sinus thrombosis [7, 20, 21].

15.2.3 Budd–Chiari Syndrome

Budd–Chiari syndrome, which is one of the most lethal forms of VBD, is seen in less than 5% of all vascular manifestations [22] (Fig. 15.2). A retrospective study including 43 BCS with BD defined "symptomatic" and "silent" clinical presentation. In case of ascites presence, mortality rate is reported as 60% within median 10 months after diagnosis. Lack of ascites or any other symptoms associated with liver failure were defined as silent presentation. In silent presentation, the disease course is insidious, and less mortality is expected [23]. In a multicenter series from Türkiye, overall mortality was found 14.8% in 61 BD patients with BCS. Majority of these 61 patients had chronic and silent presentations. Mortality rate was significantly higher in BD patients with BCS compared to BD patients without BCS ($p = 0.004$) [24]. Mortality rate was found less than 20% during follow-up in two retrospective studies [25, 26].

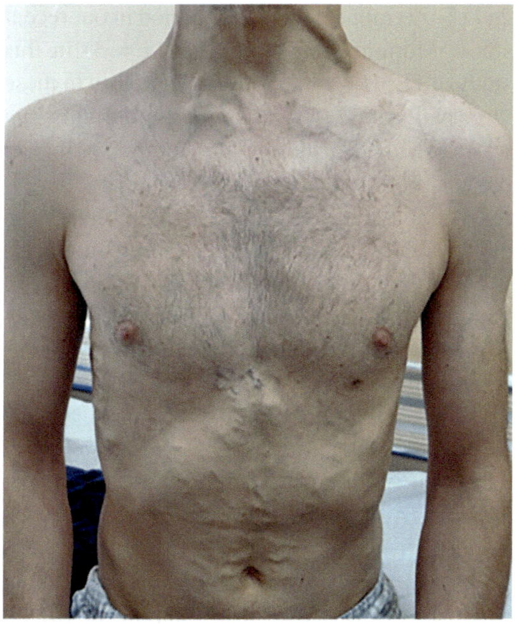

Fig. 15.2 Venous collaterals in patient with Budd–Chiari syndrome

15.2.4 Cerebral Sinus Thrombosis

About one-third of neurologic involvement in BD is cerebral sinus thrombosis (CST). It may also be accepted as a form of vascular involvement. CST generally develops in male BD patients [27]. In a multicenter retrospective study, BD was found as the cause for CST development in 108 (9.4%) of 1144 patients. Transverse sinuses were the most common involved site [28]. In a recent study from Türkiye, while venous infarction and venous hemorrhage were found less; transverse sinus thrombosis was more common in CST with BD compared to CST without BD [29]. Patients mostly present with intracranial hypertension symptoms and signs. However, patients can rarely present with fever, nausea/vomiting, seizure, and confusion [30]. In a systematic review including 290 cases of CST with BD, prognosis and response to treatment were good. Sequelae were reported in 20% of patients. Optic nerve atrophy and blindness/reduced visual acuity were the most commonly reported sequelae [31].

15.2.5 Pulmonary Arterial Involvement

Pulmonary arterial involvement (PAI) is the most frequent form of arterial involvement. It is also one of the major causes of mortality in BD. PAI was reported 5–10% among all vascular manifestations, and mostly affects young males [8, 32].

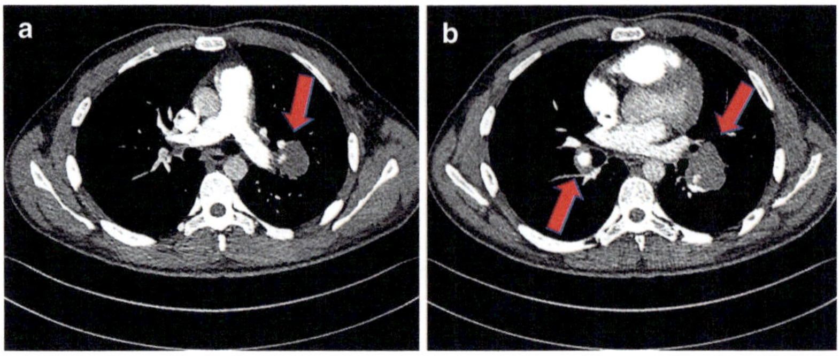

Fig. 15.3 (**a**) Aneurysmatic dilatation of left main pulmonary artery totally occluded with pulmonary thrombus. (**b**) Aneurysmatic dilatation filled with pulmonary thrombus in the left lower lobar pulmonary artery and right lower lobar pulmonary artery surrounded with thrombotic material

PAI can present as aneurysm formation, thrombosis or both. Thrombosis is defined as an inflammatory 'in situ thrombi' rather than an embolus as a result of primary inflammation of the pulmonary vessel wall. Therefore, it is tightly adherent to the vessel wall in BD [33] (Fig. 15.3). Detaching of the thrombi usually from the deep vein of the lower extremities is not expected in BD. Pulmonary thromboembolism is very rare. In early retrospective series, aneurysm formation was reported more frequently than thrombosis. Isolated "in situ" pulmonary artery thrombosis (PAT) was reported in only one-third of PAI [34–36]. However, in a recent study, aneurysmal involvement was found in only 18% of 61 BD patients with PAI. Thrombosis was found as a major presentation type of PAI [37]. In our large VBD cohort including 225 patients, pulmonary artery thrombosis was the second most common presentation of VBD (n = 78, 35%), pulmonary aneurysm formation was seen in only 3 (1.3%) patients (unpublished data). During the first presentation of thrombotic PAI, subsegmental arteries are mostly involved in BD (74.5%). Main pulmonary arterial thrombosis occurs less than 10% during the first presentation. However, segmental arterial involvement is the most frequently involved arteries during relapses [38]. Aneurysms are usually multiple and bilateral. The most frequent localization is lobar arteries [39, 40]. Hemoptysis is usually the presenting symptom of pulmonary arterial aneurysm (up to 90%). It can be massive and life threatening in half of the patients. Hemoptysis is seen less frequently in PAT. Constitutional symptoms, fever, dyspnea, cough, and chest pain may also be seen in patients with PAI [7, 34]. In our recent study including 110 BD patients with PAI, 32 (29.1%) patients were asymptomatic when PAI was detected. These patients were mostly under immunosuppressive (IS) treatment due to other disease manifestations [38]. Chronic thromboembolic pulmonary hypertension (CTEPH) is a rare complication of PAI. CTEPH developed in 9 (8.2%) of 110 BD patients with PAI during the median 24 (15–72) months follow-up period in our recent study. Mortality rate was 2.7% (n = 3) in this study. CTEPH was the cause of mortality in these three patients [38]. In early reports, mortality rate was around 25% during the follow-up in BD patients with pulmonary aneurysm. The mortality risk is associated with the size of aneurysms and systolic pulmonary artery pressure levels [32]. In the aforementioned study including 110 patients, aneurysm formation was present in only 9 (6.6%). There was no mortality in these patients during follow-up.

15.2.6 Peripheral Arterial Involvement

Peripheral arterial involvement is seen in about 5% among all vascular manifestations of BD [7, 8]. Abdominal aorta, femoral, popliteal, and carotid arteries are the most frequent involve-

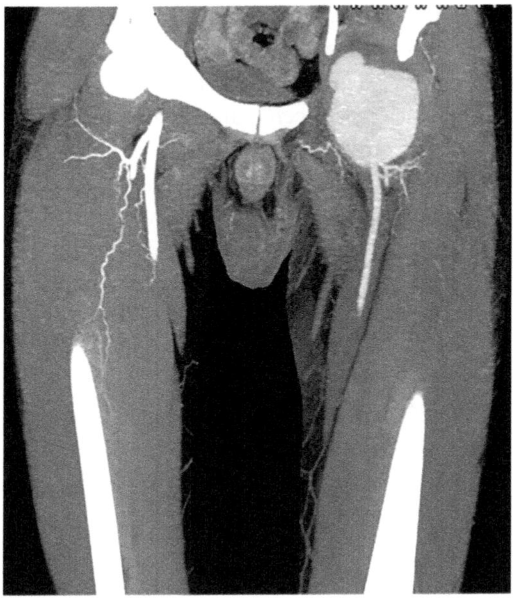

Fig. 15.4 Pseudoaneurysm formation (width: 62 mm) at posterior segment of right common femoral artery

ment sites of aneurysm formation. Aneurysm may also be seen in visceral and cerebral arteries[41]. It develops mostly in the late disease phase, on average 5–10 years after the disease-onset [7]. Aneurysm formation is the main form of peripheral arterial involvement, however thrombosis can also be seen. There is a striking male predominance similar to other vascular manifestations [42] (Fig. 15.4). Constitutional symptoms and increased acute-phase reactants are generally present in patients with peripheral arterial involvement [7]. Painful and pulsatile masses are typical presentations of peripheral aneurysms. The high risk of rupture or leakage should be kept in mind in patients with pulsatile aneurysms. Nonspecific symptoms such as back or flank pain, abdominal discomfort and constipation may be the presentation of some patients with abdominal aortic aneurysms. Abdominal aorta rupture has a high risk of mortality[43]. In retrospective case series, relapse rate was reported 20–50% during follow-up [42, 44]. Saadoun et al. reported a large series of 101 patients with arterial involvement (aorta ($n = 25$), femoral ($n = 23$) and pulmonary ($n = 21$) arteries). While relapse rate was 28% in this series, complete remission rate was 39% after a median follow-up of 7.6 years. Mortality rate was reported as 14%. The 20-year survival rate was significantly lower in patients with arterial involvement compared to patients without arterial involvement (73% vs. 89%, $p < 0.0001$) [45].

15.2.7 Cardiac Involvement

Cardiac involvement is very rare among all vascular manifestations in BD (<5%) [7]. Most frequent presentation of cardiac involvement is intracardiac thrombosis. It is mainly seen in male BD patients, and mostly localized at the right side of the heart. Patients mainly present with fever (>80% of patients). Dyspnea, chest pain and hemoptysis can also be seen in about one-third of patients. The other forms of cardiac involvements such as coronary arteritis, valve involvement (mostly in the aortic valve), pericarditis, myocarditis, endocarditis, endomyocardial fibrosis, and sinus of Valsalva aneurysms were also rarely reported [46]. Embolism from valvular lesions is unexpected due to the tightly attached structure of lesions to endocardium or myocardium. Some patients may rarely present with heart failure before BD diagnosis [47]. Coronary artery involvement is seen seldom in about 0.5% among all vascular manifestations [48]. Aneurysms or occlusion of coronary arteries present with myocardial infarction or aneurysm rupture in these cases [49]. There is very limited data for the prognosis of cardiac involvement. In a retrospective case series including 22 patients, thrombus resolved in 13 patients and thrombus size decreased in 7 patients during follow-up [46]. In a large French series, relapse developed in 8 (15%) of 52 patients during a median follow-up of 3 (1.7–4.2) years. Mortality rate was 15% in this study. The 5-year survival rate was 83.6% in BD patients with cardiac involvement [50].

15.3 Diagnostic Tools in Vascular and Cardiac Involvement of Behçet's Disease

Venous Doppler ultrasound (US) is the frequently used imaging tool to detect venous thrombosis in vascular BD, especially in lower extremities. Tutar et al. compared the diagnostic value of Doppler US and magnetic resonance (MR) venography in BD patients with chronic DVT. Doppler US showed chronic thrombotic changes in all patients. However, MR venography showed chronic changes in 93% of patients. On the other hand, MR venography showed collateral formation in 68% of patients, while collaterals were shown by Doppler US in only 25% of patients [51]. MR venography might be an alternative diagnostic option to show chronic thrombosis in the lower extremities. However, Doppler US is the first choice to detect acute thrombosis in lower extremities and portal veins in BD. Contrast-enhanced computed tomography (CT) and MR angiography can be used for the diagnosis of vena cava thrombosis [19, 52]. CT and MR angiography can also be used for diagnosis of cerebral sinus thrombosis. However, MRI is superior to CT for detection of a clot in the cortical or deep veins. Detection of the ischemic damage in the cerebral parenchyma is another advantage of MRI in BD patients with CVT [53].

For the detection of pulmonary arterial involvement, contrast-enhanced CT is the best option. MR angiography may also be used, but CT angiography is a better imaging tool for detection of small aneurysms [54, 55]. For the diagnosis of peripheral arterial involvement and aortic involvement in BD, both CT and MR angiography can be used [22]. Echocardiography is the most frequent diagnostic tool for cardiac involvement of BD; however, coronary angiography (either conventional or CT) or cardiac MR can be used in selected cases.

PET became a widely used imaging tool for especially large vessel vasculitis in recent years. It can be another option for the diagnosis of isolated aortic involvement with the vessel wall thickening and mural thrombus in BD. There are case reports detecting inflammation in pulmonary arteries, peripheral arteries, intracardiac thrombosis and cerebral sinus thrombosis [56–58]. Conventional angiography is not preferred for the diagnosis of vascular involvement in BD due to the risk of aneurysm formation at the insertion site [59]. However, it can be performed in selected cases with the need for endovascular interventions.

15.3.1 Femoral Vein Wall Thickness Measurement as a New Diagnostic Tool for Behçet's Disease

Despite the striking venous dominance in vascular involvement, there was limited data assessing the veins in BD until recently. High rates of venous insufficiency were previously reported in BD patients without vascular disease compared to controls [60–62]. Ambrose et al. first demonstrated increased vein wall thickness (VWT) in popliteal veins of BD patients [63]. Then, we recently published the first controlled Doppler US study showing increased VWT of lower extremity veins independent of vascular involvement in male BD patients. Common femoral vein (CFV), which is the largest of lower extremity veins, was chosen as the primary site of US assessment for being an easily and reliably measurable vein in daily practice. Cutoff values for right and left CFV ≥0.5 mm had high area under the receiver operating characteristic (ROC) curves (>0.8) with sensitivities of 81–82.8% and specificities of 78.4–81.1% [64, 65]. Our observations were also confirmed by other groups from Türkiye [66, 67]. When we assessed the *diagnostic performance* of CFV thickness in BD compared with multiple disease controls, increased CFV thickness was observed as a distinctive feature of BD. The cutoff value of ≥0.5 mm, determined in our first study, performed quite well against all control groups with a sensitivity and specificity (except antiphospholipid antibody syndrome) higher than >80%.

Values especially higher than 0.75 mm point out very high probability of BD [68]. Atalay et al. recently reported increased VWT both in complete and incomplete pediatric BD similar to our studies in adults [69]. We recently reported that increased VWT can be used as a diagnostic test in also suspected BD patients [70]. We also showed that intima–media thickness of CFV, as well as CFV wall thickness, is significantly increased in BD patients than healthy controls independent of major organ involvement. This data suggest that there is a full layer venous wall inflammation including intima–media layer in BD despite the lack of vascular involvement [71]. Although BD is a unique systemic vasculitis that mainly involves veins, pulmonary arteries are the most frequently involved arteries which had similar structure with systemic veins in terms of thin walls, increased compliance and low resistance. We recently found that pulmonary arterial wall thickness was significantly higher in BD with major organ involvement compared to BD patients with only mucocutaneous disease. Increased pulmonary arterial wall thickness is present only in patients with major organ involvement, possibly as a sign of more severe disease in BD [72]. The preliminary results of our ongoing prospective follow-up study assessing prognostic value of CFV thickness, suggest that mucocutaneous BD patients with higher CFV thickness may have a higher risk for the development of major organ involvement during follow-up [73].

Diagnosing BD can be a clinical challenge, especially in patients presenting with only vascular involvement with or without oral ulcers. These patients not meeting diagnostic criteria, receive BD diagnosis with "expert opinion" in countries with high prevalence of BD. Furthermore, early diagnosis is very important in cases with venous thrombosis as their management differs from that of non-inflammatory DVT, necessitating immunosuppressive use rather than anticoagulant therapy. Our aforementioned studies showed that measurement of CFV thickness with doppler ultrasound (US) can be a diagnostic test for these groups of patients with BD [68, 70].

15.4 Conclusion

Vascular BD is a complex vasculitis different from other systemic vasculitides. It involves all size veins and arteries. VBD is the main cause of mortality, also one of main causes of morbidity in especially male patients. DVT in the lower extremity is the most frequent vascular involvement type in VBD. However, recent data shows that mainly thrombotic form of pulmonary involvement is seen with increasing rate in BD. PTS was shown as an important morbidity cause in BD with DVT. Therefore, prevention of PTS should be targeted as well as prevention of relapses in daily practice during follow up of VBD. Diagnosis of vascular BD depends on the presence of other clinical features of BD after excluding other potential reasons. Diagnosing BD can be difficult in patients presenting with only vascular involvement with or without oral ulcers. In these patients, early diagnosis of BD has a critical value to prevent delay in the BD treatment. While other thrombotic diseases need anticoagulant treatment, BD patients are treated with immunosuppressive agents including glucocorticoids. Our recent studies showed that CFV thickness measurement can be a valuable, practical, and cheap diagnostic tool for BD with the sensitivity and the specificities higher than 80% for the cutoff value of 0.5 mm. However, the diagnostic accuracy of CFV measurement should also be validated in different ethnic populations.

References

1. Alibaz-Oner F, Direskeneli H. Update on the diagnosis of Behçet's disease. Diagnostics (Basel). 2022;13(1):41.
2. Jennette JC, Falk RJ, Bacon PA, et al. 2012 revised international Chapel Hill consensus conference nomenclature of vasculitides. Arthritis Rheum. 2013;65(1):1–11.
3. Ozguler Y, Esatoglu SN, Seyahi E, et al. Vascular and cardiac involvement. In: Yazici Y, et al., editors. Behçet syndrome. 2nd ed. Basel: Springer Nature Switzerland AG; 2020. p. 83–103.
4. Yazici H, Seyahi E, Hatemi G, Yazici Y. Behçet syndrome: a contemporary view. Nat Rev Rheumatol. 2018;14:107–19.

5. Ishido T, Horita N, Takeuchi M, et al. Clinical manifestations of Behçet's disease depending on sex and age: results from Japanese nationwide registration. Rheumatology (Oxford). 2017;56(11):1918–27.
6. Ryu HJ, Seo MR, Choi HJ, et al. Clinical phenotypes of Korean patients with Behcet disease according to gender, age at onset, and HLA-B51. Korean J Intern Med. 2018;33(5):1025–31.
7. Tascilar K, Melikoglu M, Ugurlu S, et al. Vascular involvement in Behcet's syndrome: a retrospective analysis of associations and the time course. Rheumatology (Oxford). 2014;53(11):2018–22.
8. Alibaz-Oner F, Karadeniz A, Ylmaz S, et al. Behçet disease with vascular involvement: effects of different therapeutic regimens on the incidence of new relapses. Medicine (Baltimore). 2015;94(6):e494.
9. Saadoun D, Wechsler B, Desseaux K, et al. Mortality in Behçet's disease. Arthritis Rheum. 2010;62:2806–12.
10. Kural-Seyahi E, Fresko I, Seyahi N, et al. The long-term mortality and morbidity of Behcet syndrome: a 2-decade outcome survey of 387 patients followed at a dedicated center. Medicine (Baltimore). 2003;82:60–76.
11. Bozkurt T, Karabacak M, Karatas H, et al. Earlier and more aggressive treatment with biologics may prevent relapses and further new organ involvement in Behçet's disease. Clin Immunol. 2023;248:109263.
12. Alibaz-Oner F, Vautier M, Aksoy A, et al. Vascular Behçet's disease: a comparative study from Türkiye and France. Clin Exp Rheumatol. 2022;40(8):1491–6.
13. Seyahi E, Cakmak OS, Tutar B, et al. Clinical and ultrasonographic evaluation of lower-extremity vein thrombosis in Behcet syndrome: an observational study. Medicine (Baltimore). 2015;94(44):e1899.
14. Alibaz-Oner F, Aldag B, Aldag M, et al. Post-thrombotic syndrome and venous disease-specific quality of life in patients with vascular Behçet's disease. J Vasc Surg Venous Lymphat Disord. 2016;4(3):301–6.
15. Ozguler Y, Hatemi G, Cetinkaya F, et al. Clinical course of acute deep vein thrombosis of the legs in Behçet's syndrome. Rheumatology (Oxford). 2020;59(4):799–806.
16. Kahn SR, Ginsberg JS. Relationship between deep venous thrombosis and the postthrombotic syndrome. Arch Intern Med. 2004;164:17–26.
17. Jung JY, Kim DY, Bang D. Leg ulcers in Behcet's disease. Br J Dermatol. 2008;158(1):178–9.
18. Aksoy A, Colak S, Yagiz B, et al. Predictors for the risk and severity of post-thrombotic syndrome in vascular Behçet's disease. J Vasc Surg Venous Lymphat Disord. 2021;9(6):1451–9.
19. Seyahi E. Behcet's disease: how to diagnose and treat vascular involvement. Best Pract Res Clin Rheumatol. 2016;30(2):279–95.
20. Kansu E, Ozer FL, Akalin E, et al. Behcet's syndrome with obstruction of the venae cavae. A report of seven cases. Q J Med. 1972;41(162):151–68.
21. Houman H, Lamloum M, Ben Ghorbel I, et al. Vena cava thrombosis in Behcet's disease. Analysis of a series of 10 cases. Ann Med Interne (Paris). 1999;150(8):587–90.
22. Bettiol A, Alibaz-Oner F, Direskeneli H, et al. Vascular Behçet syndrome: from pathogenesis to treatment. Nat Rev Rheumatol. 2023;19(2):111–26.
23. Seyahi E, Caglar E, Ugurlu S, et al. An outcome survey of 43 patients with Budd-Chiari syndrome due to Behçet's syndrome followed up at a single, dedicated center. Semin Arthritis Rheum. 2015;44(5):602–9.
24. Akyol L, Toz B, Bayındır Ö, et al. Budd-Chiari syndrome in Behçet's disease: a retrospective multicenter study. Clin Rheumatol. 2022;41(1):177–86.
25. Desbois AC, Rautou PE, Biard L, et al. Behcet's disease in Budd-Chiari syndrome. Orphanet J Rare Dis. 2014;9:104.
26. Sakr MA, Reda MA, Ebada HE, et al. Characteristics and outcome of primary Budd-Chiari syndrome due to Behçet's syndrome. Clin Res Hepatol Gastroenterol. 2020;44(4):503–12. pii: S2210-7401(19)30249-9.
27. Akman-Demir G, Serdaroglu P, Tasçi B. Clinical patterns of neurological involvement in Behçet's disease: evaluation of 200 patients. The Neuro-Behçet Study Group. Brain. 1999;122(Pt 11):2171–82.
28. Uluduz D, Midi I, Duman T, et al. Behçet's disease as a causative factor of cerebral venous inüs thrombosis: subgroup analysis of data from the VENOST study. Rheumatology (Oxford). 2019;58(4):600–8.
29. Emekli AS, Doğan FU, Gündüz T, et al. Lesion probability map in cerebral vein thrombosis due to Behçet's disease. Int J Rheum Dis. 2023;26:145–50.
30. Saadoun D, Wechsler B, Resche-Rigon M, et al. Cerebral venous thrombosis in Behçet's disease. Arthritis Rheum. 2009;61(4):518–26.
31. Aguiar de Sousa D, Mestre T, Ferro JM. Cerebral venous thrombosis in Behçet's disease: a systematic review. J Neurol. 2011;258(5):719–27.
32. Hamuryudan V, Er T, Seyahi E, et al. Pulmonary artery aneurysms in Behçet syndrome. Am J Med. 2004;117:867–70.
33. Tsukui D, Hirohata S, Kikuchi H, et al. Histopathology of pulmonary thromboembolism in a patient with Behcet's disease. Clin Exp Rheumatol. 2022;40(8):1584–7.
34. Seyahi E, Melikoglu M, Akman C, et al. Pulmonary artery involvement and associated lung disease in Behcet disease: a series of 47 patients. Medicine (Baltimore). 2012;91(1):35–48.
35. Uzun O, Akpolat T, Erkan L. Pulmonary vasculitis in Behcet disease: a cumulative analysis. Chest. 2005;127(6):2243–53.
36. Lakhanpal S, Tani K, Lie JT, et al. Pathologic features of Behcet's syndrome: a review of Japanese autopsy registry data. Hum Pathol. 1985;16(8):790–5.
37. Eroglu DS, Torgutalp M, Baysal S, et al. Clinical characteristics of pulmonary artery involvement in patients

with Behcet's syndrome: single-centre experience of 61 patients. Clin Rheumatol. 2021;40(10):4127–34.
38. Abacar K, Boncukcuoglu AE, Aksoy A, et al. Anticoagulant treatment in addition to immunosuppressives decrease the relapse rate in pulmonary involvement of Behçet's disease. J Turk Soc Rheumatol. 2023;15(Suppl):2.
39. Yuan S. Pulmonary artery aneurysms in Behçet disease. J Vasc Bras. 2014;13(3):217–28.
40. Tunaci M, Ozkorkmaz B, Tunaci A, et al. CT findings of pulmonary artery aneurysms during treatment for Behcet's disease. AJR Am J Roentgenol. 1999;172(3):729–33.
41. Chae EJ, Do KH, Seo JB, et al. Radiologic and clinical findings of Behcet disease: comprehensive review of multisystemic involvement. Radiographics. 2008;28(5):e31.
42. Tuzun H, Seyahi E, Arslan C, et al. Management and prognosis of nonpulmonary large arterial disease in patients with Behçet disease. J Vasc Surg. 2012;55:157–63.
43. Tuzun H, Beşirli K, Sayin A, et al. Management of aneurysms in Behcet's syndrome: an analysis of 24 patients. Surgery. 1997;121(2):150–6.
44. Kwon TW, Park SJ, Kim HK, et al. Surgical treatment result of abdominal aortic aneurysm in Behçet's disease. Eur J Vasc Endovasc Surg. 2008;35:173–80.
45. Saadoun D, Asli B, Wechsler B, et al. Long-term outcome of arterial lesions in Behçet disease: a series of 101 patients. Medicine (Baltimore). 2012;91(1):18–24.
46. Emmungil H, Yaşar Bilge NŞ, Küçükşahin O, et al. A rare but serious manifestation of Behçet's disease: intracardiac thrombus in 22 patients. Clin Exp Rheumatol. 2014;32(4 Suppl 84):S87–92. Epub 2014 Jul 28.
47. Lee I, Park S, Hwang I, et al. Cardiac Behcet disease presenting as aortic valvulitis/aortitis or right heart inflammatory mass: a clinicopathologic study of 12 cases. Am J Surg Pathol. 2008;32(3):390–8.
48. Fei Y, Li X, Lin S, et al. Major vascular involvement in Behcet's disease: a retrospective study of 796 patients. Clin Rheumatol. 2013;32(6):845–52.
49. Farouk H, Zayed HS, El-Chilali K. Cardiac findings in patients with Behcet's disease: facts and controversies. Anatol J Cardiol. 2016;16(7):529–33.
50. Geri G, Wechsler B, Thi Huong DL, et al. Spectrum of cardiac lesions in Behcet disease: a series of 52 patients and review of the literature. Medicine (Baltimore). 2012;91(1):25–34.
51. Tutar B, Kantarci F, Cakmak OS, et al. Assessment of deep venous thrombosis in the lower extremity in Behçet's syndrome: MR venography versus Doppler ultrasonography. Intern Emerg Med. 2019;14(5):705–11.
52. Tunaci A, Berkmen YM, Gokmen E. Thoracic involvement in Behcet's disease: pathologic, clinical, and imaging features. AJR Am J Roentgenol. 1995;164(1):51–6.
53. Bonneville F. Imaging of cerebral venous thrombosis. Diagn Interv Imaging. 2014;95(12):1145–50.
54. Esatoglu SN, Seyahi E, Ugurlu S, et al. Bronchial artery enlargement may be the cause of recurrent haemoptysis in Behcet's syndrome patients with pulmonary artery involvement during follow-up. Clin Exp Rheumatol. 2016;34(6 Suppl 102):92–6.
55. Mehdipoor G, Davatchi F, Ghoreishian H, et al. Imaging manifestations of Behcet's disease: key considerations and major features. Eur J Radiol. 2018;98:214–25.
56. Lin M, Xue Q, You X, et al. Cerebral venous sinus thrombosis caused by neuro-Behçet disease accidentally detected by 68Ga-FAPI PET/CT. Clin Nucl Med. 2021;46(12):1028–9.
57. Cho SB, Yun M, Lee JH, et al. Detection of cardiovascular system involvement in Behcet's disease using fluorodeoxyglucose positron emission tomography. Semin Arthritis Rheum. 2011;40(5):461–6.
58. Trad S, Bensimhon L, El Hajjam M, et al. 18F-fluorodeoxyglucose-positron emission tomography scanning is a useful tool for therapy evaluation of arterial aneurysm in Behcet's disease. Joint Bone Spine. 2013;80(4):420–3.
59. Bradbury AW, Milne AA, Murie JA. Surgical aspects of Behçet's disease. Br J Surg. 1994;81:1712–21.
60. Kuzu A, Köksoy C, Ozaslan C, et al. Evaluation of peripheral vascular system disorders in vascular symptom—free Behçet's disease. Cardiovasc Surg. 1996;4(3):381–3.
61. Kisacik B, Oren C, Kasifoglu T, et al. Investigation of the veins in patients with Behçet's disease with no known vascular event by Doppler ultrasonography. Rheumatol Int. 2012;32(2):303–6.
62. Alibaz-Oner F, Karatay E, Akpinar IN, et al. Evaluation of asymptomatic venous disease by venous Doppler ultrasonography in patients with Behcet's disease without overt thrombosis. Clin Rheumatol. 2014;33(2):277–80.
63. Ambrose N, Pierce IT, Gatehouse PD, et al. Magnetic resonance imaging of vein wall thickness in patients with Behçet's syndrome. Clin Exp Rheumatol. 2014;32:S99–102.
64. Alibaz-Oner F, Mutis A, Ergelen R, et al. Venous vessel wall thickness in lower extremity is increased in male Behcet's disease patients without vascular involvement. Rheumatology (Oxford). 2017;56;Suppl 3.
65. Alibaz-Oner F, Ergelen R, Mutis A, et al. Venous vessel wall thickness in lower extremity is increased in male patients with Behçet's disease. Clin Rheumatol. 2019;38(5):1447–51.
66. Tezcan D, Özer H, Gülcemal S, et al. Diagnostic performance of lower extremity venous wall thickness and laboratory findings in the diagnosis of the Behçet disease. J Clin Rheumatol. 2022;28(2):e521–7.
67. Kaymaz S, Yilmaz H, Ufuk F, et al. Ultrasonographic measurement of the vascular wall thickness and intima-media thickness in patients with Behçet's

disease with symptoms or signs of vascular involvement: a cross-sectional study. Arch Rheumatol. 2021;36(2):258–66.
68. Alibaz-Oner F, Ergelen R, Yıldız Y, et al. Femoral vein wall thickness measurement: a new diagnostic tool for Behçet's disease. Rheumatology (Oxford). 2021;60(1):288–96.
69. Atalay E, Oguz B, Sener S, et al. A new tool supporting the diagnosis of childhood-onset Behçet's disease: venous wall thickness. Rheumatology (Oxford). 2023;62(SI2):SI181–8.
70. Alibaz-Oner F, Ergelen R, Kutluğ-Ağaçkıran S, et al. Common femoral vein wall thickness measurement as a diagnostic test in suspected Behçet's disease. Rheumatology (Oxford). 2023;8:kead476.
71. Sevik G, Ergelen R, Ağaçkıran SK, et al. Intima-media thickness of common femoral vein is increased in Behçet's disease. Clin Immunol. 2023;250:109306.
72. Kutluğ Ağaçkıran S, Sünbül M, Doğan Z, et al. Pulmonary arterial wall thickness increased in Behçet's disease patients with major organ involvement: is it a sign of severity? Rheumatology (Oxford). 2023;62(3):1238–42.
73. Abacar K, Ergelen R, Temiz F, et al. Does vein wall thickness have prognostic value in Behcet's disease? A prospective follow up study [abstract]. Arthritis Rheumatol. 2022;74(Suppl 9).

Management of Cardiovascular Involvement in Behçet's Disease

16

Sinem Nihal Esatoglu
and Vedat Hamuryudan

Contents

16.1 Venous Involvement

Case Vignette *A 22-year-old male patient was diagnosed with Behçet syndrome (BS) based on a 4-year history of recurrent oral and genital ulcers and erythema nodosum. He presented with an acute-onset headache and blurred vision in both eyes. An ophthalmologic examination showed bilateral papilledema. Magnetic resonance revealed cerebral venous sinus thrombosis in the right transverse sinus and right sigmoid sinus* (Fig. 16.1). *Chest and abdomen computed tomography angiography, echocardiography, and lower extremity venous Doppler ultrasonography did not detect any other vascular involvement.*

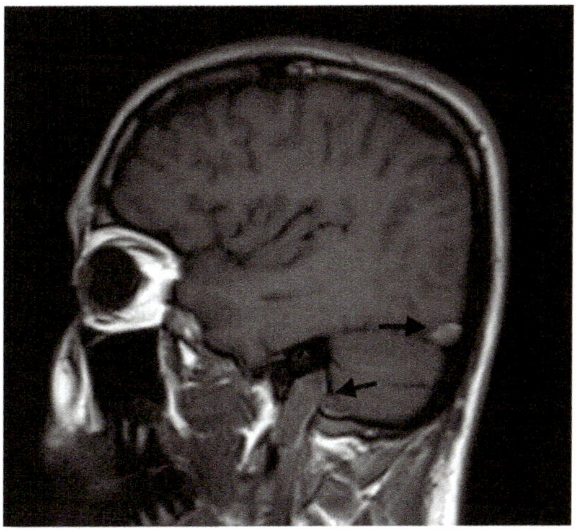

Fig. 16.1 Contrast-enhanced magnetic resonance imaging shows abnormal high signal on the T1-weighted images due to thrombosis in the right transverse sinus and right sigmoid sinus

The management of deep vein thrombosis (DVT) in BS differs from other causes of DVT and primarily involves the use of immunosuppressives. This is because vessel wall inflamma-

S. N. Esatoglu · V. Hamuryudan (✉)
Division of Rheumatology, Department of Internal Medicine, Cerrahpaşa Medical Faculty, Istanbul University-Cerrahpaşa, Istanbul, Türkiye

Behçet's Disease Research Center, Cerrahpaşa Medical Faculty, Istanbul University-Cerrahpaşa, Istanbul, Türkiye

E. Alpsoy et al. (eds.), *Behçet's Disease: An Integrated Approach*,
https://doi.org/10.1007/978-3-031-77251-1_16

tion, rather than thrombophilic factors, is thought to be the main cause of thrombosis in BS. Although we do not routinely screen BS patients for thrombophilic factors, thrombophilia testing may be considered for patients with relapsing disease despite adequate immunosuppressive therapy to guide management. The 2018 EULAR recommendations for the management of BS endorse the use of immunosuppressives, including azathioprine (AZA), cyclosporine-A, and cyclophosphamide (CYC), along with glucocorticoids for acute DVT. Monoclonal tumor necrosis factor-alpha (TNF) antibodies are reserved for cases with refractory disease. The addition of anticoagulants to immunosuppressives remains a subject of debate in the management of vascular involvement in BS, and the task force has decided to recommend its use in patients with refractory DVT with great caution, taking into consideration the potential risk of bleeding [1]. The main concern in the use of anticoagulants in BS is pulmonary artery involvement (PAI). Given that PAI and DVT in the lower extremities usually occur in the same patient, pulmonary artery aneurysm (PAA) should be excluded before starting anticoagulants even in patients who are asymptomatic for PAA. This concern also remains in patients with pulmonary artery thrombosis (PAT) as PAT may progress to PAA in some patients [2].

The EULAR recommendations on the use of immunosuppressives for venous involvement in BS were based on three retrospective studies that showed a reduction in the relapse rate of thrombosis with the use of immunosuppressives. In the initial study by Ahn and colleagues the relapse rate was 12.5% in the immunosuppressives-only group compared to 75% in the anticoagulation-alone group [3]. The second study demonstrated a thrombosis relapse rate of 5.8% in patients using immunosuppressives combined with anticoagulants, in contrast to 43.5% in those using anticoagulants alone [4]. The third study reported relapse rates of 29% in the immunosuppressives-only group, 22% in the combination group, and 92% in the anticoagulants-only group [5]. A meta-analysis of these studies demonstrated a significant decrease in the risk of relapse with the use of immunosuppressives (RR 0.17, 95% CI 0.08–0.35), whereas anticoagulants exhibited no significant reduction in relapse risk (RR 0.75, 95% CI 0.48–1.17) [6]. However, relapse rate was 20% (29/142) in the combination group and 27% (30/112) in the immunosuppressives-only group, suggesting that a type 2 error may be operative. After the release of the recommendations, three retrospective studies have been published. Two of them observed no benefit of adding anticoagulants to immunosuppressives in reducing the relapse rate of DVT [7, 8]. In the third study, direct oral anticoagulants (DOACs) were assessed in the prevention of relapses in patients with DVT [9]. In Cox analysis, DOACs with or without immunosuppressives were associated with a reduced relapse risk compared to no DOACs. Eight of the 13 relapses occurred after DOACs had been discontinued. However, this study lacked a control group and patients who discontinued DOACs during the study were used as a comparative group.

The benefit of adding anticoagulants to immunosuppressives for preventing post-thrombotic syndrome (PTS), a severe complication of DVT in the lower extremities, has been studied in three retrospective studies with conflicting results. While two studies from the Marmara group showed no benefit with the addition of anticoagulants to immunosuppressives [10, 11], the Cerrahpaşa group found a 3.8-fold increase in the development of severe PTS with the use of only immunosuppressives [12]. However, in the second study from the Marmara group, the authors observed increased recanalization and more collateral vessels in the combination group compared with the immunosuppressives-only group [10]. In the light of these retrospective studies, a definitive decision on whether to add anticoagulants to immunosuppressives in venous involvement in BS remains elusive.

Another controversial issue is the choice of immunosuppressive drug. Conventional immunosuppressive agents include AZA, methotrexate (MTX), mycophenolate mofetil (MMF), cyclosporine-A, CYC, and interferon-alpha (IFN). Among these, AZA is the most commonly preferred immunosuppressive agent for DVT in the lower extremities in BS, and CYC for venous involvement with higher morbidity and mortality such as hepatic, mesenteric, portal, and vena cava involvement [13]. In a prospective study by the Cerrahpaşa group and in a cross-sectional study from the Marmara group, IFN resulted in a higher rate of recanalization in patients with DVT in the lower extremities [10, 14]. However, due to difficulties in access, its use is limited worldwide.

Our group prospectively followed 33 patients with DVT in the lower extremities for a mean of 40.7 ± 13.4 SD months [14]. Twenty-nine patients were initially treated with AZA, two with CYC, and two with IFN. The relapse rates of 29%, 37%, and 45% at 6, 12, and 24 months, respectively, were higher than those observed in retrospective studies. In other words, 15 of the 33 patients experienced a relapse at 2 years despite AZA therapy. The effective dosage of AZA is another critical consideration in the treatment of BS. A retrospective study investigated the effectiveness of the optimal AZA dose in preventing relapse rates in 78 patients with predominantly venous involvement [15]. Relapse-free survival was significantly longer in patients receiving AZA at a dose of >2 mg/kg/day than in those receiving AZA at a dose of <2 mg/kg/day.

In the management of venous involvement in BS, the primary goal is to prevent relapses in the same vessel or at different vessels to reduce morbidity and mortality. A retrospective study from the Marmara group including 806 patients with various types of involvement showed that any major event, defined as a relapse and/or the development of de novo major organ involvement, was more common in patients receiving conventional immunosuppressives than in those treated with biologic agents including monoclonal TNF antibodies and IFN [16]. In patients with venous involvement, the high relapse rates with conventional immunosuppressives raise questions whether biologics agents might be a better option.

Among biologic agents, monoclonal TNF antibodies, especially infliximab (IFX) and adalimumab (ADA), are frequently used. Only one study has compared a biologic agent with conventional immunosuppressives. In this retrospective study of 70 patients with venous involvement, 35 patients received conventional immunosuppressives, while 35 were administered ADA, with 8 of them also receiving conventional immunosuppressives [8]. Patients treated with ADA exhibited a higher response rate, a shorter time to vascular response, and a more pronounced glucocorticoid-sparing effect compared to those treated only with conventional immunosuppressives. The Cerrahpaşa group also demonstrated a low relapse rate among 61 patients with DVT treated with IFX [17]. The remission rate was 82% and 70% at month 6 and 12, respectively. During a mean follow-up of 40 ± 28 SD months, relapse rate was only 7% and 15 of the patients were able to discontinue IFX therapy due to remission. Adding conventional immunosuppressives to biologics did not provide a benefit in the two studies. Infections, especially tuberculosis and infusion reactions are the most reported serious adverse events with IFX use.

Our current approach for the management of venous involvement, along with pulmonary and extrapulmonary artery involvement, is depicted in Fig. 16.2. It now involves the use of AZA at a dose of 2.5 mg/kg/day in combination with glucocorticoids (0.5–1 mg/kg/day) for the initial treatment of DVT in the lower extremities and superficial thrombophlebitis. Additionally, AZA is used in combination with three pulses of 1 g methylprednisolone followed by high-dose oral prednisolone (1 mg/kg/day) for the initial treatment of cerebral venous sinus thrombosis. We prefer to initiate AZA in patients with cerebral venous sinus thrombosis due to its association with thrombosis at other sites [18], and in patients with superficial thrombophlebitis due to its association with the development of DVT at different vessels [19]. In relapsed or refractory disease, monoclonal TNF antibodies are the preferred options. For venous thrombosis at other locations such as the superior vena cava, inferior vena cava, hepatic veins, portal veins, mesenteric veins, and intracardiac thrombosis, CYC or monoclonal TNF antibodies combined with high-dose glucocorticoids are administered. This includes an initial three pulses of 1 g methylprednisolone followed by high-dose oral prednisolone (1 mg/kg/day), gradually tapered after 1 month by 10 mg monthly, and then maintained

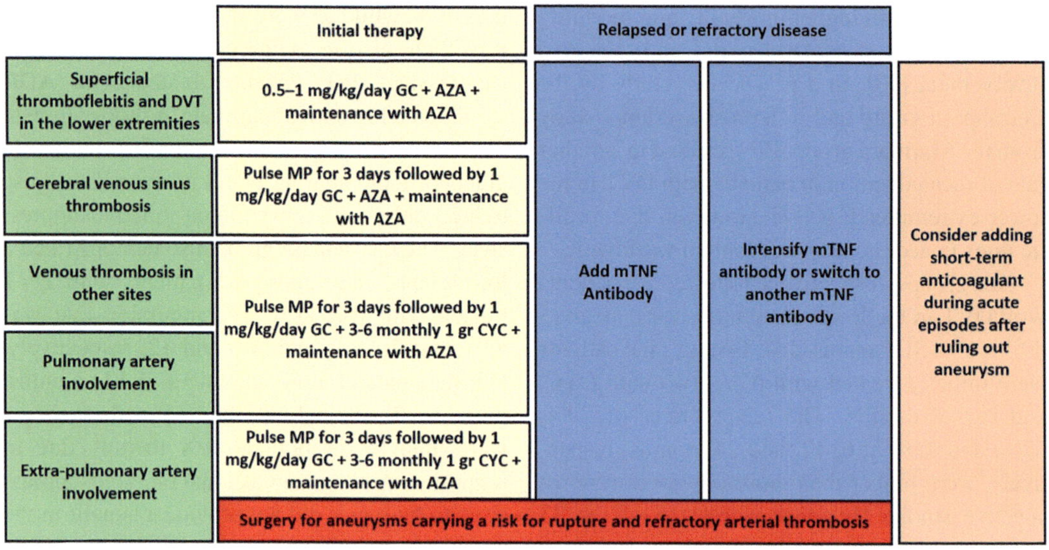

Fig. 16.2 Management of vascular involvement in Behçet syndrome. AZA: azathioprine; CYC: cyclophosphamide; DVT: deep vein thrombosis; GC: glucocorticoid (prednisolone); mTNF: monoclonal tumor necrosis factor-alpha; Pulse MP: 1 g intravenous methylprednisolone; Infliximab or adalimumab are the initial preferred agents among the mTNF antibodies

at a dose of 5 mg/day for at least 1 year. Short-duration anticoagulants may be considered in patients with DVT after ruling out aneurysms. As we have observed toxicity including malignancy and infertility in a significant proportion of patients treated with CYC [20], the use of CYC is limited to 6–12 months. AZA or monoclonal TNF antibodies in combination with AZA are used to maintain remission. In patients with relapses on monoclonal TNF antibodies, switching to another monoclonal TNF antibody, or intensification of IFX (10 mg/kg or reducing intervals to 4 weeks) or ADA (weekly dose) may be considered. MMF, MTX, and cyclosporine-A are the other options for patients intolerant to AZA. The optimal duration of immunosuppressive therapy is not known, and we do not recommend surgery for venous involvement due to the high risk of complications [21].

Venous ulcers in BS result from recurrent DVT in the lower extremities. These ulcers have a tendency to relapse and are often refractory to treatment, possibly, because they represent damage from PTS. While there is a lack of controlled data, efforts are made to manage these ulcers using immunosuppressives, along with interventions such as rest, elevation, compression stockings, wound care including dressings, and the application of topical agents and vasodilators like pentoxifylline and iloprost [17].

Follow-Up of the Case *We initiated three pulses of 1 g methylprednisolone followed by high-dose glucocorticoids, AZA, low-molecular-weight heparin, and acetazolamide. His symptoms improved with the initial therapy, and low-molecular-weight heparin and acetazolamide were discontinued at month 3. Three years later, he developed DVT in the left superficial femoral vein while on AZA and low-dose prednisolone, and IFX was added. Two years later, he had DVT in the right common iliac vein, and IFX was switched to ADA.*

16.2 Pulmonary Artery Involvement

Case Vignette *A 24-year-old male patient was diagnosed with BS due to a 2-year history of recurrent oral and scrotal ulcers, along with acne- or folliculitis-like papulopustular lesions.*

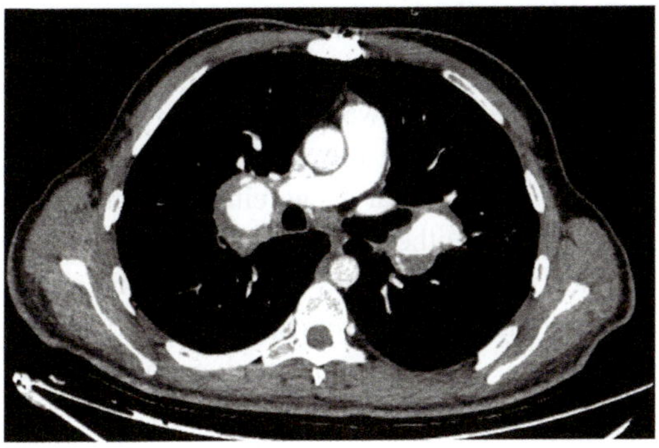

Fig. 16.3 Computed tomography scan of the chest shows bilateral pulmonary artery aneurysms

Two years later, while using colchicine, he developed bilateral DVT in the lower extremities. AZA was added to treatment, but he was lost to follow-up. Four years later, he was admitted to the emergency ward because of abundant hemoptysis that had been followed by fever and nonproductive cough for 1 week. A chest computed tomography scan revealed multiple bilateral aneurysms in the lower lobe pulmonary arteries (Fig. 16.3).

PAI, especially in the form of PAA, should be considered as a medical emergency due to its high mortality rate because of the risk of aneurysm rupture resulting in massive hemoptysis. In BS, PAI can also manifest as PAT with or without aneurysm. A previous retrospective study from our center showed that early diagnosis and early treatment were significantly associated with increased survival of patients with PAI [22].

The classical induction treatment of PAI, endorsed by the 2018 EULAR recommendations for the treatment of patients with BS, consists of high dose glucocorticoids and CYC [1]. Glucocorticoids are initially given as three consecutive daily intravenous pulses of 1 g methylprednisolone followed by prednisolone 1 mg/kg/day that is tapered down monthly by 10 mg and then maintained at a dose of 5–10 mg/day for 1–2 years. CYC is given as monthly 1 g intravenous pulses and is usually continued for 1 year. In case of good clinical response, which can be defined as amelioration of symptoms, normalization of acute phase responses and lack of radiological worsening, CYC is replaced with AZA 2.5 mg/kg/day for maintenance for several years. MMF, extrapolated from its use in other immune-mediated diseases, appears to be another choice for maintenance but experience with this agent in BS literature is limited and inconsistent [23]. In 2004, in a cohort of 26 patients with PAA we reported 1-year mortality of 15% and 5-year survival rate of 62% [22]. In 2012, in a new cohort of 47 patients the survival rate was 74% at 7 years [2]. Similarly, a retrospective study from a single center in France on 101 BS patients with arterial involvement reported that 3 of 21 patients with PAI had died during a median follow-up of 7 years [24].

CYC is by no doubt a potent drug for vascular involvement of BS but its use is associated with severe adverse events that may develop even after several years. In a retrospective study on 198 BS patients who had received at least one dose of CYC, we had observed the occurrence of short term (within 1 year following the initiation of CYC) adverse events like hemorrhagic cystitis and infections in 9% of the patients [20]. After a median follow-up of 25 years, 15 patients (8%) developed malignancies and 26 patients (30%) experienced infertility, underlining the need for safer treatment options.

Experience from observational studies has shown that monoclonal TNF antibodies, especially IFX and ADA are effective for all severe complications of BS [25]. IFX 5 mg/kg is given at weeks 0, 2, and 6, and every 6–8 weeks thereafter usually in combination with AZA 2.5 mg/kg/day. The dose can be increased to 10 mg/kg when clinically needed [26]. ADA 40 mg every other week is also an option. Until now, 6 retrospective studies, including 2 from our center, have reported 59 BS patients with PAI treated either with IFX or ADA in the English literature [17, 27–31].

A retrospective study from our center reported 122 BS patients with various vascular involvement including 38 with PAI, who have been treated with IFX between 2004 and 2022 [17]. Most of these patients were refractory to or had relapses during previous treatment with conventional immunosuppressives. IFX was combined with AZA in more than 70% of the patients. At months 6 and 12, the remission rates of the patients with PAI were 84% and 68%, respectively. IFX was discontinued in 7 patients with PAI due to remission after a mean treatment duration of 26 months. Three of them remained in remission but the remaining 4 experienced relapses between 21 and 79 months after IFX discontinuation. Two further patients with PAT died because of right heart failure as a complication of pulmonary hypertension during follow-up. Infusion reactions and infections were the main adverse events leading to withdrawal of IFX treatment. In a French study, two patients relapsed under monoclonal TNF antibody therapy, but both responded favorably to decreasing the interval between infusions [29]. Considering the favorable results obtained with IFX and ADA, along with the notorious toxicity of CYC treatment, these agents are now being started earlier following a 3–6 months induction with CYC as maintenance treatment or even used as first line replacing CYC in the treatment of PAI. In fact, Baki et al. reported the first successful use of IFX as a first-line treatment in a case of BS with PAA [32]. However, these agents should not be regarded as the final solution and patients should be closely followed up for loss of efficacy or relapses over time. In a retrospective survey we have observed development of de novo BS manifestations (a new manifestation that was not present before) in 7% of 282 BS patients including three patients who developed PAI while receiving treatment with IFX for various BS manifestations during a median follow-up of 3 years [17].

The use of anticoagulants is still a controversial issue in BS. According to the 2018 EULAR recommendations anticoagulation might be conditionally used in BS patients with refractory venous thrombosis after ruling out existing aneurysms [1]. However, almost all patients with PAI have associated venous thrombosis and/or intracardiac thrombus formation, making a clinical decision difficult. In a retrospective study from Türkiye 30 of 61 BS patients with PAI (49%) received anticoagulants in addition to immunosuppressives. Of these, 29 had isolated PAT and 1 had PAA complicated with atrial fibrillation. The relapse rate was 25% in the anticoagulation group and 55% in the non-anticoagulated group, with an absolute risk reduction of 30% and no hemorrhagic complication was observed [33]. However, relapse in this study was defined as the reoccurrence of any vascular event, either in pulmonary arteries or in other vascular structures and no detailed information was available on the site of relapse. In another retrospective study from Türkiye the use of anticoagulation was not associated with vascular relapses or anti-TNF drug survival in nine patients with PAI [28]. In a retrospective study from France on 101 BS patients with arterial involvement, including 21 patients with PAI, anticoagulation was given to 47 patients (46.5%) in addition to immunosuppressives. Anticoagulation was used in cases of arterial occlusions/stenosis and in a few cases of thrombosed aneurysms. Although no hemorrhagic complications were observed, only the use of immunosuppressives but not anticoagulation was associated with complete remission [24]. Anticoagulation, at the first instance, might perhaps appear to be reasonable for patients with isolated PAT, but in our survey of 47 PAI patients one-fourth of patients with isolated PAT developed PAA during follow-up [2].

In emergent cases presenting with massive hemoptysis endovascular embolization of the bleeding aneurysms with coils or cyanoacrylate might be lifesaving [34, 35]. A retrospective study from France reported immediate control of hemoptysis following embolization in nine BS patients along with eight additional cases from the literature [36]. Two patients developed pulmonary infarction and one patient experienced worsening of pulmonary hypertension as the complications of the procedure. Immunosuppressive treatment was continued in 15 (88%) patients. Hemoptysis recurred in seven patients after a median of 7 months following embolization which was related to bronchial artery enlargement. Embolization of the bronchial arteries was performed in four patients but this was effective in two patients. The overall 1-year mortality of the 17 patients was 24%. In our center, six patients with PAI underwent bronchial artery embolization for continuing hemoptysis that could be not explained with active PAI

[37]. One patient with severe pulmonary hypertension died 3 weeks following embolization, the remaining five patients remained under follow-up for between 5 months and 9 years. Pulmonary infarction and mild hemiparesis were short-term complications in two patients, respectively. Surgical treatment and endarterectomy will be discussed in another chapter of this book.

Follow-Up of the Case *The patient was initially treated with 1 g pulsed methylprednisolone and then underwent emergent endovascular embolization of the bleeding aneurysm with cyanoacrylate which enabled immediate control of hemoptysis. His medical treatment was continued with two additional methylprednisolone boluses followed by oral glucocorticoid and monthly 1 g CYC, which was replaced with IFX 5 mg/kg 3 months later. He remained symptom-free during his follow-up and a repeat chest computed tomography scan 1 year later revealed the complete disappearance of the aneurysms, except for a single persisting one that diminished in size. He continued to receive IFX.*

16.3 Extrapulmonary Artery Involvement (EPAI)

Arterial occlusions that are asymptomatic or causing mild ischemic symptoms and small saccular aneurysms may be managed with medical treatment only [24, 38]. However, aneurysms of the aorta and peripheral aneurysms usually need surgery or endovascular intervention due to rupture risk. Follow-up after surgery is complicated by suture dehiscence, graft thrombosis, development of aneurysms at the anastomosis site and new aneurysms [38, 39]. In order to decrease the risk of these complications, except in emergency situations, surgical intervention is usually deferred until the disease activity has been controlled with immunosuppressives that are also continued after surgery. A retrospective study from France on 23 BS patients who underwent 47 operations for arterial involvement showed that patients receiving preoperative immunosuppressives had significantly less recurrence rates (28%) compared to that observed (75%) in untreated patients [39].

Similar to PAI treatment, high-dose glucocorticoids that are tapered over several months and monthly infusions of CYC are endorsed by the 2018 EULAR recommendations for the treatment of arterial involvement [1]. Maintenance treatment is usually made with AZA for several years [40, 41]. The remission rate with this treatment was 39% in a French series of 101 patients with arterial involvement and relapses were observed in 28% of the patients during a median follow-up of 13 months [24]. The monoclonal TNF antibodies, IFX and ADA, are being increasingly used in patients with vascular involvement who are refractory to CYC [27–29]. In our center, we have treated 16 BS patients with EPAI refractory to conventional immunosuppressive treatment with IFX [17]. The remission rates with IFX added to immunosuppressive treatment were 69% at month 6 and 63% at month 12, and the relapse rate was 44%. Six patients discontinued IFX, four due to inefficacy and two due to adverse events. The response rates for EPAI in this study were lower compared to PAI and venous involvement, indicating the refractory nature of EPAI to treatment.

Observational studies suggest that tocilizumab, an IL-6 receptor inhibitor, might be beneficial in patients refractory to monoclonal TNF antibodies [42–44]. Two retrospective studies from China reported favorable results with the JAK inhibitors tofacitinib and baricitinib in the treatment of vascular BS [45, 46]. However, due to the increased risk of venous thromboembolism observed with JAK inhibitors, these satisfactory results await confirmation with further studies.

References

1. Hatemi G, Christensen R, Bang D, Bodaghi B, Celik AF, Fortune F, et al. 2018 update of the EULAR recommendations for the management of Behcet's syndrome. Ann Rheum Dis. 2018;77(6):808–18.
2. Seyahi E, Melikoglu M, Akman C, Hamuryudan V, Ozer H, Hatemi G, et al. Pulmonary artery involvement and associated lung disease in Behcet disease: a series of 47 patients. Medicine (Baltimore). 2012;91(1):35–48.

3. Ahn JK, Lee YS, Jeon CH, Koh EM, Cha HS. Treatment of venous thrombosis associated with Behcet's disease: immunosuppressive therapy alone versus immunosuppressive therapy plus anticoagulation. Clin Rheumatol. 2008;27(2):201–5.
4. Desbois AC, Wechsler B, Resche-Rigon M, Piette JC, Huong Dle T, Amoura Z, et al. Immunosuppressants reduce venous thrombosis relapse in Behcet's disease. Arthritis Rheum. 2012;64(8):2753–60.
5. Alibaz-Oner F, Karadeniz A, Ylmaz S, Balkarl A, Kimyon G, Yazc A, et al. Behcet disease with vascular involvement: effects of different therapeutic regimens on the incidence of new relapses. Medicine (Baltimore). 2015;94(6):e494.
6. Ozguler Y, Leccese P, Christensen R, Esatoglu SN, Bang D, Bodaghi B, et al. Management of major organ involvement of Behcet's syndrome: a systematic review for update of the EULAR recommendations. Rheumatology (Oxford). 2018;57(12):2200–12.
7. Alibaz-Oner F, Vautier M, Aksoy A, Mirouse A, Le Joncour A, Cacoub P, et al. Vascular Behcet's disease: a comparative study from Turkey and France. Clin Exp Rheumatol. 2022;40(8):1491–6.
8. Emmi G, Vitale A, Silvestri E, Boddi M, Becatti M, Fiorillo C, et al. Adalimumab-based treatment versus disease-modifying antirheumatic drugs for venous thrombosis in Behcet's syndrome: a retrospective study of seventy patients with vascular involvement. Arthritis Rheumatol. 2018;70(9):1500–7.
9. Vautier M, Gallien Y, Emmi G, Bettiol A, Karadag O, Bolek EC, et al. Direct oral anticoagulant for venous thrombosis in Behcet's syndrome. Autoimmun Rev. 2021;20(4):102783.
10. Aksoy A, Colak S, Yagiz B, Coskun BN, Omma A, Yildiz Y, et al. Predictors for the risk and severity of post-thrombotic syndrome in vascular Behcet's disease. J Vasc Surg Venous Lymphat Disord. 2021;9(6):1451–9.
11. Alibaz-Oner F, Aldag B, Aldag M, Unal AU, Mutis A, Toptas T, et al. Post-thrombotic syndrome and venous disease-specific quality of life in patients with vascular Behcet's disease. J Vasc Surg Venous Lymphat Disord. 2016;4(3):301–6.
12. Seyahi E, Cakmak OS, Tutar B, Arslan C, Dikici AS, Sut N, et al. Clinical and ultrasonographic evaluation of lower-extremity vein thrombosis in Behcet syndrome: an observational study. Medicine (Baltimore). 2015;94(44):e1899.
13. Hellmich B, Agueda A, Monti S, Buttgereit F, de Boysson H, Brouwer E, et al. 2018 update of the EULAR recommendations for the management of large vessel vasculitis. Ann Rheum Dis. 2020;79(1):19–30.
14. Ozguler Y, Hatemi G, Cetinkaya F, Tascilar K, Hamuryudan V, Ugurlu S, et al. Clinical course of acute deep vein thrombosis of the legs in Behcet's syndrome. Rheumatology (Oxford). 2020;59(4):799–806.
15. Girgin S, Yurumez S, Omma A, Celik S, Cemal Icacan O, Bes C, et al. Comparison of relapse rates in Behcet's disease with venous involvement on different doses of azathioprine therapy, a retrospective observational study. Int J Rheum Dis. 2021;24(4):562–6.
16. Bozkurt T, Karabacak M, Karatas H, Kutlug Agackiran S, Ergun T, Direskeneli H, et al. Earlier and more aggressive treatment with biologics may prevent relapses and further new organ involvement in Behcet's disease. Clin Immunol. 2023;248:109263.
17. Hatemi G, Tukek NB, Esatoglu SN, Ozguler Y, Taflan SS, Uygunoglu U, et al. Infliximab for vascular involvement in Behcet's syndrome. Clin Immunol. 2023;253:109682.
18. Saadoun D, Wechsler B, Resche-Rigon M, Trad S, Le Thi Huong D, Sbai A, et al. Cerebral venous thrombosis in Behcet's disease. Arthritis Rheum. 2009;61(4):518–26.
19. Seyahi E, Yurdakul S. Behcet's syndrome and thrombosis. Mediterr J Hematol Infect Dis. 2011;3(1):e2011026.
20. Gurcan M, Esatoglu SN, Hamuryudan V, Saygin D, Ugurlu S, Seyahi E, et al. Long term follow-up of Behcet's syndrome patients treated with cyclophosphamide. Rheumatology (Oxford). 2020;59(9):2264–71.
21. Dincses E, Esatoglu SN, Fresko I, Melikoglu M, Seyahi E. Outcome of invasive procedures for venous thrombosis in Behcet's syndrome: case series and systematic literature review. Clin Exp Rheumatol. 2019;37 Suppl 121(6):125–31.
22. Hamuryudan V, Er T, Seyahi E, Akman C, Tuzun H, Fresko I, et al. Pulmonary artery aneurysms in Behcet syndrome. Am J Med. 2004;117(11):867–70.
23. Ucar D, Esatoglu SN, Cerme E, Batu-Oto B, Hamuryudan V, Seyahi E, et al. Mycophenolate mofetil may be an alternative for maintenance therapy of Behcet syndrome uveitis: a single-center retrospective analysis. Rheumatol Int. 2023;43(11):2099–106.
24. Saadoun D, Asli B, Wechsler B, Houman H, Geri G, Desseaux K, et al. Long-term outcome of arterial lesions in Behcet disease: a series of 101 patients. Medicine (Baltimore). 2012;91(1):18–24.
25. Desbois AC, Vallet H, Domont F, Comarmond C, Cacoub P, Saadoun D. Management of severe complications in Behcet's disease with TNF inhibitors. Expert Opin Biol Ther. 2017;17(7):853–9.
26. Ozguler Y, Esatoglu S, Seyahi E, Melikoglu M. Vascular and cardiac involvement. In: Yazici Y, Hatemi G, Seyahi E, Yazici H, editors. Behçet syndrome. Basel: Springer Nature; 2020. p. 83–104.
27. Kehribar DY, Ozgen M. Infliximab treatment in refractory vascular Behcet's disease: a single-center experience. Vascular. 2020;28(6):829–33.
28. Aksoy A, Yazici A, Omma A, Cefle A, Onen F, Tasdemir U, et al. Efficacy of TNFalpha inhibitors for refractory vascular Behcet's disease: a multicenter observational study of 27 patients and a review of the literature. Int J Rheum Dis. 2020;23(2):256–61.
29. Desbois AC, Biard L, Addimanda O, Lambert M, Hachulla E, Launay D, et al. Efficacy of anti-TNF alpha in severe and refractory major vessel involve-

ment of Behcet's disease: a multicenter observational study of 18 patients. Clin Immunol. 2018;197:54–9.
30. Chan E, Sangle SR, Coghlan JG, D'Cruz DD. Pulmonary artery aneurysms in Behcet's disease treated with anti-TNFalpha: a case series and review of the literature. Autoimmun Rev. 2016;15(4):375–8.
31. Hamuryudan V, Seyahi E, Ugurlu S, Melikoglu M, Hatemi G, Ozguler Y, et al. Pulmonary artery involvement in Behcet's syndrome: effects of anti-Tnf treatment. Semin Arthritis Rheum. 2015;45(3):369–73.
32. Baki K, Villiger PM, Jenni D, Meyer T, Beer JH. Behcet's disease with life-threatening haemoptoe and pulmonary aneurysms: complete remission after infliximab treatment. Ann Rheum Dis. 2006;65(11):1531–2.
33. Eroglu DS, Torgutalp M, Baysal S, Colaklar A, Sezer S, Yayla ME, et al. Clinical characteristics of pulmonary artery involvement in patients with Behcet's syndrome: single-centre experience of 61 patients. Clin Rheumatol. 2021;40(10):4127–34.
34. Cantasdemir M, Kantarci F, Mihmanli I, Akman C, Numan F, Islak C, et al. Emergency endovascular management of pulmonary artery aneurysms in Behcet's disease: report of two cases and a review of the literature. Cardiovasc Intervent Radiol. 2002;25(6):533–7.
35. Durieux P, Bletry O, Huchon G, Wechsler B, Chretien J, Godeau P. Multiple pulmonary arterial aneurysms in Behcet's disease and Hughes-Stovin syndrome. Am J Med. 1981;71(4):736–41.
36. Voiriot G, Parrot A, Antoine M, Gibelin A, Haddad S, Carette MF, et al. Transcatheter embolotherapy of pulmonary artery aneurysms as emergency treatment of hemoptysis in Behcet patients: experience of a referral center and a review of the literature. Intern Emerg Med. 2018;13(4):491–500.
37. Esatoglu SN, Seyahi E, Ugurlu S, Gulsen F, Akman C, Cantasdemir M, et al. Bronchial artery enlargement may be the cause of recurrent haemoptysis in Behcet's syndrome patients with pulmonary artery involvement during follow-up. Clin Exp Rheumatol. 2016;34(6 Suppl 102):92–6.
38. Tuzun H, Seyahi E, Arslan C, Hamuryudan V, Besirli K, Yazici H. Management and prognosis of nonpulmonary large arterial disease in patients with Behcet disease. J Vasc Surg. 2012;55(1):157–63.
39. Gaudric J, Jayet J, Saadoun D, Couture T, Ferfar Y, Davaine JM, et al. Factors influencing the recurrence of arterial involvement after surgical repair in Behcet disease. J Vasc Surg. 2020;72(5):1761–9.
40. Torgutalp M, Sahin Eroglu D, Sezer S, Yayla ME, Karatas G, Uslu Yurteri E, et al. Analysis of vascular involvement in 460 patients with Behcet's syndrome: clinical characteristics and associated factors. Joint Bone Spine. 2022;89(2):105277.
41. Tascilar K, Melikoglu M, Ugurlu S, Sut N, Caglar E, Yazici H. Vascular involvement in Behcet's syndrome: a retrospective analysis of associations and the time course. Rheumatology (Oxford). 2014;53(11):2018–22.
42. Arida A, Saadoun D, Sfikakis PP. IL-6 blockade for Behcet's disease: review on 31 anti-TNF naive and 45 anti-TNF experienced patients. Clin Exp Rheumatol. 2022;40(8):1575–83.
43. Zhong H, Liu T, Liu Y, Zhang X, Zhou Y, Su Y. Efficacy and safety of tocilizumab in Behcet's syndrome with refractory arterial lesions: a single-centre observational cohort study in China. Rheumatology (Oxford). 2022;61(7):2923–30.
44. Ding Y, Li C, Liu J, Yu X, Wang Y, Shi J, et al. Tocilizumab in the treatment of severe and/or refractory vasculo-Behcet's disease: a single-centre experience in China. Rheumatology (Oxford). 2018;57(11):2057–9.
45. Wang Z, Wang X, Liu W, Wang Y, Liu J, Zhang L, et al. Baricitinib for the treatment of refractory vascular Behcet's disease. Clin Immunol. 2023;250:109298.
46. Liu J, Hou Y, Sun L, Li C, Li L, Zhao Y, et al. A pilot study of tofacitinib for refractory Behcet's syndrome. Ann Rheum Dis. 2020;79(11):1517–20.

17 Surgical Approach in Cardiovascular Involvement of Behçet's Disease

Uğur Bengisun

Contents

17.1 Introduction

Nearly a century ago, Behçet's Disease (BD), discovered as a result of Dr. Hulusi Behçet's observations on his patients, is a disease characterized by recurrent aphthous ulcers and numerous systemic involvement [1–3]. In addition to recurrent oral aphthous ulcers, BD is now known to cause genital ulcers, skin lesions, arthritis, eye, neurological, gastrointestinal, and vascular involvement [4–10].

In this article, cardiovascular pathologies in BD and their surgical and endovascular treatment methods were evaluated. The subject was analyzed by examining the medical records of 1768 patients with BD in our clinical expertise, and 2 patients with peripheral aneurysms were presented.

17.2 Vascular Involvement

Vascular pathologies in BD mostly occur in the venous system. Superficial or deep vein thrombosis develops more frequently than arterial thrombosis. In BD, arterial system involvement mostly occurs as an aneurysm. It is reported in the literature that vascular involvement is seen in 7–49% of patients with BD [3–5, 9–21]. Vascular involvement was observed at 17.1% in our clinical experience between 1976 and 2020. In our clinical observations, similar rates of vascular involvement were detected in different periods (16.8% and 17.6% in 1976–1997 and 1998–2020, respectively). Vascular involvement was detected in 17.6% (n = 312) of 1768 BD between 1998

U. Bengisun (✉)
Division of Peripheral Vascular Surgery, Department of General Surgery, İbni Sina Hospital, University of Ankara, Ankara, Türkiye

E. Alpsoy et al. (eds.), *Behçet's Disease: An Integrated Approach*,
https://doi.org/10.1007/978-3-031-77251-1_17

Table 17.1 Patients with BD with vascular involvement between 1998 and 2020 [5]

Patients with BD with vascular involvement in Ankara University $n = 312$		
Superficial and/or deep vein thrombosis	290[a]	93%
Vena cava inferior syndrome	16	
Vena cava superior syndrome	5	
Thrombosis of internal jugular vein	1	
Budd–Chiari syndrome	1	
Thrombosis of pulmonary artery	14	
Pulmonary artery aneurysm	9	
Femoral artery aneurysm	5	
Abdominal aortic aneurysm	3	
Iliac artery aneurysm	2	
Popliteal artery aneurysm	1	
Carotid aneurysm	1	
Intracardiac thrombosis	1	

[a] Number of all patients with venous involvement

and 2020. Superficial and/or deep vein thrombosis was observed in 93% ($n = 290$) of 312 patients with BD with vascular involvement (Table 17.1) [5].

In some patients, the leading and diagnostic symptom of BD is vascular involvement. Vascular involvement affects male patients more and occurs at younger ages, and the average age of onset in our clinical observations is 31.73 ± 8.61 years [5].

17.3 Venous Involvement

Venous thrombosis is frequently seen in the lower extremity veins; mostly in the superficial veins of the crural region. These are erythematous, hard, and painful lesions resembling erythema nodosum in the superficial vein segment. Although thrombosis sometimes involves a segment of the vena saphena magna or parva, the clinically more important thrombosis occurs in deep veins. Thrombosis frequently occurs in the popliteal and femoral veins. Additionally, superior and inferior vena cava, iliac veins, internal jugular veins, and hepatic veins are also affected by thrombosis. Pulmonary embolism is rare. However, thrombosis and aneurysms in the pulmonary artery are relatively common [11–17].

The pathogenesis of vascular involvement in BD is not yet fully known. Venous thrombosis in BD is associated with nonspecific vasculitis and hypercoagulability. In BD, neutrophil-predominant vasculitis is present and vasculitis affects all layers of the vascular wall and vasa vasorum, and may reveal fibrous thickening and nonspecific inflammatory infiltration in the late phase. Although various factors that may predispose patients to thrombosis have been investigated, various studies suggest that endothelial dysfunction in BD develops as a result of inflammation. This inflammation is due to the immune response and creates a predisposition to thrombosis. Hypercoagulability with excessive thrombin generation, decreased fibrinolysis, platelet hyperactivity, and formation of platelet/neutrophil complexes occurs in association with BD vasculitis. All these changes may facilitate the formation of thrombosis [3, 9–11].

Since the inflammatory process initiates venous thrombosis in patients with BD, the mainstay of treatment is immunosuppressive therapy. However, it is controversial whether immunosuppressive therapy should be used alone or immunosuppressive and anticoagulant together in the treatment of venous thrombosis in patients with BD. Conventional treatment of non-BD venous thrombosis is to prevent thrombus propagation and pulmonary embolism with anticoagulants. However, the main problem in BD is vasculitis, which involves all layers of the vessel. For this reason, some centers apply direct immunosuppressive treatment without applying anticoagulants in venous thrombosis occurring in patients with BD [4, 9, 11–13, 20].

Superficial and/or deep vein thrombosis was detected in 16.4% ($n = 290$) in our clinical observations between 1998 and 2020 (Table 17.1). Our general treatment policy in acute venous thrombosis is to combine immunosuppressive therapy with short-term anticoagulant therapy if there is no contraindication, such as bleeding or aneurysm rupture risk. In our clinical expertise, in patients with BD with arterial and venous pathology, azathioprine 2–3 mg/kg/day (administered for 5 years) and methyl-prednisolone or prednisolone (the dose is usually reduced and discontinued in 2 months) and colchicine 1–2 mg/day (given continuously) as an anti-inflammatory and immunosuppressive agent is started. We do not routinely use anticoagulants in patients with BD, except for vena cava thrombosis and hepatic vein thrombosis, but in patients with strong thrombophilia or intracardiac thrombus, we generally apply anticoagulant in the form of low molecular weight heparin.

The main causes of postthrombotic syndrome (PTS) that we frequently see in BD are chronic obstruction and valve insufficiency in the proximal veins after lower extremity venous thrombosis, as well as severe venous hypertension resulting from recurrent thrombosis. Swelling, pain, hyperpigmentation, and venous ulcers in the legs frequently occur in patients with BD who develop PTS. In this condition, which greatly impairs the quality of life, endovenous stenting can be applied for obstructions in the iliac veins and vena cava, as well as compression stockings, elastic or non-elastic compression. In the chronic phases, superior vena cava thrombosis can lead to superior vena cava syndrome, which manifests itself with edema on the face and upper body, cyanosis, venous blood loss, and respiratory distress [9, 20].

Budd–Chiari syndrome occurs in 0.3–3% of patients with BD. As a result of hepatic vein thrombosis, abdominal distension due to acid, collateral vessels in the abdominal wall, esophageal varices, and liver failure may occur. The clinical course and survival of patients with BD with Budd–Chiari syndrome is poor [7, 9].

17.4 Arterial Involvement

Arterial involvement is generally less common than venous involvement in BD. We encountered 22 cases (1.2%) with arterial involvement in the last period records of our clinical observations (Table 17.1). While arterial involvement is one-tenth of venous involvement in the region including our country, venous/arterial involvement rates are close to each other in western countries and North America. However, arterial involvement in BD is more important in terms of morbidity and mortality. The most common pathology in arterial involvement is pseudoaneurysms, in which three layers of the arterial wall are absent. Arterial occlusions are less common. The aneurysm probably develops due to local vasculitis in the vessel wall or an inflammatory process in the vasa vasorum. The inflammatory process in the vascular wall can cause the destruction of elastic fibers, which can lead to transmural necrosis of the walls of the main muscular arteries and, as a result, the formation of aneurysms [3, 9–11, 14, 15, 18].

Pulmonary artery aneurysm is the most common and dangerous complication of vascular involvement. Pulmonary artery aneurysm or dilatation may be seen in 1–2% of patients with BD [17]. It often causes hemoptysis, and in these cases, agents that increase bleeding such as anticoagulants should be avoided. Rupture of pulmonary artery aneurysm is among the greatest causes of mortality in BD. With early diagnosis, appropriate immunosuppressive treatment, and transcatheter embolization, the high mortality rate has now been reduced to 20%. In cases resistant to medical treatment, life-saving open surgical treatments such as pulmonary lobectomy may be necessary [4, 11, 16, 17].

In the peripheral arterial system, an aneurysm in BD is most commonly seen in the femoral and popliteal arteries, followed by the abdominal aorta and iliac arteries. Most aneurysms in BD are asymptomatic. However, during the activation of BD, they grow rapidly and cause compression and rupture. Most patients who develop rupture have not previously been diagnosed with or treated for BD. Peripheral artery aneurysms in patients with BD usually present with a pulsatile mass and pain. In addition to the clinical diagnosis of vascular lesions, noninvasive or minimally invasive radiological imaging methods such as arterial Doppler ultrasonography (DU) and computed tomography (CT)-angiography are primarily used (Figs. 17.1 and 17.2). Diagnostic imaging techniques that require arterial puncture are not preferred because they may lead to access site pseudoaneurysm development. Arterial aneurysms are relatively common in patients with BD and are a significant cause of mortality when rupture occurs. Therefore, surgical treatment is mandatory as soon as possible in cases of aneurysm in BD [14, 15, 18, 19].

The best treatment method for arterial aneurysms in patients with BD is still controversial. In general, the choice of treatment method in BD varies depending on the clinical symptoms and risk status of the patient. However, treatment including immunosuppressants and/or steroids is

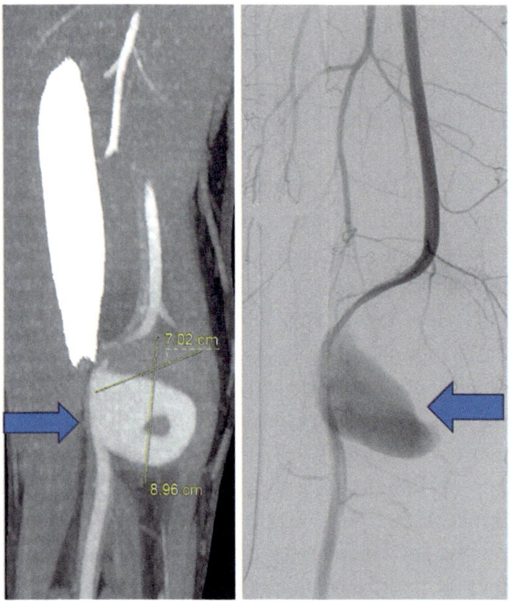

Fig. 17.1 CT-angiography (left) and Digital Subtraction Angiography (DSA) (right) images of a pseudoaneurysm (arrows) containing a partial thrombus large enough to push the femoral artery in a young male patient with BD

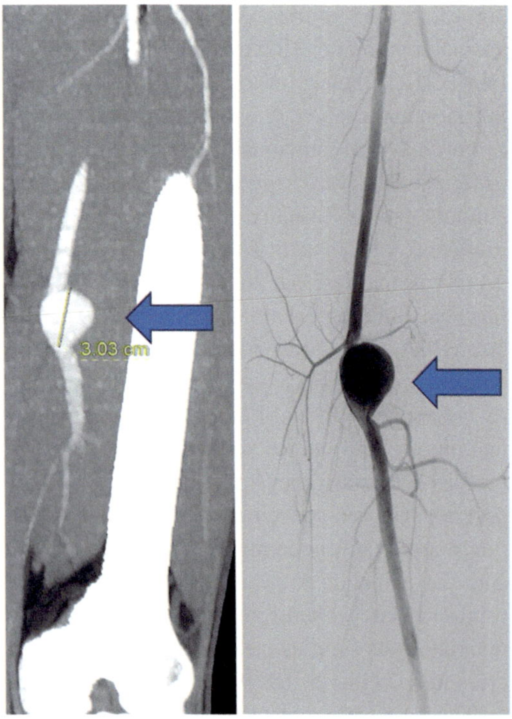

Fig. 17.2 CT-angiography (left) and DSA (right) images of simultaneous pseudoaneurysm (arrows) in the left femoral artery of the same patient with BD

essential and should be administered before endovascular and open surgery whenever possible. Surgical repair is inevitable in acute-onset and complicated patients with BD, such as aneurysm rupture. However, since morbidity and mortality rates after open surgery are still high, endovascular treatment is considered a suitable option for patients classified as high risk. In addition, since open surgical repair has less satisfactory results in terms of postoperative vascular complications (such as pseudoaneurysm and graft occlusion), endovascular therapy has been shown to be a better alternative and has become the preferred approach in most patients at high surgical risk. Endovascular treatment can be used in elective or even emergency conditions for aneurysm repair in patients with BD with appropriate anatomy. Implantation of endovascular prostheses such as stent grafts or covered stents or coil embolization can be used for this purpose (Fig. 17.3). Therefore, endovascular treatment of aneurysms with a high risk of morbidity and mortality may provide a better prognosis for patients with BD. For these reasons, endovascular procedures have become the preferred treatment method in arterial aneurysm cases. Also endovascular procedures generally have a shorter operating time, shorter hospital stay and less blood loss

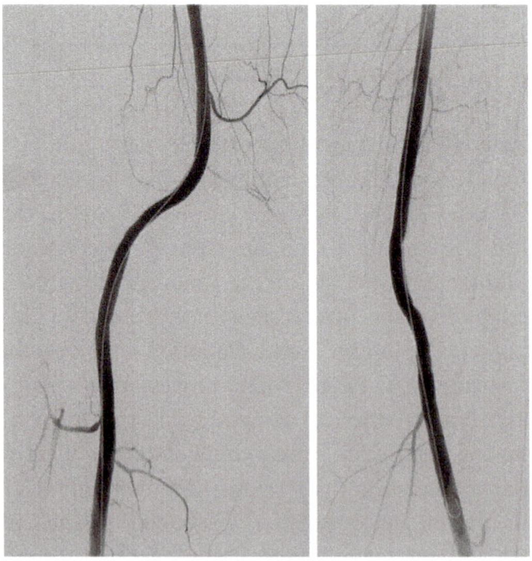

Fig. 17.3 DSA images after treatment of bilateral BD pseudoaneurysm with endoprostheses

Fig. 17.4 Treatment options in BD with vascular involvement

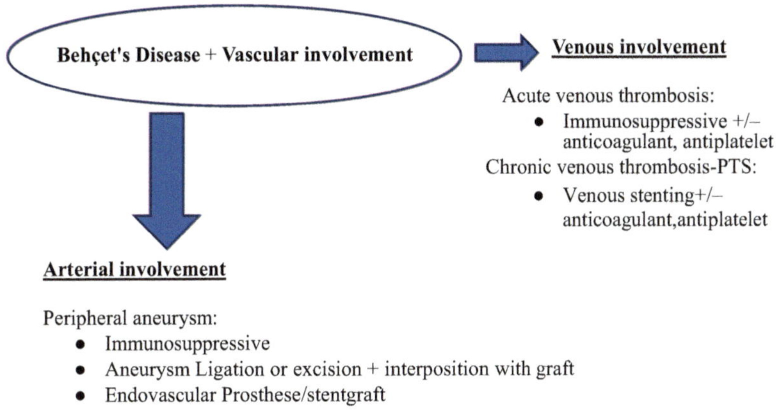

than open surgical treatment. In addition, the technical success rate in placing the endovascular prosthesis is over 90% in selected cases. On the other hand, endovascular treatment also has some limitations, mainly such as technical feasibility, endoleak and occlusion. In traditional open surgery, the vascular segment with the aneurysm is first excised or ligated. Then, revascularization should be achieved by interpositioning a vascular graft between the artery ends that are not affected by vasculitis. Performing open surgery during the period when BD is active leads to a high incidence of complications such as para-anastomotic aneurysm and graft occlusion. Thanks to the accompanying or compensatory collateral vessels, aneurysm ligation alone, without revascularization, is generally well tolerated by patients with BD [14, 15, 18–20]. The treatment algorithm in BD with vascular involvement is summarized in Fig. 17.4.

Below is the summary of two patients with BD with vascular involvement, one of whom was treated with endovascular surgery and the other with open surgery.

Case 1 A 42-year-old male patient was diagnosed with BD at the age of 34 due to oral aphthous ulcers and genital ulcers, bilateral femoral artery aneurysms, and previous deep vein thrombosis.

The patient was admitted due to BD and vascular involvement. Lower extremity DU revealed chronic thrombosis of the right popliteal and left femoral veins, as well as bilateral femoral artery aneurysms. CT angiography revealed a pseudoaneurysm containing a partial thrombus with a diameter of 7 × 7 × 10 cm in the distal part of the superficial femoral artery on the right. In addition, a pseudoaneurysm with a diameter of 2.5 × 2.4 × 3 cm was detected in the middle section of the superficial femoral artery on the left (Figs. 17.1 and 17.2). Immunosuppressive treatment, containing corticosteroids and azathioprine, was initiated along with colchicine.

Endovascular treatment was planned due to bilateral saccular aneurysms at the level of canalis adductorius (Hunter's canal) in the right and left femoral arteries. A 7 × 150 mm endoprosthesis (Gore Viabahn stent graft) was placed successfully for a large pseudoaneurysm in the right femoral artery, and a 7 × 100 mm endoprosthesis (Gore Viabahn stent graft) for a 28 mm diameter pseudoaneurysm in the left femoral artery was successfully deployed in the same session (Fig. 17.3).

Approximately 3 years after the placement of an endoprosthesis in the bilateral femoral artery pseudoaneurysm, the patient presented with complaints of genital ulcers and arthralgia in the ankles. No vascular symptoms were detected, but CT angiography showed that there was no contrast material filling in the stent grafts in the bilateral femoral artery. It was observed that both popliteal arteries were filled with collaterals developing from the bilateral deep femoral artery.

The patient, who could not visit the BD Unit in Ankara due to the Covid pandemic and was under medical control where he lived, was contacted by phone. The patient, who stopped taking immunosuppressant medications during the Covid period, reported that he was still using colchicine and acetyl salicylic acid (ASA) and that his condition was good.

Case 2 The 24-year-old male patient was admitted when he was 18 years old, complaining of swelling and pain behind his right knee. This young patient was diagnosed with BD upon detection of an aneurysm in the popliteal artery, oral aphthous ulcer, and erythema nodosum. His father also had BD.

No other systemic or vascular involvement was seen on contrast-enhanced thoracoabdominal and pelvic CT. To avoid arterial puncture and possible traumatic aneurysm, the lower extremity arterial and venous system were evaluated only with DU. DU revealed a 48 × 36 mm saccular aneurysm in the middle segment of the right popliteal artery and no other vascular pathology was detected in the lower extremity.

The patient, who was diagnosed with BD with vascular involvement, underwent popliteal artery aneurysm ligation and saphenous vein interposition under corticosteroid immunosuppression, which was started in the rheumatology department.

The patient was discharged on the fourth postoperative day with corticosteroid and ASA. The saphenous vein graft was patent and the pulse of dorsalis pedis artery (DPA) was palpable. On the tenth postoperative day, drainage was performed due to the development of a hematoma in the right groin area where the saphenous vein was removed. The patient, who received azathioprine, methyl prednisolone, colchicine and ASA treatment, had no complaints and no signs of active BD in the postoperative sixth-month examination. DU showed that the saphenous vein graft was patent.

The patient, who stopped taking medications other than ASA before Covid, did not visit the BD Unit until recently. He was contacted by phone and invited for re-examination. No vascular pathology or signs of BD were detected in the patient and he had no complaints. The patient's saphenous vein graft was patent and DPA was palpable. He was referred to the BD Unit and Rheumatology Department.

17.5 Cardiac Involvement

Cardiac involvement is not common in patients with BD. It has been reported that the main vessels of the heart, coronary arteries, conduction system, endocardium, and myocardium are involved. Intracardiac thrombus sometimes occurs as the first sign of the disease in young patients. It is mostly found in the right ventricle and with pulmonary aneurysm. Coronary artery involvement manifests as silent ischemia, unstable angina, acute myocardial infarction (MI), and even sudden cardiac death. Coronary artery stenting or coronary artery bypass surgery may be required in MI cases with BD. Immunosuppressive therapy is necessary to reduce relapses and complications in surgical or endovascular treatments of cardiac manifestations such as vascular involvement [21].

17.6 Conclusion

In BD, which is still an important health problem in certain geographical areas such as Mediterranean and East Asian countries, vascular system pathologies such as venous thrombosis and arterial aneurysm remain serious. Despite the successes in immunosuppressive and immunomodulatory drugs, the number of patients requiring open vascular surgery and endovascular treatment is not small.

Acknowledgements The author would like to thank Ms. Mine Aslan and Mr. Richard Edwards for the English editing of the article.

Conflict of Interest Statement None.

References

1. Saylan T. Life story of Dr. Hulusi Behçet. Yonsei Med J. 1997;38:327–32.
2. Behçet H, Matteson EL. On relapsing, aphtous ulcers of the mouth, eye and genitalia caused by a virus. 1937. Clin Exp Rheumatol. 2010;28(Suppl 60):S2–5.
3. Leccese P, Alpsoy E. Behçet's disease: an overview of etiopathogenesis. Front Immunol. 2019;10:1067. https://doi.org/10.3389/fimmu.2019.0106.
4. Alpsoy E, Leccese P, Emmi G, Ohno S. Treatment of Behçet's disease: an algorithmic multidisciplinary approach. Front Med. 2021;8:624795. https://doi.org/10.3389/fmed.2021.624795.
5. Boyvat A, Oktem A, Kalay Yildizhan I, Ates A, Yalcindag N, Koksoy C, et al. A comparison of adult and juvenile Behçet patients and a look at clinical trends: retrospective data from a Turkish follow-up cohort study. Dermatology. 2023;239(6):958–65. https://doi.org/10.1159/000534316.
6. Jun JB, Kim HJ, Kazmi SZ, Kang T, Kim KB, Kang MJ, et al. Significant decline in the incidence of Behçet's disease in South Korea: a nationwide population-based study (2004-2017). Arthritis Care Res (Hoboken). 2021;73(11):1689–96.
7. Bayraktar Y, Balkanci F, Bayraktar M, et al. Budd–Chiari syndrome: a common complication of Behçet's disease. Am J Gastroenterol. 1997;92:858–62.
8. Wang Y, Li S, Tang S, et al. Risk factors of cardiovascular involvement in patients with Behcet's disease. J Transl Autoimmun. 2023;6:100195.
9. Yazici H, Seyahi E, Hatemi G, Yazici Y. Behçet syndrome: a contemporary view. Nat Rev Rheumatol. 2018;14(2):107–19.
10. Vargas RM, Cruz MLN, Giarllarielli MPH, et al. Vascular involvement in Behçet's disease: the immunopathological process. J Vasc Bras. 2021;20:e20200170. https://doi.org/10.1590/1677-5449.200170.
11. Ouchi K, Narui R, Sakuma T, Ojiri H. Serious complication of anticoagulation in vessel thrombosis-associated Behçet disease. Intern Med. 2020;59(13):1615–20. Published online 2020 Mar 26. https://doi.org/10.2169/internalmedicine.4109-19.
12. Lee NH, Bae M, Jin M, Chung SW, Lee CW, Jeon CH. Characterization of venous involvement in vasculo-Behçet disease. Korean J Thorac Cardiovasc Surg. 2020;53(6):381–6.
13. Ozguler Y, Hatemi G, Cetinkaya F, et al. Clinical course of acute deep vein thrombosis of the legs in Behçet's syndrome. Rheumatology. 2020;59:799–806. https://doi.org/10.1093/rheumatology/kez352.
14. Koksoy C, Gyedu A, Alacayir I, Bengisun U, Uncu H, Anadol E. Surgical treatment of peripheral aneurysms in patients with Behçet's disease. Eur J Vasc Endovasc Surg. 2011;42:525–30.
15. Yang SS, Park KM, Park YJ, Kim YW, Do YS, Park HS, et al. Peripheral arterial involvement in Behçet's disease: an analysis of the results from a Korean referral center. Rheumatol Int. 2013;33:2101–8.
16. Tuzun H, Seyahi E, Guzelant G, et al. Surgical treatment of pulmonary complications in Behçet's syndrome. Semin Thorac Cardiovasc Surg. 2018;30(3):369–78. https://doi.org/10.1053/j.semtcvs.2018.07.008.
17. Acıcan T, Ozdemir Kumbasar O. Behçet's disease and pulmonary involvement (Turkish). J Ankara Univ Faculty Med. 2011;64(Suppl 3):39–44.
18. Eleshra A, Abdelgawwad M, Regal S, Soliman M, Khafagy T. Short-term outcome of primary stent graft for peripheral artery aneurysm in patients with Behçet disease. J Vasc Surg. 2021;73:279–84.
19. Goksel OS, Torlak Z, Çınar B, Sahin S, Karatepe C, Eren E. Midterm results with endovascular approach to abdominal aortic pathologies in Behçet's disease. Ann Vasc Surg. 2012;26(277):e5–9.
20. Alibaz-Oner F, Vautier M, Aksoy A, et al. Vascular Behçet's disease: a comparative study from Turkey and France. Clin Exp Rheumatol. 2022;40:1491–6.
21. Akkuzu G, Erdoğan A, Moustafa C, et al. A case of Behçet syndrome presenting with acute coronary syndrome. Int J Rheum Dis. 2024;27:e14852. https://doi.org/10.1111/1756.85X.14852.

18 Behçet's Disease and Nervous System Involvement

Ahmed Serkan Emekli, Tuncay Gündüz, and Gülşen Akman-Demir

Contents

18.1 Introduction

Neuro-Behçet's disease (NBD) is one of the most serious manifestations of Behçet's disease (BD) that causes long-term morbidity and mortality. In large published series, the frequency of NBD has been reported to be between 3% and 9% [1]. The frequency of NBD was found to be 13% in males and 5.6% in females in a study including patients with BD with follow-up of two decades [2]. Although some studies state that frequency is higher, this variability may be affected by geographical differences and the inclusion of primary headaches coinciding with BD [3]. The neurological involvement of BD begins between the ages of 20 and 40 and is more common in males [4]. In addition, male patients had higher morbidity and mortality in long-term disease course [2]. The NBD occurs 3–6 years after the systemic findings of BD appear [4]. However,

A. S. Emekli · T. Gündüz · G. Akman-Demir (✉)
Department of Neurology, Istanbul Faculty of Medicine, Istanbul University, Istanbul, Türkiye

E. Alpsoy et al. (eds.), *Behçet's Disease: An Integrated Approach*,
https://doi.org/10.1007/978-3-031-77251-1_18

neurological involvement may occasionally be seen as the first sign of BD in some patients [1].

The NBD is rare in childhood. The rate of neurological involvement in pediatric age (<16 years) was found to be 3.6% [5]. Cerebral venous sinus thrombosis (CVST) was detected in 88.5% of these patients diagnosed with pediatric-onset NBD [5].

The most common neurological complaint in BD is headache, which is seen in approximately 70% of patients [6]. Although headaches may be related to central nervous system (CNS) involvement, primary headaches, headaches associated with ocular inflammation, and nonstructural headaches of BD are among the most common causes of headaches in BD [6]. Of the BD patients referred to the neurology clinics due to headache, migraine was diagnosed in 46%, tension-type headache in 26%, secondary headache in one-third, and headache accompanying systemic exacerbation of BD in 13% [7].

Neurological manifestation of BD is almost always limited to CNS. The most common form is parenchymal involvement affecting the mesodiencephalic region and brainstem. Occasionally, spinal cord involvement may be seen as longitudinally extensive transverse myelitis. Non-parenchymal involvement is less common and occurs mostly in the form of CVST.

18.2 Parenchymal Neuro-Behçet's Disease

Parenchymal CNS involvement is seen as pyramidocerebellar syndrome, which occurs with brainstem and corticospinal tract findings accompanied by headache, ataxia, dysarthria, and hemiparesis, which usually develop over days to weeks [1, 3]. Parenchymal disease may be observed less frequently with sensory findings, myelopathy, sphincter dysfunction, emotional lability, cognitive-behavioral changes, and rarely with extrapyramidal findings, seizure, optic neuropathy, and cranial nerve involvement [1, 3]. Subacute meningoencephalitis is observed in 75% of patients with parenchymal involvement [4]. Clinically, the disease course may be with attacks and remissions, or it may follow a progressive course after an attack or, rarely, a progressive course without a significant attack period [8]. Although parenchymal involvement is predominantly in the brain, spinal cord involvement has been reported with a rate of 11–14% [8, 9].

18.3 Non-parenchymal Neuro-Behçet's Disease

The most common form of non-parenchymal NBD is CVST [8]. It is observed in approximately 10–20% to one-third of patients with NBD [8, 10]. It most commonly presents with intracranial hypertension syndrome consisting of headache and papilledema [8, 11]. In addition, diplopia and cranial nerve palsies may accompany one-third of patients [11]. It is thought to take weeks or months for thrombosis to develop; therefore, complaints may remain vague, and the diagnosis may be difficult [6]. In BD-related CVST, findings including the development of venous infarction, seizure, aphasia, and hemiparesis are less frequent compared to non-BD-related CVST [8, 11]. Since it pathophysiologically resembles vascular BD more than parenchymal NBD, its association with parenchymal involvement is very rare, and peripheral vascular involvement may accompany [12, 13].

Rarely, involvement in the form of aseptic meningitis without parenchymal lesions may be observed [8]. Vertebral artery dissection, large vessel occlusion, and aneurysms are also rare involvements of NBD [8, 10, 14].

Neurological disease caused by intracranial hypertension due to superior vena cava syndrome and cerebral embolism due to cardiac complications of BD are considered secondary neurologic involvement [1].

18.4 Other Clinical Features

Some patients with BD may develop a neurobehavioral syndrome, including euphoria, disinhibition, psychomotor agitation, and paranoid or obsessive thoughts [1]. In studies consisting of neuropsychological examinations of patients with NBD, memory impairment in the form of recalling difficulties and frontal dysfunction with findings such as apathy and disinhibition were found [15, 16].

In a group of patients with BD who had no neurologic complaints, neurologic examination findings might be detected, and some patients in this group may have mild neurologic attacks during the course of the disease [8]. In patients with silent or subclinical neurologic involvement, mortality and morbidity are significantly lower [17].

In addition, peripheral nervous system involvement, such as polyneuropathy and myositis, may be observed very rarely [8, 12], as well as optic neuropathy.

18.5 Diagnosis

In neurological patients with recurrent oral or genital ulcers, uveitis, or other systemic BD symptoms, it is crucial to consider NBD. The NBD has characteristic disease patterns. The recognized neurological syndromes include parenchymal and non-parenchymal syndromes of NBD, as described above. International Consensus Recommendations criteria have been established for the diagnosis of NBD (Table 18.1) [18]. According to these criteria, it has been stated that a valid criterion for BD should be fulfilled, a recognized neurological syndrome should be supported by neuroimaging or cerebrospinal fluid (CSF) findings, and the existing neurological syndrome should not be explained by another condition in order to make a diagnosis of "definite NBD" [18]. If the systemic criteria for BD are not met, and if the patient has a "typical" parenchymal or non-parenchymal neurological presentation, then a diagnosis of "probable NBD" can be made.

18.6 Neuro-Imaging Findings

Magnetic resonance imaging (MRI) is the most sensitive method to demonstrate parenchymal NBD lesions. In parenchymal NBD, lesions during an attack appear iso/hypointense on T1-weighted imaging and hyperintense on T2-weighted and FLAIR imaging [14]. In contrast-enhanced T1-weighted imaging, contrast enhancement is observed in a region much smaller than the size of the lesion detected in T2 and FLAIR images. The most commonly affected parenchymal structures are the rostral pons, mesencephalon, and diencephalic region (Fig. 18.1) [19–21]. The lesions in the posterior leg of the internal capsule and corticospinal tract are typical for parenchymal NBD [22]. Parenchymal NBD lesions are thought to be caused by thrombosis of small veins in the brainstem [21]. Lesions are distributed asymmetrically in the acute and subacute periods and extend around long fiber tracts. The typical water-flow-like image in coronal MRI formed by the lesions has been named

Table 18.1 International Consensus Recommendations Criteria for NBD [Adapted from Kalra et al. [18]]

Definite NBD: The following three criteria must be met
1. Fulfill the ISG[a] criteria for BD
2. The objective neurological finding with the recognized syndrome in BD is supported by the presence of characteristic and relevant abnormalities in either or both of the following
(a) Neuroimaging
(b) CSF
3. Lack of a better explanation of neurological findings
Probable NBD: One of the following criteria must be met in the absence of a better explanation for the neurologic findings
The presence of neurologic syndrome and systemic BD findings as in definite NBD and ISG criteria are not met
The occurrence of an uncharacteristic neurological syndrome within the scope of a diagnosis of BD supported by ISG criteria

[a]ISG (International Study Group. 1990) or other current or future accepted criteria. *NBD* Neuro-Behçet's disease, *BD* Behçet's disease, *CSF* cerebrospinal fluid.

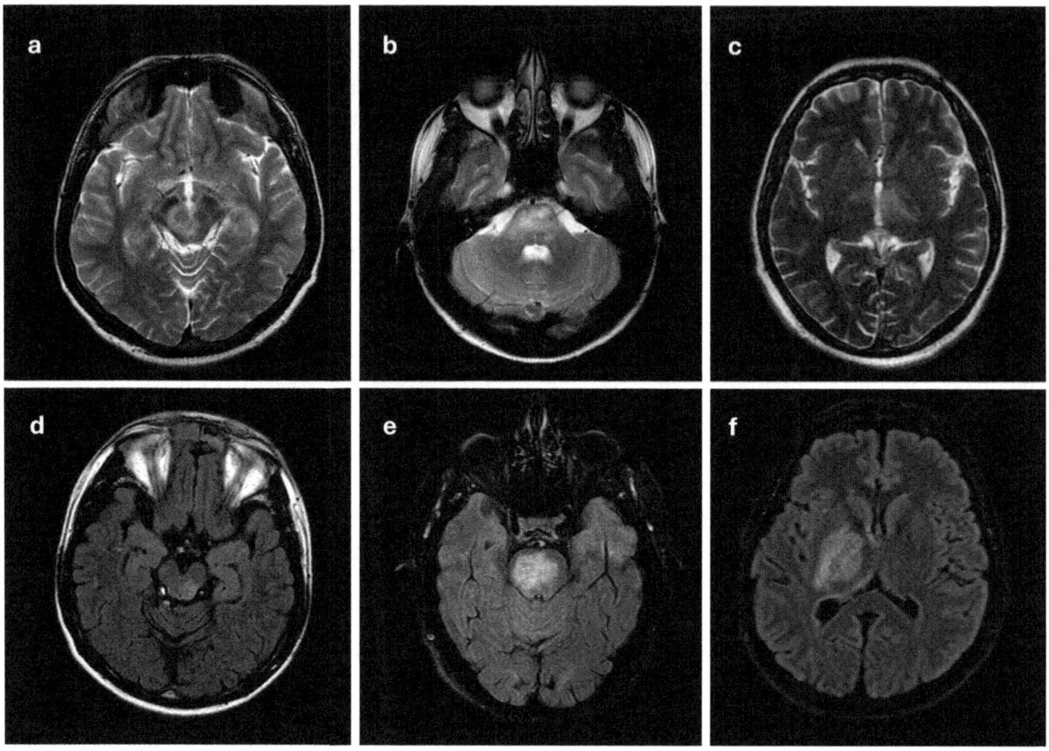

Fig. 18.1 Acute attack lesions of patients with parenchymal neuro-Behçet's disease. Axial T2-weighted hyperintense lesions in (**a**) right mesencephalon, (**b**) pons, (**c**) left thalamus and internal capsule, axial FLAIR imaging hyperintense lesions in (**d**) left posterior mesencephalon, (**e**) pons, (**f**) right thalamus and internal capsule

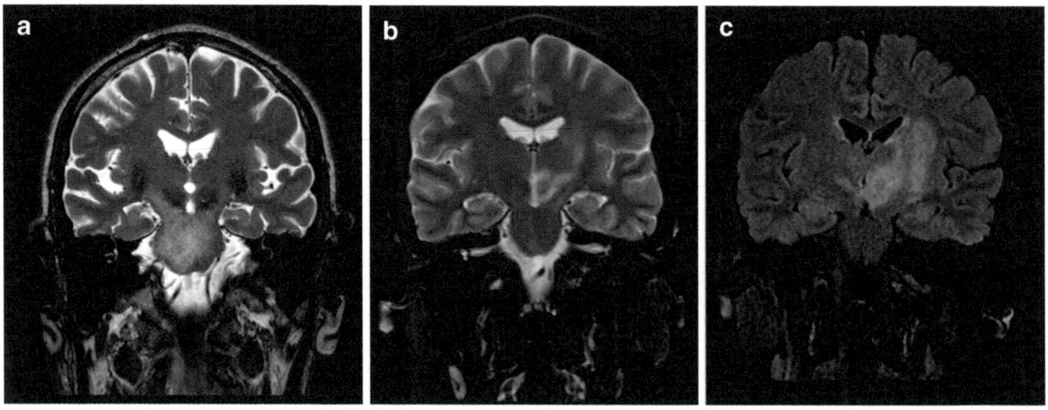

Fig. 18.2. (**a**, **b**) Coronal T2 and (**c**) FLAIR images of three different patients with parenchymal neuro-Behçet's disease. Note the typical water-flow-like appearance of lesions from the diencephalic region to the brainstem ("cascade sign")

"cascade sign" (Fig. 18.2) [3]. In long-term follow-up, these lesions are replaced by small, scattered lesions and atrophy [23]. Regression or disappearance of the lesions suggests that the underlying cause is inflammation and edema [20]. Hemispheric white matter is not a typical

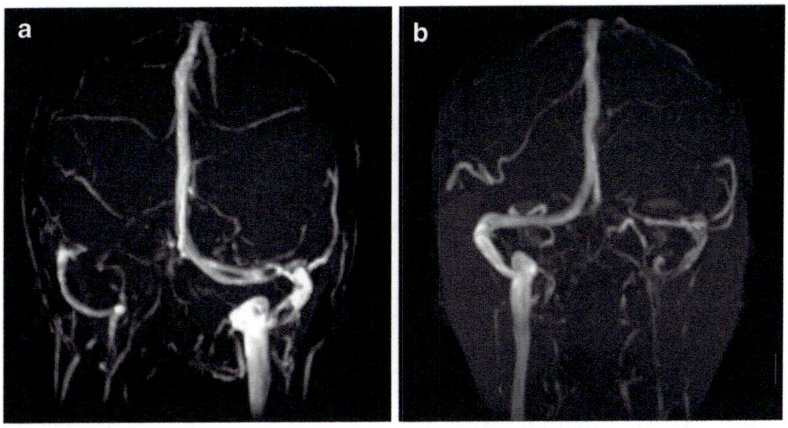

Fig. 18.3 (**a**) Right and (**b**) left transverse sinus thrombosis in patients with non-parenchymal neuro-Behçet's disease

lesion localization for parenchymal NBD. Parenchymal brain lesions in atypical locations might be seen in patients with BD with cyclosporine exposure [19, 24]. The pattern of neuropsychological impairment in parenchymal NBD, which is frequently attributed to frontal cognitive networks, may be due to alteration in frontal association tracts observed by diffusion tensor imaging that otherwise appear structurally normal [25].

MRI findings of parenchymal NBD in the acute phase are remarkably distinguishable from other inflammatory diseases of the CNS, however, this rate decreases significantly in chronic parenchymal NBD [26]. In addition, brainstem atrophy is highly specific for parenchymal NBD in patients without cortical atrophy [26]. Brainstem atrophy on initial imaging of parenchymal patients with NBD is associated with a progressive course [27]. Furthermore, late age of onset is a worse prognostic factor [19]. A severe and progressive disease course may be predicted by corticospinal lesions in the acute period, necessitating aggressive treatment. It is interesting to note that females having a higher incidence of brainstem lesions and pathergy test status might exert influence on lesion lateralization [19].

Spinal involvement is less common than brain involvement in parenchymal NBD. Long-segment (three segments and above) myelopathy findings may be observed in spinal cord involvement. The cervical and dorsal spinal cord is most commonly affected [9]. In spinal cord involvement, a pattern in which a hyperintense ring surrounding a central hypointense region with or without contrast enhancement is called the "bagel sign" [28]. Another pattern described is the motor neuron pattern in which anterior horn cells are symmetrically involved [28].

The preferred imaging modalities for diagnosing CVST are brain MRI and magnetic resonance venography. Patients with BD are more likely to have transverse sinus thrombosis (Fig. 18.3) [29]. It is a common mistake to interpret an atresic transverse sinus as dural sinus thrombosis; this should be avoided. In addition, hemorrhage and venous infarction are less frequent in CVST patients with BD compared with other etiologies [29].

18.7 Laboratory Findings

Cerebrospinal fluid (CSF) studies have an important place in the diagnosis of both parenchymal and non-parenchymal involvement. CSF examination performed during an acute parenchymal NBD attack usually reveals inflammatory findings [8, 12]. Although the pleocytosis in CSF is less than one hundred per cubic millimeter, up to one thousand may be found [3, 8]. In the early period, neutrophilic pleocytosis predominates, however, lymphocytic cell predominance is observed in the late period [8]. The frequency of detection of oligoclonal bands in CSF has been found below 20% [8, 30]. In CSF examinations of patients with CVST, the number of cells and protein level is generally normal, but elevated intracranial pressure is found [8, 18].

It has been reported that CSF interleukin-6 (IL-6) levels are increased in acute and chronic progressive NBD and are associated with disease activity and prognosis [31, 32]. Patients with elevated CSF IL-6 levels also had higher CSF cell counts and total protein levels, and these three characteristics were associated with poor long-term (>3 years) disease outcome [31].

18.8 Differential Diagnosis

Neuro-Behçet's disease should be included in the differential diagnosis with many other conditions due to its diversity in clinical and laboratory findings. Although multiple sclerosis (MS) is most commonly included in the differential diagnosis, stroke at a young age, sarcoidosis, tuberculosis and infections, brainstem gliomas and malignancies are also among the diseases that should be considered in the differential diagnosis (Table 18.2). In addition, it should be taken into consideration that rare diseases such as Vogt-Koyanagi-Harada, Reiter, Eales', Susac, Cogan, and Neuro-Sweet syndrome, may cause both eye and CNS involvement [1, 10].

Headaches, motor symptoms, and cognitive-behavioral abnormalities are more common in parenchymal NBD compared to MS; while sensory presentation, optic neuritis, internuclear ophthalmoplegia, and spinal and cerebellar findings are more common in MS [18]. In parenchymal NBD, CSF exhibits a higher cell count, with neutrophils possibly predominating; in MS, cells are typically rare, and lymphocytes are predominant [18]. Barkhof criteria have a value in the distinction between parenchymal NBD and MS. Barkhof-negative patients showed typical large lesions involving the brainstem, diencephalon, and basal ganglia regions and symptoms indicating brainstem involvement. On the other hand, Barkhof-positive patients have classical MS-like lesions, fulfilled the McDonald criteria, have fewer brainstem symptoms, are female-dominant, have more frequent attacks, have normal CSF cell counts, and rates of oligoclonal bands in CSF are similar to patients with MS [33]; these patients should be considered as having MS, rather than NBD.

Table 18.2 Differential diagnosis of parenchymal Neuro-Behçet's disease

Multiple sclerosis
Stroke at a young age
Neurosarcoidosis
Central nervous system tuberculosis
Brainstem gliomas
Primary central nervous system lymphoma
Primary and secondary central nervous system vasculitis
Vogt-Kayanagi-Harada syndrome
Reiter syndrome
Susac syndrome
Eales' disease
Cogan's syndrome
Neuro-sweet syndrome

Adapted from Siva et al. [10]

18.9 Treatment

Neuro-Behçet's disease attacks exhibit an apparent activation of the inflammatory cascade, similar to exacerbations in systemic BD [31, 34]. Prominent contrast-enhancing lesions on MRI and pleocytosis in CSF further confirm this finding. Early therapy is crucial due to the potential for serious damage to neural tissue resulting from the involvement of innate immune cells during parenchymal NBD attack. Unfortunately, there is insufficient evidence regarding the treatment and preventive measures for NBD. Knowledge and practices usually originate from small case studies and individual experience.

18.9.1 Acute Attack Treatment

High-dose intravenous methylprednisolone (IVMP) is commonly administered during the acute phase of neuro-Behçet's attacks, similar to other rheumatologic disorders [35]. In general, the below-mentioned treatment approach is similar for both parenchymal and non-parenchymal NBD involvements. During the attack period, if there are no contraindications, 1 g/day methylprednisolone infusion therapy can be administered for 5–7 days. Immediately thereafter, oral 32 mg/day methylprednisolone should be administered with a gradual tapering over 6 months. We also recommend high-dose IVMP once a week for at least 4 weeks. The extended use of steroid therapy aims to prevent a potential severe relapse with disastrous outcomes. Patients typically begin to show a response to this treatment protocol within 1–2 weeks based on our clinical experience [36]. In unresponsive patients, intravenous cyclophosphamide (CYC) at a dosage of 0.5–1 g per month may be an effective alternative [35, 37]. The European Alliance of Associations for Rheumatology, EULAR, similarly recommends the initiation of high-dose IVMP followed by oral corticosteroids in acute parenchymal NBD attacks, and the initiation of infliximab in cases of poor response [36]. In centers with easy access to anti-TNF-α (antitumor necrosis factor-α) therapies, this approach may be a good alternative to CYC, an agent that can have serious side effects.

Acute parenchymal NBD commonly manifests with mesodiencephalic involvement, which may result in symptoms including significant somnolence, behavioral changes, and difficulties with swallowing. In addition, epileptic seizures may occasionally develop during the initial days. Therefore, nasogastric catheterization to prevent aspiration, antipsychotics for agitation or disinhibited behavior, or antiepileptic drugs for seizures may be necessary during this period. If these symptoms develop, they are likely to improve over time with high-dose IVMP treatment. Anticoagulation use in the setting of acute CVST is controversial. Since CVST due to BD is mainly an inflammatory event, corticosteroids will suppress the intravascular inflammation and thrombus propagation. Anticoagulants may be added to corticosteroids if needed. On the other hand, avoiding anticoagulation may be reasonable to prevent potential coincidental pulmonary aneurysmatic hemorrhages [36].

18.9.2 Prophylactic Treatment

18.9.2.1 Immunosuppressants

Although randomized controlled trials are lacking, oral immunosuppressive medications, including azathioprine (AZT), mycophenolate mofetil (MMF), and methotrexate are the preferred drugs to prevent a new relapse of NBD. AZT, a purine analog-antimetabolite, is typically used as the initial treatment in our clinic. It exerts its anti-inflammatory properties by targeting quickly proliferating activated lymphocytes. The maximum recommended dosage for NBD is 2–2.5 mg/kg/day [35, 37]. Some patients may encounter hepatotoxicity characterized by a sudden and significant increase in liver enzymes. Therefore, it is crucial to administer AZT in 50 mg/day increments every 15 days to mitigate this side effect. MMF is a suitable alternative as an initial treatment or for individuals unable to use AZT. At a maximum dose of 2 g/day, this drug has a relatively safe side effect profile and is recommended as the initial therapy by the Japanese National Research Committee for Behçet's Disease [38]. As AZT, it is also safe to initiate treatment with MMF at 500 mg dosage increases weekly. Methotrexate is the final oral medication in this category, acting as a purine/pyrimidine analog and inhibiting DNA synthesis. Evidence from retrospective studies has shown that it is effective in preventing NBD. The suggested dosage for first-line treatment of NBD is between 12.5 and 20 mg/day [35, 36, 38]. Monitoring of blood counts and liver function tests for at least 3 months is recommended for all three oral agents.

Some patients with NBD may not respond to first-line conventional oral immunosuppressants or may suffer a severe attack from the outset and recover with sequelae. In such patients, before the widespread use of biologics, the most appropriate treatment was monthly intravenous CYC infusion. CYC, an alkylating chemotherapeutic agent, is a highly effective immunosuppressant at a dose of 0.5–1 g per month and may provide long-term remissions in NBD [38]. Due to the potential for teratogenicity and malignancy in the long term, CYC should be employed for limited time periods or replaced with biological treatment as soon as possible. Cyclosporine should not be used in the treatment of NBD, since it may trigger parenchymal involvement [24].

18.9.2.2 Biological Agents

Research on the immunopathogenesis of BD addresses cytokines, including TNF, interleukin-1 (IL-1), and IL-6, which play a significant role in the innate immune response. Agents that block these cytokines are highly effective in controlling BD and NBD activity [39, 40].

No randomized controlled trials have been conducted on TNF-α inhibitors in NBD. Monoclonal antibody drugs like infliximab, etanercept, and adalimumab bind to soluble or transmembrane TNF-α, blocking its interaction with TNF-α receptors 1 and 2 on the cell surface. Therefore, the prevention of nuclear factor kappa B (NF–κB) end-pathway-driven inflammation within the cell occurs in this way [41, 42]. Typically, infliximab medication is initiated early in the treatment course for cases that do not respond to first-line treatments. Infliximab treatment begins with a dosage of 5 mg/kg at weeks 0, 2, and 6, then continues with intravenous infusions every 8 weeks. If patients do not respond to the initial treatment or experience a relapse or disability progression, they can be switched to adalimumab (40 mg s.c. every 2 weeks) or etanercept (50 mg s.c. every week). Retrospective studies demonstrate that these biological agents are highly effective and show a favorable side effect profile [35–37]. However, caution should be exercised with regard to opportunistic infections, especially tuberculosis, and prophylactic antituberculosis treatment should be given to prevent possible reactivation of tuberculosis in the presence of quantiferon or PPD positivity. Subcutaneously administered agents are easier to use and have better patient compliance as they can be administered by the patient.

Interleukin-1 plays an integral part in the development of BD. While anti-IL-1 receptor blockers like anakinra and canakinumab have shown high efficacy in treating BD, there is a lack of evidence of their effectiveness in NBD [36, 37]. It is reasonable to assume that they will be highly effective.

Interleukin-6 levels are shown to be significantly elevated in CSF during exacerbations of parenchymal NBD and decrease with treatment, suggesting that IL-6 plays a crucial role in the pathophysiology of NBD [31, 39]. Successfully treated cases of treatment-refractory NBD with tocilizumab also support this perspective [43, 44]. Currently, IL-6 antagonists are being used in cases of NBD not responding to anti-TNF agents.

Evidence-based data is still required for the treatment of NBD. The scarcity of the NBD is a significant challenge in carrying out randomized controlled studies. Reported case series and retrospective observational studies offer crucial insights into the optimal treatment. Yet, there are substantial deficiencies in the "treat-to-target" strategy, which involves assessing therapy response and identifying the best response through monitoring disease activity markers [45].

18.10 Prognosis

Neurological manifestations in BD are among the most severe clinical manifestations and may lead to substantial disabilities. Prompt diagnosis and early delivery of effective treatment are crucial in preventing disability while improving the prospects for recovery. Parenchymal NBD causes the most severe disability in the long run, while severe CVST may give rise to parenchymal damage and chronic elevated intracranial pressure, requiring a ventriculoperitoneal shunt.

Akman-Demir et al. reported in their seminal study that one-third of 162 parenchymal NBD patients experienced recovery with significant disability, and the mean time to severe dependability or death was around 10 years [8]. A recent review indicates that around 80% of cases of parenchymal NBD begin with an attack, with 70% of these cases not experiencing another attack, whereas 30% either continue to have attacks or progress to a more severe phase [46]. In our clinic, the meantime to the second attack was 5.4 ± 0.7 years for 167 patients with parenchymal NBD and 13.7 ± 1.3 years for the 89 patients with CVST (unpublished data).

Overall, the data suggest that a significant proportion of parenchymal patients with NBD either have relapse or progression or recover with residual cognitive or physical neurological sequelae. Today's more efficient diagnostic methods and the ability to initiate powerful biological treatments early on may alter the typical progression of NBD. Markers are still required to forecast disease activity and prognosis.

18.11 Conclusions

Neurological involvement is a severe and feared manifestation in patients with BD; however, with early diagnosis and early effective treatment options, it can be controlled without further damage. Over-diagnosis is an important risk in patients with suspected NBD; in such cases, expert opinion should be sought. Class I evidence is still needed for the treatment of NBD.

References

1. Saip S, Akman-Demir G, Siva A. Neuro-Behçet syndrome. Handb Clin Neurol. 2014;121:1703–23.
2. Kural-Seyahi E, Fresko I, Seyahi N, Ozyazgan Y, Mat C, Hamuryudan V, et al. The long-term mortality and morbidity of Behçet syndrome: a 2-decade outcome survey of 387 patients followed at a dedicated center. Medicine (Baltimore). 2003;82:60–76.
3. Kürtüncü M, Tüzün E, Akman-Demir G. Behçet's disease and nervous system involvement. Curr Treat Options Neurol. 2016;18:19.
4. Al-Araji A, Kidd DP. Neuro-Behçet's disease: epidemiology, clinical characteristics, and management. Lancet Neurol. 2009;8:192–204.
5. Uluduz D, Kürtüncü M, Yapici Z, Seyahi E, Kasapçopur O, Özdoğan H, et al. Clinical characteristics of pediatric-onset neuro-Behçet disease. Neurology. 2011;77:1900–5.
6. Uygunoglu U, Saip S, Siva A. Behçet's disease and neuro-Behçet's syndrome. EMJ Neurol. 2018;6:77–85.
7. Aykutlu E, Baykan B, Akman-Demir G, Topcular B, Ertas M. Headache in Behçet's disease. Cephalalgia. 2006;26:180–6.
8. Akman-Demir G, Serdaroglu P, Tasçi B. Clinical patterns of neurological involvement in Behcet's disease: evaluation of 200 patients. Brain. 1999;122:2171–81.
9. Yesilot N, Mutlu M, Gungor O, Baykal B, Serdaroglu P, Akman-Demir G. Clinical characteristics and course of spinal cord involvement in Behçet's disease. Eur J Neurol. 2007;14:729–37.
10. Siva A, Saip S. The spectrum of nervous system involvement in Behçet's syndrome and its differential diagnosis. J Neurol. 2009;256:513–29.
11. Yesilot N, Bahar S, YIlmazer S, Mutlu M, Kurtuncu M, Tuncay R, et al. Cerebral venous thrombosis in Behçet's disease compared to those associated with other etiologies. J Neurol. 2009;256:1134–42.
12. Siva A, Kantarci OH, Saip S, Altintas A, Hamuryudan V, Islak C, et al. Behçet's disease: diagnostic and prognostic aspects of neurological involvement. J Neurol. 2001;248:95–103.
13. Tunc R, Saip S, Siva A, Yazici H. Cerebral venous thrombosis is associated with major vessel disease in Behçet's syndrome. Ann Rheum Dis. 2004;63:1693–4.
14. Borhani-Haghighi A, Kardeh B, Banerjee S, Yadollahikhales G, Safari A, Sahraian MA, et al. Neuro-Behcet's disease: an update on diagnosis, differential diagnoses, and treatment. Mult Scler Relat Disord. 2020;39:101906.
15. Öktem-Tanör Ö, Baykan-Kurt B, Hakan Gürvit I, Akman-Demir G, Serdaroğlu P. Neuropsychological follow-up of 12 patients with neuro-Behcet disease. J Neurol. 1999;246:113–9.
16. Gündüz T, Emir Ö, Kürtüncü M, Mutlu M, Tumaç A, Akca Ş, et al. Cognitive impairment in neuro-Behcet's disease and multiple sclerosis: a comparative study. Int J Neurosci. 2012;122:650–6.
17. Yesilot N, Shehu M, Oktem-Tanor O, Serdaroglu P, Akman-Demir G. Silent neurological involvement in Behçet's disease. Clin Exp Rheumatol. 2006;24:S65–70.
18. Kalra S, Silman A, Akman-Demir G, Bohlega S, Borhani-Haghighi A, Constantinescu CS, et al. Diagnosis and management of neuro-Behçet's disease: international consensus recommendations. J Neurol. 2014;261:1662–76.
19. Emekli AS, Ersözlü E, Emekli MA, Gündüz T, Kürtüncü M. Lesion distribution pattern of parenchymal neuro-Behçet's disease using probability mapping. Mult Scler Relat Disord. 2022;58:103457.
20. Akman-Demir G, Bahar S, Coban O, Tasci B, Serdaroglu P. Cranial MRI in Behçet's disease: 134 examinations of 98 patients. Neuroradiology. 2003;45:851–9.
21. Koçer N, Islak C, Siva A, Saip S, Akman C, Kantarci O, et al. CNS involvement in neuro-Behcet syndrome: an MR study. Am J Neuroradiol. 1999;20:1015–24.
22. Lee SH, Yoon PH, Park SJ, Kim DI. MRI findings in neuro-Behçet's disease. Clin Radiol. 2001;56:485–94.
23. Gerber S, Biondi A, Dormont D, Wechsler B, Marsault C. Long-term MR follow-up of cerebral lesions in neuro-Behçet's disease. Neuroradiology. 1996;38:761–8.
24. Akmar-Demir G, Ayranci O, Kurtuncu M, Vanli EN, Mutlu M, Tugal-Tutkun I. Cyclosporine for Behçet's uveitis: is it associated with an increased risk of neurological involvement? Clin Exp Rheumatol. 2008;26:84–90.
25. Gündüz T, Server S, Küçükali Cİ, Özyurt O, Akman Demir G, Kürtüncü M. Diffusion tensor imaging in parenchymal neuro-Behçet's disease. Noropsikiyatri Ars. 2024;61:39–46.
26. Çoban O, Bahar S, Akman-Demir G, Taşçı B, Yurdakul S, Yazıcı H, et al. Masked assessment of MRI findings: is it possible to differentiate

neuro-Behcet's disease from other central nervous system. Neuroradiology. 1999;41:255–60.
27. Farahangiz S, Sarhadi S, Safari A, Borhani-Haghighi A. Magnetic resonance imaging findings and outcome of neuro-Behçet's disease: the predictive factors. Int J Rheum Dis. 2012;15:142–9.
28. Uygunoglu U, Zeydan B, Ozguler Y, Ugurlu S, Seyahi E, Kocer N, et al. Myelopathy in Behçet's disease: the bagel sign. Ann Neurol. 2017;82:288–98.
29. Emekli AS, Doğan FU, Gündüz T, Sezgin M, Ekizoğlu E, Yeşilot N, et al. Lesion probability map in cerebral vein thrombosis due to Behçet's disease. Int J Rheum Dis. 2023;26:145–50.
30. Saruhan-Direskeneli G, Yentür SP, Mutlu M, Shugaiv E, Yesilot N, Kürtüncü M, et al. Intrathecal oligoclonal IgG bands are infrequently found in neuro-Behçet's disease. Clin Exp Rheumatol. 2013;31:25–7.
31. Akman-Demir G, Tüzün E, Içöz S, Yeşilot N, Yentür SP, Kürtüncü M, et al. Interleukin-6 in neuro-Behçet's disease: association with disease subsets and long-term outcome. Cytokine. 2008;44:373–6.
32. Hirohata S, Kikuchi H, Sawada T, Nagafuchi H, Kuwana M, Takeno M, et al. Clinical characteristics of neuro-Behcet's disease in Japan: a multicenter retrospective analysis. Mod Rheumatol. 2012;22:405–13.
33. Akman-Demir G, Mutlu M, Kiyat-Atamer A, Shugaiv E, Kurtuncu M, Tugal-Tutkun I, et al. Behçet's disease patients with multiple sclerosis-like features: discriminative value of Barkhof criteria. Clin Exp Rheumatol. 2015;33:S80–4.
34. Ishido M, Horita N, Takeuchi M, Shibuya E, Yamane T, Kawagoe T, et al. Distinct clinical features between acute and chronic progressive parenchymal neuro-Behçet disease: meta-analysis. Sci Rep. 2017;7:1–8.
35. Kürtüncü M, Altunrende B, Akman G. Treatment of neuro-Behçet's disease. In: Tüzün E, Kürtüncü M, editors. Neuro-Behçet's Dis Pathog Clin Asp Treat. Springer: Cham; 2021. p. 123–49.
36. Sota J, Capuano A, Emmi G, Iannone F, Cantarini L, Hatemi G, et al. Therapeutic approach to central nervous system involvement of Behçet's disease. Semin Arthritis Rheum. 2023;61:152206.
37. Alibaz-Oner F, Direskeneli H. Advances in the treatment of Behcet's disease. Curr Rheumatol Rep. 2021;23:47.
38. Hirohata S, Kikuchi H, Sawada T, Okada M, Takeno M, Kuwana M, et al. Recommendations for the management of neuro-Behçet's disease by the Japanese National Research Committee for Behçet's disease. Intern Med. 2020;59:2359–67.
39. Tong B, Liu X, Xiao J, Su G. Immunopathogenesis of Behcet's disease. Front Immunol. 2019;10:1–12.
40. Gül A. Pathogenesis of Behçet's disease: autoinflammatory features and beyond. Semin Immunopathol. 2015;37:413–8.
41. Pedersen J, Coskun M, Soendergaard C, Salem M, Nielsen OH. Inflammatory pathways of importance for management of inflammatory bowel disease. World J Gastroenterol. 2014;20:64–77.
42. Webster JD, Vucic D. The balance of TNF mediated pathways regulates inflammatory cell death signaling in healthy and diseased tissues. Front Cell Dev Biol. 2020;8:1–14.
43. Karabulut Y. Use of non-TNF biologics for the treatment of neuro-Behçet's disease: literature review and 2 refractory cases of monoclonal anti-TNFs treated with tocilizumab. Eur J Rheumatol. 2021;8:223–7.
44. Liu J, Yan D, Wang Z, Yang Y, Zhang S, Wu D, et al. Tocilizumab in the treatment of severe and refractory parenchymal neuro-Behçet's syndrome: case series and literature review. Ther Adv Musculoskelet Dis. 2020;12:1759720X2097190.
45. Fragoulis GE, Bertsias G, Bodaghi B, Gul A, van Laar J, Mumcu G, et al. Treat to target in Behcet's disease: should we follow the paradigm of other systemic rheumatic diseases? Clin Immunol. 2023;246:109186.
46. Kidd DP. Neurological involvement by Behçet's syndrome: clinical features, diagnosis, treatment and outcome. Pract Neurol. 2023;23:386–400.

19 Gastrointestinal Manifestations in Behçet's Disease

M. Enver Dolar

Contents

19.1 Introduction

Behçet's disease (BD) is a chronic, relapsing inflammatory disease involving multiple organs, characterized by oral ulcers, genital ulcers, uveitis, skin manifestations, arthritis, and vascular, neurologic, and gastrointestinal involvement. Intestinal BD is diagnosed when there is a typical ulcerative lesion in the gastrointestinal tract in patients with BD [1–6]. There is confusion about the terminology used to describe this intestinal involvement. Among the terms used are "intestinal BD," "entero-BD," and "intestinal lesions associated with BD," with the various terms possibly due to a lack of standardized diagnostic criteria. But currently, Japanese and Korean diagnostic criteria are proposed to detect gastrointestinal (GI) involvement. The etiology and

M. E. Dolar (✉)
Department of Gastroenterology, Bursa Uludağ Üniversitesi Tıp Fakültesi, Bursa, Türkiye
e-mail: edolar@uludag.edu.tr

E. Alpsoy et al. (eds.), *Behçet's Disease: An Integrated Approach*,
https://doi.org/10.1007/978-3-031-77251-1_19

pathogenesis of BD is clearly unknown. The disease course is characterized by relapsing–remitting patterns and presents with a range of diverse clinical manifestations. Abdominal pain, nausea, vomiting, diarrhea, and gastrointestinal bleeding are the most common symptoms. BD may involve any portion of the alimentary tract and different GI organs. GI manifestations of BD are associated with notable morbidity and mortality and decreased quality of life. The frequency of intestinal involvement in patients with BD is reported between 0% and 60% depending on the diagnostic criteria used, age groups and geographical location and the prevalence is high in East Asian countries, including Korea and Japan [1–7].

19.2 Epidemiology of GI Involvement of BD

The reported incidence of gastrointestinal Behçet's disease (GIBD) varies widely, and virtually all available data on the incidence of GIBD are based on the experience of different and separate clinical disciplines. Different reports have used different diagnostic criteria to diagnose the primary condition. However, some studies have assessed the incidence of GIBD based on GI symptoms alone, without endoscopic or radiological confirmation. Countries with a high prevalence of BD are found along the silk route, in the Mediterranean region (especially in Türkiye), in the Middle East, and the Far East. The frequency of GI involvement varies between 0% and 60% depending on the diagnostic criteria used, age groups and geographical location [1–5]. It demonstrates regional disparities, with rates ranging from around 0–4.0% in Türkiye, India, and Saudi Arabia, 10% in China, 38–53% in the UK, and 50–60% in Japan [5–10]. While BD is diagnosed frequently among patients aged 20–30 years the onset of GIBD is generally in the fourth or early fifth decade. On the other hand, it can be seen at any age. Its juvenile BD accounts for 3–7% of all cases of GIBD [3]. The male-to-female ratio of GIBD has been reported to be 1:1 in Türkiye and to be slightly higher in Korea and Japan (1.2–2:1). Whether males with GIBD have more severe disease, as is the case with many other manifestations of BD, is not known, but a Korean study found no difference in the frequency of severe GI disease between males and females [3, 10].

19.3 Pathogenesis and Pathophysiology of Intestinal BD

The specific mechanisms driving the pathogenesis of intestinal BD remain unidentified. There are multiple theories and mechanisms currently being studied to explain the development of GIBD. The widely accepted hypothesis posits that a complex interplay of environmental factors and genetic susceptibility leads to immune dysfunction, resulting in an inflammatory disorder with features of both autoimmune and autoinflammatory conditions [3, 11, 12].

Genetic factors Some studies have specifically investigated the genetic susceptibility loci associated with intestinal involvement in BD and few genetic factors associated with the phenotype of intestinal BD have been identified [3, 11–13].

Environment Research has indicated that cessation of smoking can reduce the frequency and severity of oral ulcers in BD and that nicotine patches can reduce the frequency and severity of oral ulcers in BD. However, no evidence is available on the possible effects of smoking on bowel disease in BD, as is the case for IBD. Despite a sharp and steady increase in IBD prevalence globally, including in previously low-prevalence regions such as Asia and Africa, there appears to be no similar trend in the prevalence of BD/GIBD. This could indicate that environmental factors, such as chemical toxins and other nongerm antigens, are not as important in the pathogenesis of GIBD as they are in IBD [3, 14].

Intestinal Permeability Intestinal permeability increased according to some reports. It is unclear if this constitutes a primary event or is secondary to bowel inflammation and ischemia. As such, the relevance of this finding to the disease mechanism remains uncertain [3].

Immunological abnormalities The gastrointestinal tract serves as a significant gateway for various environmental stimuli that cause immune reactions. Susceptibility genes identified through *Genome-Wide Association Studies (GWAS)* indicate that abnormal immunological responses may be involved in BD's pathogenesis. Also intestinal BD has been linked with abnormal innate immune responses [3, 4, 11–13]. Another possible explanation for GIBD is that it indicates an immune response to potential infectious agents in the gut. M cells, which are optimized for adhering to and transporting antigens, have a crucial role as portals for potential pathogenic agents in gut-associated lymphoid tissue [3, 4]. The expression of intercellular adhesion molecule-1 (ICAM-1) is strong in the majority of venules with inflammatory changes in GIBD [3]. It is considered that chronic and persistent hypoxia originating from the intestinal wall is the underlying cause of ulcer formation [3, 11, 15–17]. Additionally, a study of peripheral blood lymphocytes reported the involvement of activated CD8+ T cells in the pathogenesis of GIBD. Recent research indicates that T cell immune responses in GIBD are skewed toward Th1 dominance due to Txk-expressing Th1 cells. T1-associated cytokines may also play a critical role in the pathogenesis of the disease. Th1 cells in BD patients release cytokines, including INF-α, IFN-y, IL-12, TNF-α, IL-2, and IL-18. indicating distorted Th1 responses [3, 4, 16, 17]. Elevated levels of cytokines, such as IL-8 and TNF-α, in the bloodstream activate polymorphonuclear cells and the endothelial surface. The effectiveness of anti-TNF-α monoclonal antibodies indicates the significance of TNF-α in the development of intestinal Behcet's disease [1–3, 15–17].

19.4 Clinical Manifestations of Intestinal BD

BD is considered a chronic relapsing disease with multiple organ system involvement. Clinical manifestations of intestinal Behçet's disease (BD) exhibit a variety of symptoms, ranging from mild abdominal discomfort to severe abdominal pain, diarrhea, and weight loss accompanied by bleeding (hematochezia or melena), an abdominal mass, weight loss fistula, and perforations. The location and pattern of pain often correlates with the location of the pathology. In a similar pattern to Crohn's disease (CD), a common pain pattern in GIBD is cramping pain in the right lower quadrant in patients with ulcers in the ileocecal area. Gastrointestinal symptoms typically arise between 4 and 6 years after oral ulceration. However, in some cases, intestinal lesions may precede extraintestinal symptoms. The clinical course of intestinal BD is heterogeneous. Over a 5-year follow-up of patients with intestinal BD, the disease remained mildly active in the majority of cases (72%), while the rest (28%) reported multiple relapses or persistent symptoms [1, 3, 4, 18]. Deep ulcers are responsible for the most prevalent intestinal complications, including severe bleeding and perforation. As a result, intestinal lesions have been identified as a determinant associated with a poor prognosis in BD patients, leading to emergency abdominal surgery and bowel resection.

19.5 Patterns of GI Involvement in BD

BD can affect any of the digestive organs, from the mouth to the anus [4]. The involvement of the oral cavity, esophagus, stomach, duodenum, jejunum, ileum, colon, pancreas, liver, and biliary system may occur within the gastrointestinal system. Intestinal BD typically involves the ileocecal area, but similar to CD, although small bowel involvement in GIBD is less common than in CD, recent studies of small bowel involvement using capsule endoscopy have shown that lesions such as erythema, erosions and ulcers can occur in the small bowel, with erythema seen in >90% of patients [1]. Intestinal area is frequently affected, displaying mural findings. The most typical findings are mural ulcerations with a polypoid mucosal surface with involvement of the terminal ileum and ileocecal valve and are less common in the colon, usually excluding the rectum. Diffuse involvement of the colon in less than 15% of cases has been reported. Unlike orogenital ulcers, perianal ulcers are rarely seen in GIBD [3]. In rare instances, the mesentery may also be impacted, which can result in fibrofatty proliferation. Gastrointestinal BD may lead to neutrophilic phlebitis, which causes mucosal ulcerations. Alternatively, it can affect large vessels such as the mesenteric arteries, resulting in ischemia and infarction of the gastrointestinal segments [1–6].

19.6 Diagnosis of Intestinal Behçet's Disease

The diagnosis and management of intestinal BD lesions are not standardized. BD should be considered as a possible diagnosis in patients presenting with right-sided lower abdominal pain and blood-filled stool. In addition, severe abdominal symptoms can occur in patients due to ileus, perforation/penetration, and massive hemorrhage. The diagnosis of GIBD usually requires two steps: (1) The patient should have BD. (2) Intestinal lesions for which no other explanation can be discerned must be identified. Patients who meet that two criteria are diagnosed with intestinal BD. For example, GIBD can be diagnosed if there is a typically oval-shaped deep punched-out ulcer in the ileocecal area, and clinical findings meet BD diagnostic criteria, with the exclusion of infectious enterocolitis, intestinal tuberculosis (I-TB), CD, and other possible causes, including NSAID (nonsteroidal anti-inflammatory drug) colitis. Some GI ulcers in BD patients are difficult to differentiate from those seen in IBD and I-TB. The latter point is especially important in geographies in which BD and I-TB are both common [3]. It should be kept in mind that esophagus and small intestine may also be involved in GIBD. To aid in the differential diagnosis, formal guidelines have been proposed. One such set is a consensus-based practice guideline for the diagnosis and treatment of GIBD using a modified Delphi approach, as proposed in Japan [19]. Based on this, Intestinal BD is diagnosed by the presence of a typical gastrointestinal lesion, consisting of a large, typically oval or round ulcer in the terminal ileum or ulcerations or inflammation in the small or large intestine in patients who meet the Japanese diagnostic criteria of BD [19]. On the other hand, not all patients with GIBD fulfill the systemic BD criteria at the time of colonoscopic evaluation, and systemic manifestations may sequentially develop over a period of many years. Based on this, new diagnostic criteria for GIBD were developed, reflecting temporal changes in systemic manifestations of BD. In this scheme, the patients are categorized into four groups for the diagnosis of GIBD: definite, probable, suspected, and nondiagnostic. They suggested that systemic BD patients with typical ileocecal ulcers should be diagnosed as having "definite intestinal BD," patients with typical ileocecal ulcer and oral ulcers and patients with systemic BD and atypical ulcers should be diagnosed as having "probable intestinal BD," and patients with typical ileocecal ulcers without any BD symptoms should be diagnosed with "suspected intestinal BD" (Fig. 19.1) [20]. The overall sensitivity, specificity, positive predictive value, negative predictive value, and accuracy of the diagnosis probability of these criteria were 99%, 83%, 86%, 98%, and 91%, respectively [20]. Nevertheless, diagnosing patients who are not previously diagnosed with BD and do not present any symptoms can be challenging [21, 22].

Considering the multi-organ involvement in BD, studies have been performed to characterise the clinical and biochemical independent risk factors for the development of GI involvement

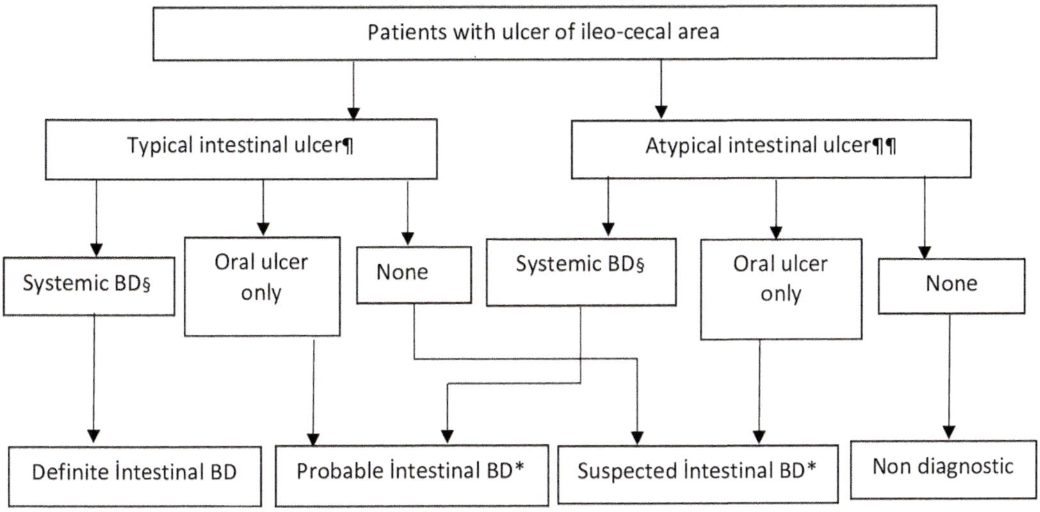

Fig. 19.1 Algorithm for the diagnosis of intestinal Behçet's syndrome based on the type of ileocolonic ulcerations and clinical manifestations. §Complete, incomplete, and suspected subtypes of systemic Behçet's syndrome were classified according to the diagnostic criteria of the Research Committee of Japan; *Close follow-up is necessary; ¶Typical: <5 ulcers, oval in shape, deep, discrete borders located in ileocecal region; ¶¶Atypical: Ulcerations that do not satisfy all criteria for typical. (Adapted from Cheon et al. [20])

and include male gender, Behçet's Disease Current Activity Form (BDCAF) (≥2), ESR (≥15 mm/H), CRP (>10 mg/L), HGB (<130 g/L), and IL-6 (>7 pg/ml) [22, 23].

19.7 Severity of Intestinal BD

Determining the activity of the disease is of great importance for managing the patient, making the treatment plan and predicting prognosis. Disease activity index for intestinal Behçet's disease (DAIBD) is currently used to determine the severity of intestinal BD, but has not been fully validated. Remission is defined as having a score below 19, whereas mild disease is indicated by scores between 20 and 39, moderate disease by scores ranging from 40 to 74, and severe disease by a score equal to or greater than 75 (Table 19.1) [24]. Despite the weak association between endoscopic severity and DAIBD, intestinal ulcers, especially those categorized as crater-like, could serve as a valuable predictor of disease severity. In intestinal Behçet's disease (BD), disease activity is monitored through the assessment of biomarkers. C-reactive protein (CRP) is commonly utilized to evaluate inflammation degree and disease activity [21–25]. Also fecal calprotectin (FC) and fecal lactoferrin (FL) may be useful for screening BD patients who may have small bowel lesions. Patients with small intestinal lesions were found to have significantly higher levels of FC and FL [26, 27]. Direct evaluation of disease activity in intestinal lesions can be conducted by examining ulcerative findings and endoscopic healing. Additionally, monitoring disease activity can be achieved through the use of DAIBD. In a study, the effectiveness of the DAIBD in moni-

Table 19.1 Disease activity index for intestinal Behcet's disease

Item	Score
General well-being for 1 week	
Well	0
Fair	10
Poor	20
Very poor	30
Terrible	40
Fever	
< 38°C	0
> 38°C	10
Extraintestinal manifestations[a]	5 per item
Abdominal pain in 1 week	
None	0
Mild	20
Moderate	40
Severe	80
Abdominal mass	
None	0
Palpable mass	10
Abdominal tenderness	
None	0
Mildly tender	10
Moderately or severely tender	20
Intestinal complications[b]	10 per item
No. of liquid stools in 1 week	
0	0
1–7	10
8–21	20
22-35	30
>36	40

Adapted from Cheon [24]

[a]Score 5 for oral ulcer, genital ulcer, eye lesion, skin lesion, or arthralgia; score 15 for vascular involvement or central nervous system involvement

[b]Fistula, perforation, abscess, or intestinal obstruction

toring changes over time was demonstrated by evaluating changes in score as improved (>20), somewhat improved (10–19), no change (−9 to 10), somewhat worsened (−14 to −11) and worsened (<−15) [24].

19.8 Diagnostic Modalities

Biochemistry There are no laboratory findings characteristic of intestinal BD. Blood biochemistry tests do not indicate any specific features, but they may demonstrate elevated levels of inflammation, including CRP, hypoalbuminemia and anemia, depending on the severity of the illness, nutritional status and level of illness. ESR and CRP showed poor performance as markers of disease activity in patients with full and possible forms of GIBD. In addition, CRP is usually not markedly elevated in GIBD unless it is elevated due to other manifestations of GIBD [3, 22, 25]. Therefore, very high levels of CRP in a patient with GIBD may indicate complications such as stricture, fistula, perforation and abscess formation. A high level of CRP has been reported to be a negative prognostic factor [3, 22, 25]. It has been proposed that *anti-Saccharomyces cerevisiae* antibodies (ASCA), a well-known hallmark of CD, could be also high in patients with BD and GIBD. Intestinal tuberculosis, on the other hand, can also be associated with high ASCA levels [22, 25]. Patients with small intestinal lesions were found to have significantly higher levels of FC and FL, and it may be useful for screening BD patients who may have small bowel lesions. It has been reported to have a cutoff value of FC 70–120 μg/g and FL 17 μg/g for intestinal lesions in BD patients [25–27]. FC is also demonstrating its correlation with disease activity and it has the potential to become a noninvasive biomarker for mucosal healing [3, 22]. Although human leukocyte antigens (HLA), especially HLA-B*51, are the most closely related genetic factor in BD, they are positive in only 32–53% of patients in different geographies. In patients with GİBD, the rate of HLA-B51 positivity varies between 20% and 35% and this rate is slightly lower than in BD [1, 3, 22].

Endoscopy Upper endoscopy should be performed in patients with symptoms in the upper GI tract. *Esophageal involvement is relatively rare, occurring in only 5–11% of cases (4).* The middle part of the esophagus is often the site of esophageal lesions. Various forms of esophageal lesions have been documented, such as erosions, aphthous, linear, or perforating ulcers, widely spreading esophagitis, dissection of the mucosa, varices, and stenosis. Usually, a diagnosis of this condition requires biopsy and cultures to differentiate it from infectious (cytomegalovirus and herpes virus) or malignant conditions. It is important to note that involvement may not be correlated with systemic disease activity, disease duration, or any other aspect of the disease. Additionally, in over 50% of cases, esophageal involvement is accompanied by other gastrointestinal symptoms, mainly jejunal and ileocolonic ulcers. Furthermore, rare but serious complications such as strictures, bleeding, fistulas, or perforations have been reported [3–6, 22]. *The stomach is likely the least affected organ in BD. Ulcers may be found in the stomach or duodenum alone or in both organs at the same time. Rare manifestations include pyloric stenosis and gastroparesis (2).* In cases where intestinal involvement is suspected, a colonoscopy is essential. Typical colonoscopic findings in patients with intestinal BD and previous gastrointestinal surgery were found to be single or multiple deep ulcers with discrete margins in the ileocecal area or at anastomotic sites (Fig. 19.2a). The disease was further classified as localized single, localized multiple, multisegmental and diffuse based on the location and distribution of the lesions, with the localized single type being the most common finding [2]. The incidence of gastrointestinal manifestations in patients with BD was found to be approximately 12–18% in the ileocecal region and 3–5% in the esophagus. Conversely, 96% of patients with intestinal BD have been shown to have ulcerative lesions in the ileocecal regions. In the report of intestinal BD, 12% of patients present with lesions in the ascending colon, 10% in the cecum, 61% in the terminal ileum, and 42% in the ileocecal valve [20, 21]. Regarding the morphology and number of ulcerative lesions in patients with intestinal BD, volcano-shaped ulcers make up 50–83% of cases, with round and geographic ulcers also observed. In patients, 72–76% of ulcers are 1 cm or larger in diameter, and 50–67% are single ulcers [22]. Wireless capsule endoscopy or double balloon endoscopy should be considered in symptomatic patients with negative conventional endoscopic procedures (gastroscopy/colonoscopy) and reasonable clinical indicators such as high CRP levels, stool calprotectin positivity, and/or the existence of unexplained iron deficiency. Capsule endoscopy has a major role in detecting small bowel lesions including reddened lesions, erosions, and ulcers. It also has a role in following up and detecting the efficacy of remission [2, 22, 28]. Diagnosing intestinal BD based on endoscopic biopsy is challenging due to the absence of specific mucosal findings.

Imaging Barium studies can reveal the specific characteristics of vasculitis that affects the gastrointestinal tract. It also help to determine the size of these lesions in cases where significant ulcers are detected. The characteristic radiological findings include single or multiple discrete, button or ring-shaped lesions with marked thickening of the surrounding mucosal folds. The double contrast technique is considered greater diagnostic value [3]. Computed Tomography (CT) is beneficial in evaluating intestinal BD, and

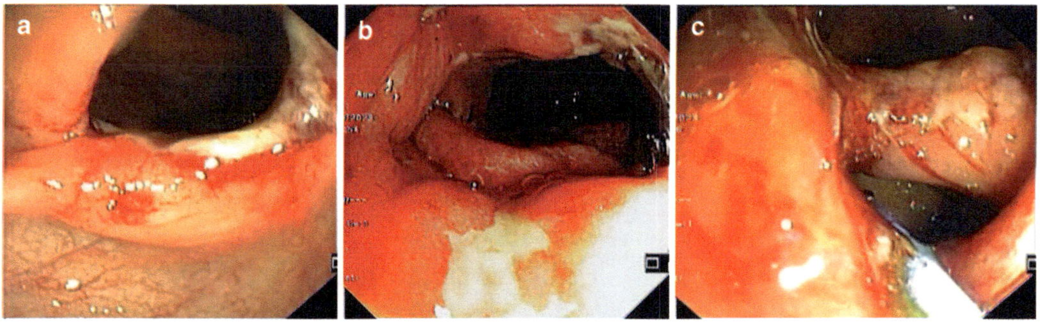

Fig. 19.2 Gastrointestinal lesions in Behçet syndrome (BD), Crohn's disease (CD), and Intestinal tuberculosis (I-TB) (**a**) A typical giant oval-shaped deep punched-out ulcer in the ileocecal area of a patient with BD; (**b**) Longitudinal ulcers in the ileocecal area of a patient with CD. (**c**) Annular ulcers in the ileocecal area of patients with active I-TB. (Private collection)

it is suggested for diagnostic use and early detection of complications and for ruling out other abdominal pathological conditions. The evaluation of intestinal BD may reveal intestinal wall thickening, inflammatory masses, penetration and perforation, and contrast-enhanced CT may help in assessing the disease state. Contrast-enhanced CT can be used as the primary diagnostic tool for patients suspected to have abscess formation, or perforation, with severe right lower abdominal pain or inflammatory masses. Magnetic Resonance Imaging (MRI) can also be useful to visualise bowel wall thickening and inflammatory masses [4, 6, 18, 22]. CT and MR enterography show promise in the diagnosis of GIBD. Furthermore, CT and MR enterography may be useful in differentiating intestinal BD, intestinal tuberculosis and CD [22]. CT, MRI, and abdominal ultrasonography have low sensitivity in morphological identification of intestinal ulcerative lesions and require gastrointestinal angiography and endoscopy or interpretation of surgical specimens for definitive identification. MR enterography has potential as a radiation-free substitute for identifying the origin of nonspecific gastrointestinal symptoms in patients diagnosed with BD. Intestinal BD presents several findings on MR enterography that are also seen in CD and is categorized as a diagnosis of exclusion. In patients without a confirmed diagnosis of BD, the presence of a polypoid pattern on the intestinal surface may help diagnose intestinal Behçet's disease rather than CD. Stenosis formation, long segment disease and involvement of more proximal ileal segments favour small bowel CD [22, 29]. Although abdominal ultrasonography has limited usefulness for evaluating the bowel and is influenced by the operator's skill level and gastrointestinal gas presence, it enables visualization of intestinal wall thickening and inflammatory masses and is minimally invasive. Clinics use it extensively to avoid unnecessary re-endoscopies and obtain information about the bowel wall and surroundings. Ultrasonography can also be used for GIBD follow-up by considering the relative changes in the bowel wall thickness and Doppler activity as indicators of inflammation.

19.9 Differential Diagnosis of Intestinal BD

Intestinal BD should be differentiated from CD, intestinal tuberculosis, nonsteroidal anti-inflammatory drug (NSAID)-induced small

Table 19.2 Comparison of GIBD and CD characteristics

	GIBD	CD
Extraintestinal involvement		
Oral ulcers	100%[a]	20%
Genital ulcer/genital scar	95%/~60%[a]	4%[c]/No case
Nodular lesion	50%[a]	2–10%
Arthritis	20%	5%
Venous thrombosis	15%[a]	<1%
Eye involvement	45%[a]	3–6%[d]
Neurologic involvement	5%[a]	<1%
Intestinal involvement		
Ileocecal	50–90%	40–60%
Rectal	<1%	10%
Upper GI	1%	5%
Perianal	1%[b]	10–15%
Complications		
Perforation/fistula/stricture	25–50%/5–10%[b]/8%	2%/20–30%/17%
Pyoderma gangrenosum	<1%	1–10%
Laboratory assessment		

(continued)

Table 19.2 (continued)

	GIBD	CD
ASCA (IgA or IgG)	28–49%	62–41%
Distribution and endoscopic morphology of intestinal ulcers	Round, focal, isolated	Longitudinal, diffuse, segmental
Histopathology morphology of intestinal ulcers	Perivasculitis with neutrophil and lymphocyte infiltration	Non-caseating granuloma
Granuloma (in mucosal biopsy)	<1%	10–15%
Medical treatment	5-Aminosalicylic acid, systemic steroids, thiopurines, anti-TNF-α agents (infliximab, adalimumab)	5-Aminosalicylic acid, systemic steroids, thiopurines anti-TNF-α agents (infliximab, adalimumab, certolizumab pegol), anti-IL-12/23 mAb (ustekinumab), anti-α4β7 integrin mAb (vedolizumab)

Adapted from Park and Cheon [1] and Cheon et al. [3]

BD Behcet's disease, *CD* Crohn's disease, *ASCA* anti-Saccharomyces cerevisiae antibody, *TNF* tumor necrosis factor, *IL* interleukin, *mAb* monoclonal antibody

[a]Prominently less in females

[b]No anal fistula formation

[c]History based; no real description of typical genital ulcer

[d]Rarely progress to blindness

bowel ulcers and simple ulcers. Intestinal BD has gained a reputation as the "great mimic" because of its clinical and extraintestinal similarities with inflammatory bowel disease (especially CD) and intestinal tuberculosis. Table 19.2 summarizes the common and least common gastrointestinal symptoms associated with intestinal BD and CD, as well as common extraintestinal manifestations [1, 3]. During endoscopic imaging, intestinal BD usually presents as a round or oval perforated ulcer with clearly defined borders in the ileocecal region. Deep ulcerative lesions are sometimes referred to as "volcano-shaped ulcers." Diseases with ulcerative lesions in the ileocecal region include CD and intestinal tuberculosis. CD can be recognized by the characteristic endoscopic appearance of longitudinal ulcerations and cobblestone appearance. Compared with CD, findings suggestive of BD include round or oval ulcers, presence of five or fewer ulcers, dense lesion distribution and irregular geographical ulcers (Fig. 19.2b). However, without these characteristic lesions, it may be difficult to differentiate intestinal BD and CD based on endoscopic findings alone, and therefore systemic symptoms and other clinical/laboratory findings should also be considered [3, 4, 18, 22, 30]. The exclusion of active intestinal tuberculosis is crucial when determining treatment policies and when using TNF-α inhibitors. Endoscopic images of intestinal tuberculosis may vary in presentation, but typical findings include ring-shaped ulcers and scarred areas with discoloration (Fig. 19.2c). Therefore, careful diagnosis is necessary. Medical interviews and physical examinations, as well as chest X-rays and chest computed tomography (CT), are utilized for the differential diagnosis of intestinal tuberculosis. Interferon-gamma release testing (QuantiFERON, T-SPOT), and Mantoux testing may also aid in diagnosis. To distinguish between intestinal Behçet's disease and simple ulcers based solely on endoscopic and pathological findings is challenging. Currently, differentiating between simple ulcers and intestinal Behçet's disease depends on the presence or absence of clinical features of systemic Behçet's disease. However, clinical manifestations of BD can arise after a delayed duration, and subsequent follow-up may reveal that a patient satisfies the diagnostic criteria for intestinal BD. NSAID-triggered small intestinal ulcers seldom exhibit volcano-shaped ulcerative lesions in the ileocecal region; however, a differential diagnosis from intestinal BD may be necessary in the rare instances of multiple ulcerative lesions caused by NSAID therapy [22, 31]. When formulating a differential diagnosis, it is crucial to consider the patient's previous use of internal

NSAIDs and the observed improvement or regression of ulcerative lesions upon discontinuation. It is also necessary to differentiate between intestinal Behçet's disease and nonspecific multiple small bowel ulcers, a condition in which multiple ulcerative lesions occur in the ileum [22, 28]. Figure 19.1 shows the algorithm for differential and definitive diagnosis of intestinal BD [20]. On the other hand, it is important to remember that not all patients with GIBD meet the criteria for systemic BD at the time of colonoscopy, and systemic symptoms may develop sequentially over many years [3, 20, 21].

19.10 Management and Therapy

19.10.1 Medical Therapy

The goal of management of BD is to tailor medical therapy to the level of clinical severity in order to achieve and maintain remission as well as to prevent surgical intervention. A clinical scoring tool known as the disease activity index of Behcet's disease (DAIBD) is used to separate patients into varying levels of clinical severity ranging from quiescent (least severe) to severe [32]. The different medical therapies and the evidence for their use are described in Table 19.3 [2]. Two types of treatment modalities have been proposed for BD: top-down treatment (starting medical therapy initially with biological agents or a combination of a biological agent and an immunomodulator) and step-up treatment (starting initial treatment with corticosteroids and 5-ASA and adding azathioprine and biological agents in resistant cases) [3]. The algorithm for the treatment of intestinal BD are described in Fig. 19.3 [21]

Sulfasalazine or 5-ASA In mild to moderate cases, 5-ASA or the class of aminosalicylates and sulfasalazine (a prostaglandin inhibitor) are often used to induce remission and to maintain remission once it has been achieved. Sulfasalazine or 5-ASA has been shown to be effective in treating intestinal or esophageal BD in some uncontrolled studies and case series and the usual dose of 5-ASA is 2–4 g/day [3, 33–35]. In various retrospective studies, 32% of patients treated with sulfasalazine or 5-ASA monotherapy experienced a clinical relapse and 57% maintained clinical remission after 1 year of treatment. Risk factors for clinical relapse included older age at diagnosis, higher CRP and higher disease activity index score (DAIBD). In a cohort using the size of GI mucosal ulcers (aphthous lesions) as a measure of endoscopic activity, 2–4 g/day of 5-ASA derivatives was observed to heal ulcers in 62% of patients over a follow-up period of 64 months. When DAIBD was used as a disease activity and remission assessment tool in a study a first-line treatment, 5-ASA and steroid followed by AZA did achieve 67% remission rate at week 8. In

Table 19.3 Treatment modalities for Behcet's disease

Disease severity (DAIBD score)	Medical therapy	Highest level of evidence
Mild–moderate (20–39)	ASA	Retrospective cohort study, expert opinion
Moderate–severe (40–75)	CS	Retrospective cohort study, expert opinion, case reports
Moderate–severe (CS resistant)	Anti-TNF agent (adalimumab, infliximab)	Retrospective cohort study, qualitative systematic review (meta-synthesis), expert opinion, case reports
Moderate–severe (CS and anti-TNF resistant)	Immunomodulators (AZA, MTX, thiopurines)	Retrospective cohort study
Other	Thalidomide, tacrolimus	Thalidomide (case series) Tacrolimus (case report)

Adapted from Nguyen et al. [2]
DAIBD disease activity index of Behcet's disease, *CS* corticosteroids, *ASA* aminosalicylates

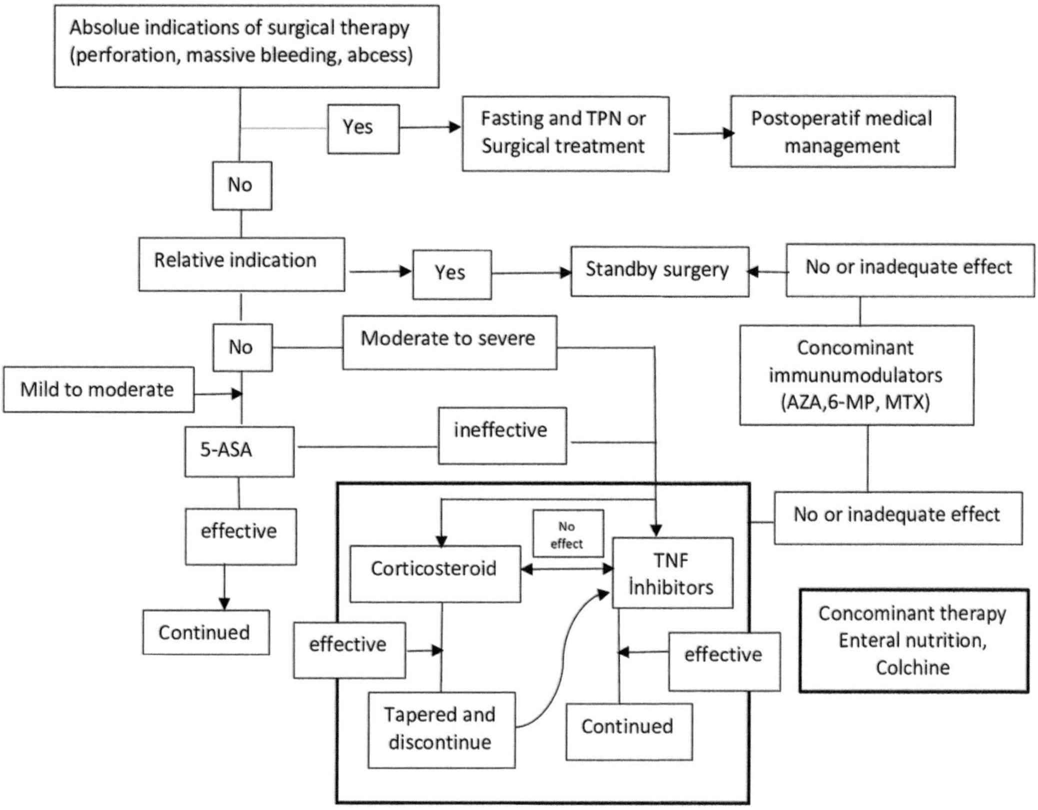

Fig. 19.3 Algorithm for the treatment of intestinal BD. 5-ASA, 5-aminosalicylic acid; 6-MP, 6-mercaptopurine; AZA, azathioprine; MTX, methotrexate; TNF, tumor necrosis factor; TPN, total parenteral nutrition. (Adapted from Watanabe et al. [21])

another study, relapse rates after the remission achievement were found around approximately 8%, 22%, 31%, and 47% at 1-, 3-, 5-, and 10-year follow-up, under 5-ASA, respectively. Therefore, ASA or sulfasalazine monotherapy is only appropriate in patients with mild to moderate disease, as the risk of relapse is significantly increased at high levels of disease activity [33, 34].

Biological Agents There is increasing evidence of efficacy of anti-tumor necrosis factor-a (TNF-a) drugs such as infliximab and adalimumab in studies with biologics to find effective treatments for intestinal BD. Furthermore, new biologics targeting cytokines such as anakinra, a recombinant interleukin (IL)-l receptor antagonist; canakinumab, a human anti-IL-1beta monoclonal antibody (mAb); and tocilizumab, a humanized anti-IL-6 receptor mAb are being actively investigated. The most studied are infliximab and adalimumab, which have been approved for the treatment of intestinal BD in several countries. According to Japanese consensus statements, anti-TNF-α mAbs should be considered a standard treatment intestinal BD [1, 31, 37]. The recently updated 2018 European League Against Rheumatism recommendations for BD management also recommend anti-TNF-α mAbs for severe or refractory intestinal BD [33]. Retrospective and prospective studies showed that TNF-inhibitor agents induced both clinical and endoscopic remission in patients with intestinal BD. A study also found that when corticosteroids are used in combination with TNF-inhibitor agents, there was a significantly increased ulcer healing rate on endoscopy which could be another option prior to moving onto third-line agents [33, 38]. Infliximab and adalimumab are thought to have a similar efficacy and safety profile in intestinal BD and the overall frequency of adverse events was similar on patients with IBD [38, 39]. Therefore, both infliximab and adalimumab can be useful in the therapeutic approach for managing patients with intestinal BD, especially those who do not respond to conventional treatment. In addition, patients who fail treatment with infliximab or adalimumab may be switched to another anti-TNF-a [40]. Independent predictors of a sustained response to infliximab treatment on multivariate analysis were old age (>40 years) at diagnosis, female sex, longer (>5 years) disease duration, concurrent use of an immunomodulator, and remission achievement at week 4 [1, 38–40]. The infliximab is effective in the rapid induction and maintenance of remission in intestinal BD. There have been several case reports on clinical remission and rapid ulcer improvement after infliximab treatment [1, 38–41]. In a retrospective, multicenter study of patients with active, moderate-to-severe intestinal BD, the clinical response rate at weeks 2, 4, 30, and 54 following infliximab infusion was aproximately 75%, 64%, 50%, and 39%, respectively [38–40]. The efficacy of infliximab was also shown in a retrospective, single-center cohort study of patients with intestinal BD refractory to conventional medical treatment, the clinical response rate was aproximately 80%, 64%, 50% and the clinical remission rate was aproximately 27%, 36%, and 38% at week 10, month 12, and month 24, respectively [41]. More recently, in the first prospective, multicentre study reported improvement in clinical symptoms and a decrease in C-reactive protein levels at week 2. Complete symptom-free response was observed in aproximately 36%, 64%, and 80% at weeks 2, 30, and 54, respectively, and healing or scarring of the main intestinal ulcer was detected in 82% of patients at week 14 [42]. The latest prospective cohort study with patients with intestinal BD reported a steroid-free remission rate of 60% at week 30. The rate of mucosal healing was 60% at week 14, and the clinical response rate was 100% and 90% at weeks 14 and 30, respectively [43]. The outcomes of all these studies suggest that infliximab is effective in the rapid induction and maintenance of remission in intestinal BD. The evidence for the effectiveness of infliximab in combination with immunomodulators or in the postoperative setting is insufficient. Combination therapy with infliximab and methotrexate was shown to be effective in a retrospective, single-center study on patients with refractory intestinal BD in achieving short-term remission and long-term response up to 244 months. The ileocecal ulcers diminished by 50% at 6 months and by 90% at 12 months [42]. In another study, the concomitant use of azathioprine did not significantly improve the clinical response to infliximab [3, 42]. Remission with adalimumab has been documented in several case reports [44, 45, 46]. In the first prospective multicentre study of adalimumab in patients with intestinal BD was found that complete remission was achieved in 20% of patients at weeks 24 and 52 with clinical response rates of 45% and 60%, respectively. According to the results of a 100-week follow-up study, 60% and 40% of patients showed clinical response at 52 and 100 weeks, respectively, and complete remission was achieved in 20% and 15% of patients [46, 47]. Etanercept, an anti-TNF agent that is not effective in inflammatory bowel disease, was used in patient with GIBD who did not respond to conventional therapy. Significant improvement was seen in the healing rate of buccal and genital ulcers, remission rate of ocular lesions, skin lesions and abdominal symptoms, healing rate of intestinal ulcers, and improvement rate of ESR and CRP. The ulcer healing rate was reported to be superior with etanercept (89%) compared to the combination of corticosteroids and methotrexate (51%). The relapse rate was also significantly reduced in etanercept treatment. Etanercept treatment, in contrast to conventional therapy, can result in better curative effect and less adverse reactions in intestinal BD [1, 2, 34, 47]. Golimumab may be an effective and safe treatment opportunity in patients with intestinal BD. Golimumab administered in combination with disease-modifying antirheumatic drugs (DMARDs) has provided better results than monotherapy [36, 48]. anakinra or canakinumab treatment showed complete remission in 43% of patients with intestinal BD after 12 months of treatment. No serious side effects were observed in patients receiving canakinumab, and both anakinra and canakinumab may be effective and safe treatments for intestinal BD. Tocilizumab was found to be effective in 80% of patients with BD and clinical symptoms and endoscopic findings improved, including patients with intestinal involvement [1, 34, 49].

Immunomodulating agents Immunomodulating agents such as azathioprine and methotrexate are recommended as third-line agents in patients with moderate to severe BD that are corticosteroid-dependent or corticosteroid and TNF-α inhibitors resistant. Thiopurines also have some utility in reducing rates or recurrence after surgery [1–4]. It is recommended at a dose of 2–2.5 mg/kg/day as in IBD. In a retrospective study, maintenance therapy with azathioprine had a beneficial effect on the reoperation rate after surgery. In a other retrospective study the rate of clinical and endoscopic remission with azathioprine was 65% within the follow-up period. In this study the indications for AZA use were either the presence of a large ulcer (>1 cm) or being refractory to 5-ASA in case of mild disease [3, 50]. In another retrospective study in which the first-line treatment modalities were 5-ASA and corticosteroids, which were followed by azathioprine if the remission could not be achieved, the remission rate at week 8 was reported as 67%. The relapse rates after induction of remission with azathioprine were approximately 6%, 44%, and 52% at 1, 3, and 5 years, respectively [50]. Infliximab and methotrexate combination therapy has been shown to induce short-term remissions and long-term responses for up to 24 months in patients with refractory intestinal BD. The ileocecal ulcers diminished by 50% at 6 months and by 90% at 12 months [1, 42].

19.10.2 Endoscopic Therapy

Obstruction and fibrotic strictures rarely occur and can be adequately treated using balloon dilation. GI bleeding is a serious and common complication of GIBD. The spraying of absolute ethanol has been shown to be effective in a case series from Japan. The effect of ethanol is thought to be achieved through the decrease or disappearance of neutrophils or mononuclear cells from ulcer surface. However, any kind of local treatment which is in use in IBD clinics has the potential for treating GIBD [3].

19.10.3 Surgical Treatment

Intestinal BD is often refractory to conventional treatment and may require surgical management. Perforation and massive GI bleeding are absolute indications for surgery, whereas abdominal abscess, fistula, and stricture can be possible indications. In patients with intestinal BD, the incidence of intestinal perforation, fistula, stricture, and abscess was 13%, 7.5%, 7%, and 3.5%, respectively [2]. The cumulative operation rate is approximately 30% at 5 years and 40% at 10 years [33, 34]. Optimal surgical procedures and the length of normal bowel to be resected are still controversial. Some reports suggest that a more extensive surgical resection such as hemicolectomy with as much as 60–100 cm of ileal resection is preferable. However, others recommended a more conservative approach, resecting only grossly involved segments of bowel, since there seems to be no difference in the rate of recurrences after either modality. Intestinal lesions, usually at the ileocecal area, tend to recur at the anastomosis site, and often require multiple operations because of perforations and fistula formation [3, 33, 34]. The patients who have a high risk of recurrence are more likely to end up receiving surgical management, including patients with GI symptoms at the initial presentation, patients with volcano-type and deep intestinal ulcers, and patients who failed to achieve complete remission during the initial treatment [2].

19.11 Prognosis and Follow-Up

Gastrointestinal involvement in Behçet's disease is often associated with an unfavourable prognosis, with higher morbidity and mortality compared to patients without GI complications. Deep ulcers in intestinal BD may result in severe complications like perforation, gastrointestinal bleeding and obstruction, thus predicting a poor prognosis. Relapses were more probable in patients with intestinal ulcers located in the ileocaecal and colorectal regions, or in those with poor compliance. A recent study reported a relapse rate of approximately 20% during long-term follow-up, regardless of the treatment method used [2, 50]. Intestinal lesions frequently recur (25–78%) after medical treatment. Several studies have reported that the cumulative recurrence rate in patients with GIBD is 25% 2 years after diagnosis, increasing to 49% after 5 years [3]. GI involvement can cause serious complications, including perforation, fistula, and hemodynamically significant GI bleeding, which may require surgery. Repeated surgeries may be necessary for certain patients [2]. Cumulative surgery rates were reported as 7% and 28% 2 years after the initial diagnosis and 15% and 32% after 5 years in two separate studies. Post-operative recurrence can occur at a relatively early stage, often within 2 years, and the cumulatively recurrence rate is as high as 30–75% over 2 years and 50–70% for 5 years [1, 22, 50, 51]. There are some poor prognostic factors, including lack of remission after initial medical treatment and prominent GI symptoms at the time of diagnosis. Furthermore, the shape of the intestinal ulcer is associated with prognosis, with typical volcano-type ulcers requiring surgery more frequently. Ocular disease and extensive disease involving the ileum together with the presence of ASCA have also been suggested as poor prognostic markers. Recurrence rates are also relatively high in patients operated as a result of perforation or fistula formation [3, 51]. Currently, endpoints for treatment are not well established in regard to whether the goal should be to aim for ulcer healing on endoscopy or simply clinical remission. Studies have shown correlation between endoscopic ulcer healing and clinical improvement and also between patients with endoscopic recurrence and clinical recurrence. Given that endoscopic ulcer healing and recurrence both correlate with clinical improvement and also may have predictive value in risk stratifying post-surgical patients for relapse, conducting regular surveillance endoscopy may have utility in determining which patients may require escalation in medical therapy; however, currently there are no established guidelines for surveillance [2]. As in any other chronic bowel inflammation, like IBD, assessment of flares in the follow-up of endoscopically confirmed GIBD with the help of symptoms, acute phase and stool calprotectin level which is a more sensitive and reliable method of stool leucocyte assessment more convenient way compared to repeating colonoscopy. The initial baseline fecal calprotectin level at the time of colonoscopy may provide an opportunity for a clearer clinical assessment at baseline and at follow-up. Any increase or decrease relative to previous measurements later during follow-up may increase the sensitivity of the assessment. Fecal calprotectin and acute phase reactants have a supporting role in predicting the frequency and necessity of repeat endoscopy, recurrences and remissions, and identifying asymptomatic patients with the potential for complicated ulcers [3].

References

1. Park Y, Cheon JH. Update on the treatment of Behcet's disease of the small bowel with biologic agents. Curr Gastroenterol Rep. 2020;22:24.
2. Nguyen A, Upadhyay S, Javaid MA. Behçet's disease: an in-depth review about pathogenesis, gastrointestinal manifestations, and management. Inflamm Intest Dis. 2021;6:175–85.
3. Cheon JH, Celik AF, Kim WH. Behçet's disease: gastrointestinal involvement. In: Yazıcı Y, Yazıcı H, editors. Behçet's syndrome. New York: Springer; 2014. p. 165–88.
4. Tadakazu H, Naganuma M, Matsuoka K, et al. Diagnosis and management of intestinal Behçet's disease. Clin J Gastroenterol. 2014;7:205–12.
5. Gürler A, Boyvat A, Türsen U. Clinical manifestations of Behçet's disease: an analysis of 2147 patients. Yonsei Med J. 1997;38:423–7.
6. Skef W, Hamilton MJ, Arayssi T. Gastrointestinal Behcet's disease: a review. World J Gastroenterol. 2015;21(13):3801–12.
7. Davatchi F, Chams-Davatchi C, Shams H, et al. Behcet's disease: epidemiology, clinical manifestations, and diagnosis. Expert Rev Clin Immunol. 2017;13(1):57–65.

8. Davatchi F, Shahram F, Chams-Davatchi C, et al. Behcet's disease: from east to west. Clin Rheumatol. 2010;29(8):823–33.
9. Kim DK, Yang SK, Byeon JS, et al. Clinical manifestations and course of intestinal Behçet's disease: an analysis in relation to disease subtypes. Intest Res. 2015;3(1):48–54.
10. Tursen U, Gurler A, Boyvat A. Evaluation of clinical findings according to sex in 2313 Turkish patients with Behçet's disease. Int J Dermatol. 2003;42:346–51.
11. Salmaninejad A, Zamani MR, Shabgah AG, et al. A. Behcet's disease: an immunogenetic perspective. J Cell Physiol. 2019;234:8055–74.
12. Kim SW, Jung YS, Ahn JB, et al. Identification of genetic susceptibility loci for intestinal Behçet's disease. Sci Rep. 2017;7:39850.
13. Mizuki N, Meguro A, Ota M, et al. Genome-wide association studies identify IL23R–IL12RB2 and IL10 as Behcet's disease susceptibility loci. Nat Genet. 2010;42:703–6.
14. Soy M, Erken E, Konca K, Ozbek S. Smoking and Behçet's disease. Clin Rheumatol. 2000;19:508–9.
15. Hayasaki N, Ito M, Suzuki T, et al. Neutrophilic phlebitis is characteristic of intestinal Behçet's disease and simple ulcer syndrome. Histopathology. 2004;45(4):377–83.
16. Suzuki Y, Hoshi K, Matsuda T, et al. Increased peripheral blood gamma delta+ T cells and natural killer cells in Behçet's disease. J Rheumatol. 1992;19(4):588–92.
17. Harzallah O, Kerkeni A, Baati T, et al. Oxidative stress: correlation with Behçet's disease duration, activity and severity. Eur J Intern Med. 2008;19(7):541–7.
18. Jung YS, Cheon JH, Park SJ, et al. Clinical course of intestinal Behcet's disease during the first five years. Dig Dis Sci. 2013;58(2):496–503.
19. Kobayashi K, Ueno F, Bito S, et al. Development of consensus statements for the diagnosis and management of intestinal Behçet's disease using a modified Delphi approach. J Gastroenterol. 2007;42(9):737–45.
20. Cheon JH, Kim ES, Shin SJ, et al. Development and validation of novel diagnostic criteria for intestinal Behcet's disease in Korean patients with ileocolonic ulcers. Am J Gastroenterol. 2009;104:2492–9.
21. Watanabe K, Tanida S, Inoue N, et al. Evidence-based diagnosis and clinical practice guidelines for intestinal Behcet's disease 2020 edited by Intractable Diseases, the Health and Labour Sciences Research Grants. Gastroenterol. 2020;55:679–700.
22. Hou C-c, Ye J-f, Ma H-f, et al. Clinical characteristics and risk factors of intestinal involvement in Behçet's syndrome patients: a cross-sectional study from a single center. Orphanet J Rare Dis. 2021;16:132.
23. Davatchi F, Assaad-Khalil S, Calamia KT, et al. The International Criteria for Behcet's Disease (ICBD): a collaborative study of 27 countries on the sensitivity and specificity of the new criteria. J EurAcad Dermatol Venereol JEADV. 2014;28:338–47.
24. Cheon JH, Han DS, Park JY, et al. Development, validation, and responsiveness of a novel disease activity index for intestinal Behcet's disease. Inflamm Bowel Dis. 2011;17:605–13.
25. Kiafar M, Faezi ST, Kasaeian A, et al. Diagnosis of Behçet's disease: clinical characteristics, diagnostic criteria, and differential diagnoses. BMC Rheumatol. 2021;5(1):2.
26. Hayashida M, Miyoshi J, Mitsu T. Elevated fecal calprotectin and lactoferrin associated with small intestinal lesions in patients with Behçet disease. J Gastroenterol Hepatol. 2020;35(8):1340–6.
27. Kim DH, Park Y, Kim B. Fecal calprotectin as a non-invasive biomarker for intestinal involvement of Behçet's disease. J Gastroenterol Hepatol. 2017;32(3):595–601.
28. Arimoto J, Endo H, Kato T, et al. Clinical value of capsule endoscopy for detecting small bowel lesions in patients with intestinal Behçet's disease. Dig Endosc. 2016;28(2):179–85.
29. Peker E, Erden A, Erden İ, et al. Intestinal Behçet disease: evaluation with MR Enterography-a case control study. AJR. 2018;211:767–75.
30. Ye JF, Guan JL. Differentiation between intestinal Behçet's disease and Crohn's disease based on endoscopy. Turk J Med Sci. 2019;9:42–9.
31. Hisamatsu T, Ueno F, Matsumoto T, et al. The 2nd edition of consensus statements for the diagnosis and management of intestinal Behcet's disease: indication of anti-TNFalpha monoclonal antibodies. J Gastroenterol. 2014;49:156–62.
32. Cheon JH, Han DS, Park JY, et al. Development, validation, and responsiveness of a novel disease activity index for intestinal Behçet's disease. Inflamm Bowel Dis. 2011;17(2):605–13.
33. Hatemi G, Christensen R, Bang D, et al. 2018 update of the EULAR recommendations for the management of Behçet's syndrome. Ann Rheum Dis. 2018;6:808–18.
34. Kun H, Dong W. The treatment principles and targets for intestinal Behcet's disease. Ther Adv Gastroenterol. 2023;16:1–10.
35. Cheon JH, Kim WH. An update on the diagnosis, treatment, and prognosis of intestinal Behcet's disease. Curr Opin Rheumatol. 2015;27(1):24–31.
36. Sugimura N, Mizoshita T, Sugiyama T, et al. Real-world efficacy of adalimumab and infliximab for refractory intestinal Behçet's disease. Dig Liver Dis. 2019;1(7):967–71.
37. Vallet H, Riviere S, Sanna A, et al. Efficacy of anti-TNF alpha in severe and/or refractory Behcet's disease: multicenter study of 124 patients. J Autoimmun. 2015;62:67–74.
38. Inoue N, Kobayashi K, Naganuma M, et al. Long-term safety and efficacy of adalimumab for intestinal Behcet's disease in the open label study following a phase 3 clinical trial. Intest Res. 2017;5(3):395–401.
39. Sugimura N, Mizoshita T, Sugiyama T, et al. Real-world efficacy of adalimumab and infliximab for refractory intestinal Behcet's disease. Dig Liver Dis. 2019;51(7):967–71.

40. Hibi T, Hirohata S, Kikuchi H, et al. Infliximab therapy for intestinal, neurological, and vascular involvement in Behcet disease: efficacy, safety, and pharmacokinetics in a multicenter, prospective, open-label, single-arm phase 3 study. Medicine. 2016;95(24):e3863.
41. Zou J, Ji DN, Shen Y, et al. Mucosal healing at 14 weeks predicts better outcome in low-dose infliximab treatment for Chinese patients with active intestinal Behcet's disease. Ann Clin Lab Sci. 2017;7(2):171–7.
42. Iwata S, Saito K, Yamaoka K, et al. Efficacy of combination therapy of anti-TNF-alpha antibody infliximab and methotrexate in refractory entero-Behcet's disease. Mod Rheumatol. 2011;21(2):184–9.
43. van Laar JA, Missotten T, van Daele PL, et al. Adalimumab: a new modality for Behcet's disease? Ann Rheum Dis. 2007;66(4):565–6.
44. De Cassan C, De Vroey B, Dussault C, et al. Successful treatment with adalimumab in a familial case of gastrointestinal Behcet's disease. J Crohns Colitis. 2011;5(4):364–8.
45. Ariyachaipanich A, Berkelhammer C, Nicola H. Intestinal Behcet's disease: maintenance of remission with adalimumab monotherapy. Inflamm Bowel Dis. 2009;15(12):769–71.
46. Tanida S, Inoue N, 19 K, et al. Adalimumab for the treatment of Japanese patients with intestinal Behcet's disease. ClinGastroenterol Hepatol. 2015;13(5):940–8.e3.
47. Ma D, Zhang CJ, Wang RP, et al. Etanercept in the treatment of intestinal Behcet's disease. Cell Biochem Biophys. 2014;69(3):735–9.
48. Vitale A, Emmi G, Lopalco G, et al. Long-term efficacy and safety of golimumab in the treatment of multirefractory Behcet's disease. Clin Rheumatol. 2017;36(9):2063–9.
49. Cantarini L, Vitale A, Scalini P, et al. Anakinra treatment in drug-resistant Behcet's disease: a case series. Clin Rheumatol. 2015;34(7):1293–301.
50. Jung YS, Cheon JH, Hong SP, et al. Clinical outcomes and prognostic factors for thiopurine maintenance therapy in patients with intestinal Behcet's disease. Inflamm Bowel Dis. 2012;18(4):750–7.
51. Jung YS, Yoon JY, Lee JH, et al. Prognostic factors and longterm clinical outcomes for surgical patients with intestinal Behcet's disease. Inflamm Bowel Dis. 2011;17:1594–602.

How Should We Diagnose Behçet's Disease

20

Ayşe Boyvat

Contents

20.1 Introduction

Behçet's disease (BD) was initially described by Prof. Hulusi Behçet as a distinct entity characterized by recurrent oral and genital aphthous ulcerations and iridocyclitis [1]. However, over time, it has become apparent that the disease is not limited to these three symptoms alone but displays a remarkably heterogeneous clinical spectrum, including mucocutaneous, arthritic, ocular, vascular, neurologic, and gastrointestinal manifestations. Subsequently, the diagnostic challenge of BD surfaced, as there was an absence of pathognomonic clinical, histopathologic, or laboratory findings. The diagnosis primarily relies on clinical manifestations requiring the exclusion of other potential causes. However, the wide clinical spectrum of the disease, the interval between the initial manifestation of the disease and the other manifestations, which may take years in some patients, as well as the course of the disease characterized by remissions and exacerbations, cause difficulties in the diagnosis of BD. Moreover, there is considerable geographical variation in both disease prevalence and manifestations.

HLA-B51 is the strongest genetic association of BD, and its positivity ranges around 40–80% in patients with BD among different ethnic populations [2–4]. The higher prevalence of HLA-B51 in BD compared to the healthy population underscores the significant role of genetic factors in the disease's pathogenesis. Despite its

A. Boyvat (✉)
Dermatology and Venereology, Ankara University, Faculty of Medicine, Ankara, Türkiye
e-mail: boyvat@medicine.ankara.edu.tr

E. Alpsoy et al. (eds.), *Behçet's Disease: An Integrated Approach*,
https://doi.org/10.1007/978-3-031-77251-1_20

importance, HLA B-51 positivity has only a limited value as a diagnostic test on account of its high frequency among the general population, particularly in countries along the ancient Silk Road, where BD is more prevalent [2–4].

20.2 Pathergy Test

Pathergy reaction is defined as a cutaneous hypersensitivity reaction to trauma induced by an intradermal prick. Pathergy reaction is the only diagnostic tool and is one of the criteria in the diagnosis of BD. However, the sensitivity of the test shows significant geographic differences. While a positive pathergy test is found in 60–70% of patients with BD in Türkiye, Iran, and Japan, the sensitivity rates are much lower, around 5–15%, in North America and Northern Europe [5].

While the pathergy test has traditionally been regarded as specific for Behçet's disease, it can also be positive in some other disorders such as Sweet's syndrome, pyoderma gangrenosum, Crohn's disease, and A20 haploinsufficiency [5]. Furthermore, recent studies indicate a decline in the positivity rate and the diagnostic value of the pathergy test in the last few decades, possibly attributable to the use of less traumatic needles and changes in skin microbiota [5–8].

20.3 Evolution of Diagnostic Criteria

As the diagnosis of BD depends on proper history taking and characteristic clinical manifestations, diagnostic criteria were developed for BD over the years to provide more objectivity to the diagnosis.

The initial set of criteria, proposed by Curth in 1946 [9], was followed by numerous others [10–24] (Table 20.1). The primary reason for the proposal of a large number of diagnostic criteria sets was likely the diversity of the disease phenotype among patients, induced primarily by factors such as gender, ethnicity, and/or country of residence. This diversity restricted the universal acceptance of the criteria sets and likely accounted for variations in the performance of the same diagnostic criteria set in studies conducted across different countries.

Table 20.1 Evolution of diagnostic criteria for Behçet's disease [9–24]

1946	Curth [9]
1969	Mason and Barnes [10]
1971	Hewitt [11]
1972	Behçet's syndrome Research Committee of Japan [12]
1974	Hubault and Hamza [13]
1974	O'Duffy [14]
1980	Cheng and Zhang [15]
1985	Dilşen [16]
1987	Behçet's syndrome research Committee of Japan (revised) [17]
1990	International Study Group for Behçet's Disease [18]
1993	Iran traditional tree [19]
1993	Iran classification tree [20]
2003	Dilşen (revised) [21]
2004	Korea [22]
2014	International Criteria for Behçet's Disease [23]
2016	Concensus Criteria for Paediatric Behçet's Disease [24]

By the end of the 1980s, nine sets of criteria had been proposed from different countries, and there was no consensus on any of them. Each of these criteria sets has its own list of clinical findings and rules for diagnosing BD. Although the symptoms and signs included in them are somewhat similar, they are assigned different values and scores. In most of these criteria, clinical features were divided into major and minor features based on the prevalence of the features, not their clinical severity. Consequently, common clinical hallmarks such as oral aphthous ulcers, genital ulcers, skin manifestations, ocular involvement, and the positivity of the pathergy test were classified as major features. In contrast, vascular, gastrointestinal, and neurological involvements—despite being the most severe manifestations of BD and life-threatening—were considered minor features due to their lower sensitivity. However, none of the criteria mentioned above achieved worldwide acceptance. In the 1980s, clinicians from different countries were using their own criteria for the diagnosis of their patients, and the classification of patients entered into studies.

To overcome this problem, the International Study Group (ISG) for Behçet's Disease was formed in 1985 with the aim of reviewing the existing criteria and agreeing on a new set of internationally accepted diagnostic criteria. The group, comprised of scientists from seven countries, expressed their main aim as 'obtaining an agreed set of diagnostic criteria to be quoted in all future published work, to enable comparisons between studies, and to be used as a basis for multicenter collaborative studies.' Twelve centers from seven countries participated in the study, and the research was conducted on 914 patients with BD and 308 controls.

According to the ISG Criteria published in 1990, the presence of recurrent oral aphthous ulceration more than three times in a year is mandatory. Additionally, any two of the following manifestations—recurrent genital ulceration, eye involvement, cutaneous manifestations, and a positive pathergy test—are required for the diagnosis (Table 20.2). Although thrombophlebitis, deep venous thrombosis, arterial, and neurologic involvement all exhibited high specificity, they were not included in the criteria due to their lower sensitivity [23]. ISG criteria were found to have 95% sensitivity and 98% specificity against the control group, and it has been the most commonly used criteria set for diagnosis.

While the ISG criteria have been validated across different ethnic groups [25], a notable limitation arises from its failure to include major organ involvements, such as vascular, neurologic, and gastrointestinal involvement. Patients with vascular or neurologic involvement may not fulfill the criteria even if they exhibit oral aphthous ulceration and one other clinical hallmark of BD, such as genital ulceration, skin manifestations, ocular involvement, and pathergy test positivity. Many authors have expressed their concerns, primarily focused on the possibility that the diagnosis of patients with early systemic involvement may be missed using the ISG criteria [26]. Thus, a delay in reaching an accurate diagnosis could lead to an unfavorable prognosis with negative therapeutic outcomes. While emphasized by two authors from the International study group, Barnes and Yazıcı, that 'International classification criteria have been developed to ensure comparability of groups of patients entered into clinical and laboratory studies, and not to be used in the diagnosis of individual patients' [27], the criteria have frequently been misinterpreted by many clinicians. The fulfillment of the criteria has been erroneously considered a requirement for the diagnosis of BD and the initiation of proper treatment.

In subsequent years, there have been efforts to improve study group criteria, leading to the development of additional criteria. The Iran classification tree, distinct from the traditional format, allows for early suspicion of BD when only two features are present [20]. In Iran criteria (traditional format), the value of ocular manifestation was doubled [19]. Dilşen criteria introduced thrombophlebitis as an additional criterion [21], and the Korean criteria doubled the value of genital ulceration while adding ileocolonic ulceration

Table 20.2 International Study Group Criteria for Behçet's disease [18]

Recurrent oral ulceration	Minor aphthous, major aphthous or herpetiform ulceration observed by physician or patient, which recurred at least three times in one 12-month period
Plus two of	
Recurrent genital ulceration	Aphthous ulceration or scarring, observed by physician or patient
Eye lesions	Anterior uveitis, posterior uveitis, or cells in the vitreous on slit lamp examination or retinal vasculitis observed by an ophthalmologist
Skin lesions	Erythema nodosum observed by physician or patient, pseudofolliculitis, or papulopustular lesions, or acneiform nodules observed by physician in a postadolescent patient, not on corticosteroid treatment
Positive pathergy test	Read by the physician within 24–48 h

[a]Findings applicable only in the absence of other clinical explanations

Table 20.3 International Criteria for Behçet's Disease- point score system: scoring ≥4 indicates Behçet's disease diagnosis [23]

Sign/symptom	Points
Ocular lesions	2
Genital aphthosis	2
Oral aphthosis	2
Skin lesions	1
Neurological manifestations	1
Vascular manifestations	1
Positive pathergy test[a]	1[a]

[a]Pathergy test is optional and the primary scoring system does not include pathergy testing. However, where pathergy testing is conducted, one extra point may be assigned for a positive result

[22]. In all of these criteria, the presence of oral ulcerations was not deemed mandatory, recognizing that some patients may not exhibit oral ulcers at the onset of the disease.

In 2014, a new set of criteria, the International Criteria for Behçet's disease (ICBD), was published. The criteria were derived from a collaborative study involving 2556 clinically diagnosed BD patients and 1163 controls from 27 countries. The ICBD criteria are based on a point score system, incorporating mucocutaneous lesions, ocular involvement, vascular manifestations, and neurological manifestations. Oral and genital ulcerations, as well as ocular lesions, each receive 2 points, while other manifestations are assigned one point. Pathergy test is optional, recognizing that it is not routinely performed in all countries and its positivity varies in different populations. However, if the pathergy test is performed, its positivity is scored as one point. A total score of 4 or more is required for classification as BD (Table 20.3) [23].

The ICBD criteria offer the advantage of facilitating earlier diagnosis and treatment, particularly for patients with vascular and neurologic involvement. The criteria exhibit a higher sensitivity (94.8%) compared to the ISG criteria (85.0%). However, the specificity (90.5%) is slightly lower (90.5% versus ISG's 96%). The potential limitation is the risk of overdiagnosis, especially in the regions where BD is infrequently seen. Patients with recurrent oral and genital ulcerations due to various dermatologic diseases may be mistakenly labeled as BD. In addition, individuals with features of spondyloarthropathy could be incorrectly diagnosed as BD.

20.4 Consensus Classification of Pediatric Behçet's Disease

Behçet's disease has pediatric onset in 4–26% of cases. In pediatric cases, the diagnosis of BD may be challenging as the manifestations of BD may resemble the manifestations of autoinflammatory diseases, inflammatory bowel diseases, and immunodeficiencies. With the objective to propose a new consensus classification for pediatric BD (PEDBD), a prospective study was carried out on 219 patients with BD from 42 centers in 12 countries. All of the patients had the first symptom of the disease before age 16 and fulfilled the criteria established by the expert committee. In the new PEDBD classification, published in 2016, contrary to ISG criteria, oral aphthous ulceration is not mandatory, and the pathergy test is not included. The exclusion of the pathergy test was due to the large variation in the rate of positivity in the pediatric population. Oral aphthous ulceration, genital ulceration, skin lesions, ocular involvement, vascular involvement, and neurologic involvement each carry equal weight, scoring one point each (Table 20.4). Patients with ≥3 scores are categorized as BD [24]. The new international PEDBD classification was shown to have a higher sensitivity (91.7%) and lower specificity (42.9%) compared to the ISG criteria, and the addition of the pathergy test did not improve performance. However, recent studies on pediatric BD reported lower sensitivity rates for PEDBD criteria, ranging between 35.8 to 76% [6, 28–31]. The sensitivity of ICBD criteria was reported to be higher

Table 20.4 Consensus classification of paediatric Behçet's disease (BD) [24]

Item	Description	Value/item
Recurrent oral aphthosis	At least three attacks/year	1
Genital ulceration or aphthosis	Typically with scar	1
Skin involvement	Necrotic folliculitis, acneiform lesions, erythema nodosum	1
Ocular involvement	Anterior uveitis, posterior uveitis, retinal vasculitis	1
Neurological signs	With the exception of isolated headaches	1
Vascular signs	Venous thrombosis, arterial thrombosis, arterial aneurysm	1

Three of six items are required to classify a patient as having pediatric BD

than that of ISG and PEDBD criteria [28–32]. Exclusion of the pathergy test in the PEDBD criteria and the absence of vascular and neurologic involvements in the ISG criteria were considered to be the main reasons for lower sensitivities.

20.5 Organ-Specific Diagnostic Approaches

Diagnosing BD poses a challenge, especially in early cases where major organ involvement, such as uveitis or vascular involvement, precedes the characteristic mucocutaneous manifestations. To address these diagnostic complexities, various approaches have been employed to identify and diagnose specific disease manifestations of BD.

Early diagnosis of BD uveitis is crucial, given its status, as it is one of the most severe causes of noninfectious uveitis that can potentially lead to blindness. Uveitis is reported as the initial manifestation in 6–20% of patients, posing a diagnostic challenge as extraocular manifestations have not yet emerged. In a recent study conducted by Tugal–Tutkun, involving nine centers across five countries, efforts were made to identify the most characteristic manifestations of BD uveitis. The study aimed to develop a diagnostic algorithm facilitating early detection and prompt treatment, regardless of the presence of extraocular manifestations. The algorithm, published in 2021, highlighted specific variables that demonstrated high accuracy in diagnosing ocular involvement in Behçet's disease. These included the presence of superficial retinal infiltrate or its sequel, retinal nerve fiber layer defect, signs of occlusive retinal vasculitis, and diffuse retinal capillary leakage observed through fluorescein angiography. In addition, the absence of granulomatous anterior uveitis or choroiditis in patients with vitritis contributed to the diagnostic criteria [33].

Another alternative approach has been taken to diagnose Neuro-Behçet's disease (NBD) in early cases. In 2014, expert consensus recommendations were published for the diagnosis and management of NBD with the objective of helping clinicians dignose patients with NBD, and differentiate the disease from other mimickers [34]. The specific manifestations of NBD, including the characteristic clinical, neuroimaging, and cerebrospinal fluid findings were outlined through an extensive literature review and consultations with an international advisory panel, followed by a Delphi exercise. International consensus recommendations criteria for the diagnosis of NBD has two levels of certainty; definite NBD was defined as characteristic neurological findings in patients who fulfill ISG criteria, and probable NBD was defined as the presence of characteristic neurological findings suggesting NBD without satisfying ISG criteria or noncharacteristic neurological findings for NBD occurring in the context of ISG criteria.

The prevalence of gastrointestinal involvement varies widely between countries, ranging from 3% to 30% of the patients. Although gastrointestinal involvement is not included in any of the diagnostic criteria sets due to low sensitivity, it is known to be more common in Far East countries like Japan and Korea. Diagnosing intestinal

BD is challenging, especially when gastrointestinal manifestations appear early in the course of the disease before fulfillment of diagnostic criteria. In 2009, 13 experts from three universities in Korea developed a diagnostic criterion for intestinal BD using a modified Delphi method [35]. Patients with fewer than five ileocecal ulcers that were oval in shape, deep with discrete borders were classified as having typical ulcers. Ulcerations that did not satisfy all the characteristic features were classified as atypical. Based on the morphological findings during colonoscopy and the presence of extraintestinal manifestations, the patients were categorized into four groups; definite, probable, suspected and nondiagnostic for intestinal BD. Although histological evidence of vasculitis confirms the diagnosis of intestinal BD, it was not included in the criteria as it was not commonly observed.

Similarly, according to the diagnostic algorithm for intestinal BD compiled by the Japanese Society for Behçet's Disease, patients with right abdominal pain and bloody stool and endoscopically confirmed ileocecal deep ulcers are classified as intestinal BD, suspected BD, or simple ulcer depending on fulfillment of diagnostic criteria defined by the BD Research Committee of Japan [36], following exclusion of Crohn's disease, intestinal tuberculosis, and nonsteroid anti-inflammatory induced ulcers [36, 37].

20.6 Venous Wall Thickness as a New Diagnostic Tool

Alongside efforts to revise and improve the diagnostic criteria, research is also ongoing to find a reliable diagnostic tool to support BD diagnosis. Recently, venous wall thickness has been proposed as a candidate for a new diagnostic criterion.

In 2014, Ambrose et al. reported the results of a feasibility study investigating the potential usefulness of high-resolution MRI in identifying patients with vascular inflammation. The study, conducted on five patients with BD (with/without vascular involvement) and seven healthy controls, revealed increased popliteal vein wall thickness in patients with BD compared to controls [38].

Later, in 2019, Alibaz-Oner et al. evaluated venous wall thickness in lower extremity veins in male patients with BD with Doppler ultrasound, a cost-effective, noninvasive, and easier way to perform vascular assessment. All venous wall measurements were found to be significantly higher in BD compared to ankylosing spondylitis and healthy controls [39].

In a subsequent study, including female patients, the authors compared BD with multiple disease controls, including ankylosing spondylitis, systemic vasculitis, antiphospholipid syndrome, and venous insufficiency. The venous wall thickness was found to be significantly higher in the lower extremity veins of patients with BD.

Recent research encompassing both adult and pediatric patients with BD has confirmed an elevation in vessel wall thickness among patients with BD, irrespective of vascular involvement. The increased thickness has been linked to persistent low-level chronic venous inflammation, suggesting a potential association with thrombosis. The findings from these studies highlight the significant diagnostic potential of the common femoral vein (CFV) thickness measurement, indicating its practical value for identifying BD. However, it's noteworthy that the cut-off value, as well as the sensitivity and specificity values for CFV, varied across different studies [32, 40–43]. Differences in the study populations and the operator-dependent nature of Doppler US may have contributed to these variations. However, the diagnostic value of this finding awaits testing in further studies in other disease groups and in different ethnic groups.

20.7 Conclusion

Until a highly sensitive and specific diagnostic feature or laboratory test for BD is identified, today's diagnosis is still primarily based on clinical manifestations and depends on the experience of the clinician. Diagnostic/classification criteria are helpful for disease diagnosis, particularly in countries where BD is not prevalent. However, it is important to emphasize that diagnostic/classification criteria were developed primarily to ensure comparability in studies conducted on BD and not for bedside diagnosis. Diagnostic difficulties may arise, especially in the early course of the disease, before patients meet the diagnostic criteria. Given the wide clinical spectrum of the disease, there will always be patients who do not meet the criteria, regardless of the set of diagnostic criteria used. The experience and judgment of the physician remain the most crucial factors in diagnosing BD. Patients suspected of having BD should be carefully monitored for the development of other manifestations, even if they do not fulfill the diagnostic criteria.

References

1. Behcet H. Uber rezidivierende aphthosa, durch ein Virus verüsachte Geschewüre am Mund, am Auge und an den Genitalien. Dermatol Wochenschr. 1937;109:1152–7.
2. Kotter I, Gunaydin I, Stubiger N, Yazici H, Fresko I, Zouboulis CC, et al. Comparative analysis of the association of HLA-B*51 suballeles with Behcet's disease in patients of German and Turkish origin. Tissue Antigens. 2001;58(3):166–70.
3. Pirim I, Atasoy M, Ikbal M, Erdem T, Aliagaoglu C. HLA class I and class II genotyping in patients with Behcet's disease: a regional study of eastern part of Turkey. Tissue Antigens. 2004;64(3):293–7.
4. Mizuki N, Meguro A, Tohnai I, Gul A, Ohno S, Mizuki N. Association of Major Histocompatibility Complex Class I Chain-Related Gene a and HLA-B alleles with Behcet's disease in Turkey. Jpn J Ophthalmol. 2007;51(6):431–6.
5. Ergun T. Pathergy phenomenon. Front Med (Lausanne). 2021;8:639404.
6. Boyvat A, Oktem A, Kalay Yildizhan I, Ates A, Yalcindag N, Koksoy C, et al. A comparison of adult and juvenile Behcet patients and a look at clinical trends: retrospective data from a Turkish follow-up cohort study. Dermatology. 2023;239(6):958–65.
7. Davatchi F, Chams-Davatchi C, Ghodsi Z, Shahram F, Nadji A, Shams H, et al. Diagnostic value of pathergy test in Behcet's disease according to the change of incidence over the time. Clin Rheumatol. 2011;30(9):1151–5.
8. Direskeneli H, Mumcu G. A possible decline in the incidence and severity of Behcet's disease: implications for an infectious etiology and oral health. Clin Exp Rheumatol. 2010;28(4 Suppl 60):S86–90.
9. Curth HO. Recurrent genito-oral aphthosis and uveitis with hypopyon (Behcet's syndrome). Arch Dermatol Syphilol. 1946;54:179–96.
10. Mason RM, Barnes CG. Behcet's syndrome with arthritis. Ann Rheum Dis. 1969;28(2):95–103.
11. Hewitt J, Escande JP, Manesse S. Revision of the diagnostic criteria of Behcet's syndrome. Presse Med (1893). 1971;79(20):901.
12. BsDRCo J. Behçet's disease: guide to diagnosis of Behçet's disease (1972). Jpn J Ophthalmol. 1974;18:291–4.
13. Hubault AH, M. La Maladie de Behçet en 1974. In: Seze Sea, editor. L'actualite Rhumatologique Paris. 15. Paris: Expension Scientifique; 1974. p. 43–55.
14. O'Duffy JD. Criteres proposes pour la diagnostic maladie Behçet et notes the rapeutiques. Rev Med. 1974;36:2371–9.
15. Cheng SPZ, X.Q. Some special clinical manifestations of Behçet's disease and review of literature. Chin J Int Med. 1980;19:15–22.
16. Dilsen NKM, Aral O. Our diagnostic criteria of Behcet's disease—an overview. In: Lehner TB, CG, editor. Recent advances in Behcet's disease. International congress and symposium series 103: London Royal Society of Medicine Services 1986. p. 177–180.
17. Mizushima Y. Revised diagnostic criteria for Behcet's disease in 1987. Ryumachi. 1988;28(1):66–70.
18. Criteria for diagnosis of Behcet's disease. International study group for Behcet's disease. Lancet. 1990;335(8697):1078–80.
19. Davatchi FS, Shahram F, Akbarian M. Accuracy of existing diagnosis criteria for Behcet's disease. In: Wechsler BG, Godeau P, editors. Behcet's disease Excerpta Medica international congress series 1037. Amsterdam: Excerpta Medica; 1993. p. 225–8.
20. Davatchi FS, Shahram F, Akbarian M, et al. Classification tree for the diagnosis of Behcet's disease. In: Wechsler BG, Godeau P, editors. Behcet's disease Excerpta Medica international congress series 1037. Amsterdam: Excerpta Medica; 1993. p. 245–8.
21. Dilşen N. About diagnostic criteria for Behcet's disease: our new proposal. In: Bang DL, Lee ES, Lee S, editors. Behçet's disease. Seoul: Design Mecca Publishing Co; 2003. p. 101–4.
22. Chang HK, Lee SS, Bai HJ, Lee YW, Yoon BY, Lee CH, et al. Validation of the classification criteria commonly used in Korea and a modified set of preliminary criteria for Behcet's disease: a multi-center study. Clin Exp Rheumatol. 2004;22(4 Suppl 34):S21–6.
23. The International Criteria for Behçet's Disease (ICBD): a collaborative study of 27 countries on the sensitivity and specificity of the new criteria. J Eur Acad Dermatol Venereol. 2014;28(3):338–47.
24. Kone-Paut I, Shahram F, Darce-Bello M, Cantarini L, Cimaz R, Gattorno M, et al. Consensus classification criteria for paediatric Behcet's disease from a pro-

spective observational cohort: PEDBD. Ann Rheum Dis. 2016;75(6):958–64.
25. O'Neill TW, Rigby AS, Silman AJ, Barnes C. Validation of the international study group criteria for Behcet's disease. Br J Rheumatol. 1994;33(2):115–7.
26. Mignogna MD, Fedele S, Lo RL. International diagnostic criteria and delay of diagnosis in Behcet's disease. J Rheumatol. 2000;27(11):2725.
27. Barnes CG, Yazici H. Behcet's syndrome. Rheumatology (Oxford). 1999;38(12):1171–4.
28. Kurt T, Aydin F, Sezer M, Tekgoz PN, Tekin ZE, Celikel E, et al. Performance of diagnostic criteria in pediatric Behcet's disease. Rheumatol Int. 2022;42(1):127–32.
29. Shahram F, Nadji A, Akhlaghi M, Faezi ST, Chams-Davatchi C, Shams H, et al. Paediatric Behcet's disease in Iran: report of 204 cases. Clin Exp Rheumatol. 2018;36(6 Suppl 115):135–40.
30. Batu ED, Sonmez HE, Sozeri B, Butbul Aviel Y, Bilginer Y, Ozen S. The performance of different classification criteria in paediatric Behcet's disease. Clin Exp Rheumatol. 2017;35 Suppl 108(6):119–23.
31. Gallizzi R, Pidone C, Cantarini L, Finetti M, Cattalini M, Filocamo G, et al. A national cohort study on pediatric Behcet's disease: cross-sectional data from an Italian registry. Pediatr Rheumatol Online J. 2017;15(1):84.
32. Atalay E, Oguz B, Sener S, Ozcan HN, Sag E, Kaya Akca U, et al. A new tool supporting the diagnosis of childhood-onset Behcet's disease: venous wall thickness. Rheumatology (Oxford). 2023;62(SI2):SI181–SI8.
33. Tugal-Tutkun I, Onal S, Stanford M, Akman M, Twisk JWR, Boers M, et al. An algorithm for the diagnosis of Behcet disease uveitis in adults. Ocul Immunol Inflamm. 2021;29(6):1154–63.
34. Kalra S, Silman A, Akman-Demir G, Bohlega S, Borhani-Haghighi A, Constantinescu CS, et al. Diagnosis and management of Neuro-Behcet's disease: international consensus recommendations. J Neurol. 2014;261(9):1662–76.
35. Cheon JH, Kim ES, Shin SJ, Kim TI, Lee KM, Kim SW, et al. Development and validation of novel diagnostic criteria for intestinal Behcet's disease in Korean patients with ileocolonic ulcers. Am J Gastroenterol. 2009;104(10):2492–9.
36. Watanabe K, Tanida S, Inoue N, Kunisaki R, Kobayashi K, Nagahori M, et al. Evidence-based diagnosis and clinical practice guidelines for intestinal Behcet's disease 2020 edited by intractable diseases, the health and labour sciences research Grants. J Gastroenterol. 2020;55(7):679–700.
37. Kobayashi K, Ueno F, Bito S, Iwao Y, Fukushima T, Hiwatashi N, et al. Development of consensus statements for the diagnosis and management of intestinal Behcet's disease using a modified Delphi approach. J Gastroenterol. 2007;42(9):737–45.
38. Ambrose N, Pierce IT, Gatehouse PD, Haskard DO, Firmin DN. Magnetic resonance imaging of vein wall thickness in patients with Behcet's syndrome. Clin Exp Rheumatol. 2014;32(4 Suppl 84):S99–102.
39. Alibaz-Oner F, Ergelen R, Mutis A, Erturk Z, Asadov R, Mumcu G, et al. Venous vessel wall thickness in lower extremity is increased in male patients with Behcet's disease. Clin Rheumatol. 2019;38(5):1447–51.
40. Kaymaz S, Yilmaz H, Ufuk F, Utebey AR, Cobankara V, Karasu U, et al. Ultrasonographic measurement of the vascular wall thickness and intima-media thickness in patients with Behcet's disease with symptoms or signs of vascular involvement: a cross-sectional study. Arch Rheumatol. 2021;36(2):258–66.
41. Alibaz-Oner F, Direskeneli H. Update on the diagnosis of Behcet's disease. Diagnostics (Basel). 2022;13(1)
42. Seyahi E, Gjoni M, Durmaz ES, Akbas S, Sut N, Dikici AS, et al. Increased vein wall thickness in Behcet disease. J Vasc Surg Venous Lymphat Disord. 2019;7(5):677–84 e2.
43. Alibaz-Oner F, Ergelen R, Yildiz Y, Aldag M, Yazici A, Cefle A, et al. Femoral vein wall thickness measurement: a new diagnostic tool for Behcet's disease. Rheumatology (Oxford). 2021;60(1):288–96.

Pathology of Skin Manifestations in Behçet Disease

21

Cuyan Demirkesen

Contents

21.1 Introduction

Behçet disease (BD) has a diverse range of skin manifestations, which can provide valuable diagnostic insights. This chapter delves into the pathology of skin manifestations to have a better understanding of the nature and pathogenesis of the disease and the underlying mechanisms. BD has no strict pathognomonic features on histopathology, however, it has a wide range of microscopic changes.

Skin involvement of BD is diverse, including oral and genital/extragenital ulcers, papulopustular lesions, erythema nodosum (EN)-like lesions, superficial thromboflebitis, pathergy test [1, 2]. Other reported associations of BD are Sweet's syndrome-like lesions, pyoderma gangrenosum-like lesions, erythema multiforme-like lesions, pernio-like lesions, neutrophilic eccrine hidradenitis, bullous lesions due to necrotizing vasculitis, and palpable purpura [3, 4]. The skin lesions often present with a cyclical pattern, mirroring the relapsing-remitting nature of the disease. Notably, the severity and distribution of cutaneous manifestations can vary widely between individuals, making accurate diagnosis a complex task.

C. Demirkesen (✉)
Department of Pathology, Medical School of Acıbadem University, Istanbul, Turkiye
e-mail: cuyan.demirkesen@acibadem.edu.tr

E. Alpsoy et al. (eds.), *Behçet's Disease: An Integrated Approach*,
https://doi.org/10.1007/978-3-031-77251-1_21

21.2 Oral Ulcers

Histopathology of oral ulcers are similar to the lesions of idiopathic recurrent aphthous stomatitis (RAS). The squamous epithelium is replaced by a necrotic, fibropurulent exudate. There is variable infiltration of lymphocytes, neutrophils, histiocytes, and in later stages plasma cells [Fig. 21.1]. Vascular proliferation with swollen endothelial cells is usually prominent. Partial occlusion of the vascular lumen and rarely leukocytoclastic vasculitis have been reported [1]. The number of mast cells is relatively increased compared to RAS and mucosa from healthy controls [5]. Expression patterns of cytokeratins (CK) are changed in oral apthous lesion in BD, accordingly CK1, CK6, and CK16 were found to be upregulated, whereas alpha6 integrin and BCL-2 were downregulated [6]. The upregulation of CD3 and gammadelta T-cell expression and other adhesion molecules including CD44, CD86, CD58 (LFA-3), VCAM-1, and intercellular adhesion molecule-1 (CD54) was also observed [6]. The authors suggest that these data may point out T cell-mediated keratinocyte activities in the pathogenesis of oral lesions in BD.

In direct immunoflourescence evaluation C3 and C1q, as well as IgM and IgG were detected in the vessel walls [7, 8]. These findings questioned if oral aphthous lesions of BD were actually an immune complex vasculitis.

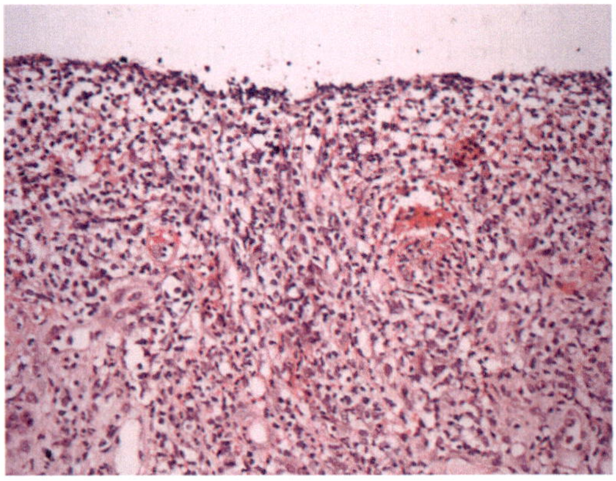

Fig. 21.1 Oral aphthous ulcer in a patient with Behçet disease: Underneath the complete loss of squamous epithelium, there is neutrophil-rich infiltration with vascular changes in the mucosa (H&Ex200)

21.3 Genital/Extragenital Ulcers

The histopathologic features are similar to oral aphthous lesions of BD. Various vascular changes has been described such as lymphocytic vasculitis, leukocytoclastic vasculitis, thickening of the vessel walls, endothelial swelling and a tendency for obliteration particularly in small arteries and capillaries in genital ulcers [1]. However, it is still not clear whether these vascular changes are a phenomenon secondary to the intense inflammation or related to BD.

21.4 Papulopustular Lesions

Papulopustular lesions have a wide range of histopathologic features, from leukocytoclastic vasculitis to a less dense neutrophilic vascular reaction [9]. Follicular involvement, resembling deep suppurative folliculitis or acne vulgaris, may be evident. In these lesions, a neutrophil-predominating infiltrate around the hair follicle, with or without destruction of the follicular epithelium and sebaceous gland, is the most common finding [Fig. 21.2]. There may be intrafollicular abscess formation along with infundibular plugging by keratin and sebaceous material (comedone). Small vessel thickening and deposition of fibrinoid material in the vessel wall may accompany, more likely to be secondary to acute inflammation rather than a true neutrophilic vascular reaction [Fig. 21.3] [1, 9].

Non-follicular papulopustular lesions reveal superficial or deep neutrophilic infiltration, mainly around vessels [Fig. 21.4]. There may be pustule formation in these lesions. Vasculitis is detected in some lesions, which are considered to represent true vasculitis by some authors [10].

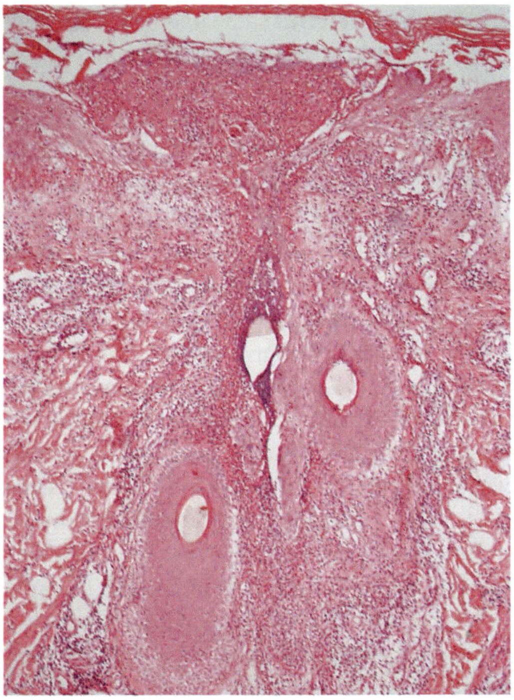

Fig. 21.2 Papulopustular lesion with follicular involvement: Neutrophil-predominating infiltrate around the hair follicle, destroying the follicular epithelium (H&Ex100)

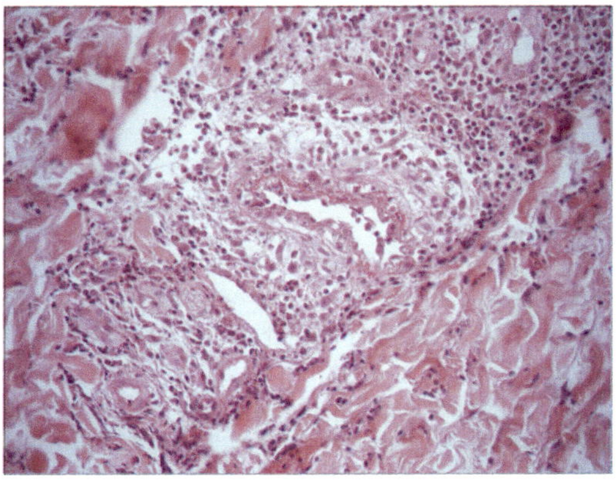

Fig. 21.3 Neutrophilic vascular reaction in the adjacent dermis: Deposition of fibrinoid material, together with neutrophils in the vessel wall (H&Ex200)

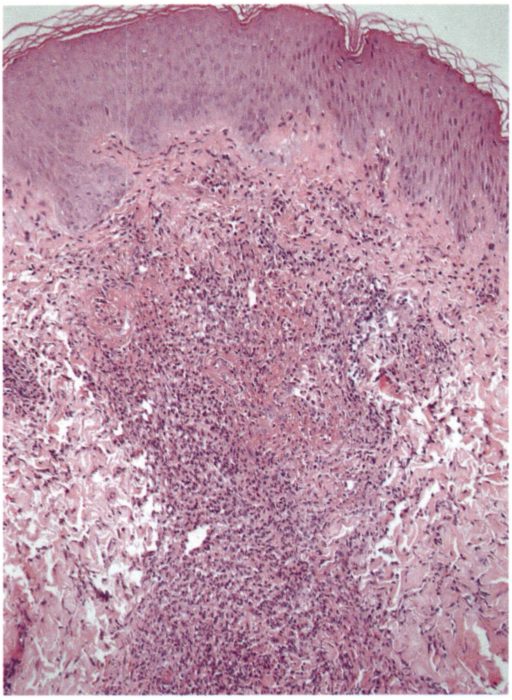

Fig. 21.4 Non-follicular papulopustular lesion (H&Ex200)

21.5 Erythema Nodosum (EN)-like Lesions

Although EN can be seen in patients with BD, panniculitis due to BD differ from classical EN. It is characterized by neutrophil-predominating infiltrate mainly in lobules [Fig. 21.5]. A neutrophilic vasculitis, involving mostly arterioles and venules, can be detected in almost half of the cases [Fig. 21.6] [11, 12]. Lymphocytic vasculitis has been documented by some authors, as well [13]. It is indicated that vasculitis is important in the pathogenesis of these lesions [12]. Some authors suggest that the presence of severe vasculitis, especially phlebitis, in these lesions may be an indicator of the involvement of the gastrointestinal tract in BD [14].

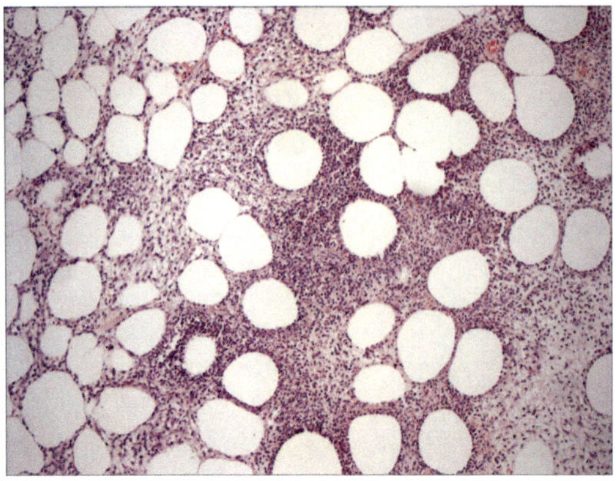

Fig. 21.5 Neutrophilic lobular panniculitis in Behçet disease (H&Ex100)

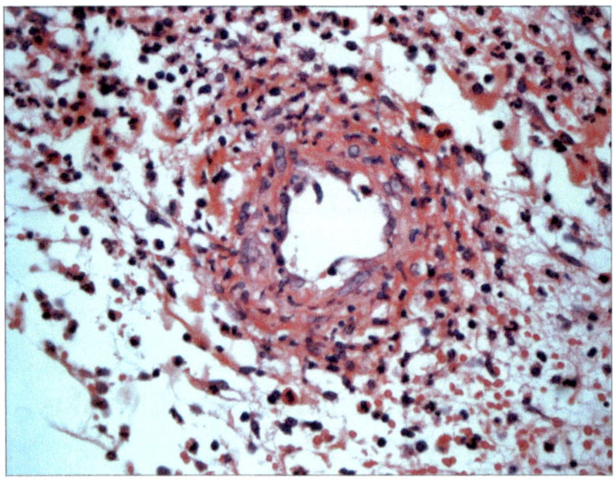

Fig. 21.6 Neutrophilic vasculitis, involving a small vessel, together with neutrophilic lobular panniculitis (H&Ex400)

Necrobiosis and leukocytoclasia usually accompany neutrophilic infiltration. Endothelial cells are often enlarged, and extravasated erythrocytes can be evident, especially in those lesions with vasculitis. The histiocytic granuloma is infrequent.

The lobular panniculitis, seen in BD, closely mimics nodular vasculitis, but the infiltrate is neutrophil predominating, especially in early lesions in BD [15]. On the other hand, it can be easily distinguished from EN [11, 12].

There have been several studies of adhesion molecules expression in the EN-like lesions, but no consistent pattern has been demonstrated yet [16–20].

21.6 Superficial Thrombophlebitis

Some patients present with tender, erythematous nodular lesions, resembling EN-like lesions of BD clinically, however veins are involved resulting in superficial thrombophelibitis. The lesions of superficial thrombophlebitis are linear lesions but may be confused with EN-like lesions when the short vein segment is involved.

The pathologic findings are seen mainly in the small to medium-sized veins in the upper subcutaneous fat tissue, In early lesions, neutrophil-predominating infiltrate is seen in the vessel walls, extending to the surrounding fat tissues [Fig. 21.7]. Later on, lymphocytes predominate in later stages. The walls show fibrous thickening in old lesions. Thrombus is often present in the lumina of the affected veins, after a while they become organized and recanalized. Deeper veins may also be involved.

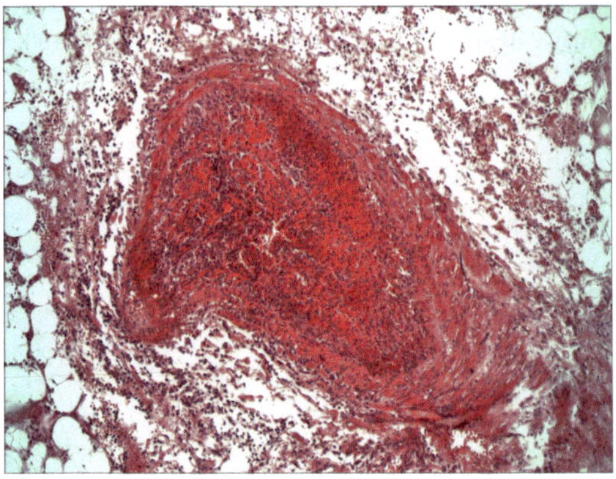

Fig. 21.7 Superficial thrombophlebitis in a patient with Behçet disease: Neutrophil-predominating infiltrate in a medium-sized vein, with a thrombus in the lumen (H&Ex200)

21.7 Pathergy Test

In response to a needle-prick, positive reactions manifesting as a papule or pustule are seen, as a result of dermal inflammation, composed of mainly neutrophils, detected starting after 12 h, becoming denser at 24 h [21, 22]. The pathergy test is one of the major features and diagnostic criteria of the disease, but it can be seen in other diseases such as Sweet's syndrome, Crohn's disease, pyoderma gangrenosum, etc. [23]. Although the precise mechanism of pathergy has not yet been entirely elucidated, it is considered as an exaggerated cutaneous inflammatory response.

Various histopathologic findings related to pathergy tests have been reported [24–27]. Perivascular or periadnexial infiltration of lymphocytes, plasma cells, histiocytes, and neutrophils with varying densities were detected in biopsies taken 24 h after the test [Fig. 21.8]. Inflammatory infiltrate is mainly in the dermis but sometimes extends to the subcutaneous fat tissue. Leukocytoclastic vasculitis and Sweet-like vasculitis were observed in some lesions [Fig. 21.9] [25]. Lymphocytic vascular reaction was also documented [27]. In a study, together with perivascular lymphohistiocytic infiltration, blood vessel thickening and erythrocyte extravasation were found to be significantly higher in patients with BD compared with control groups [26]. Intraepidermal pustules may occur at the point of pathergy stimulus.

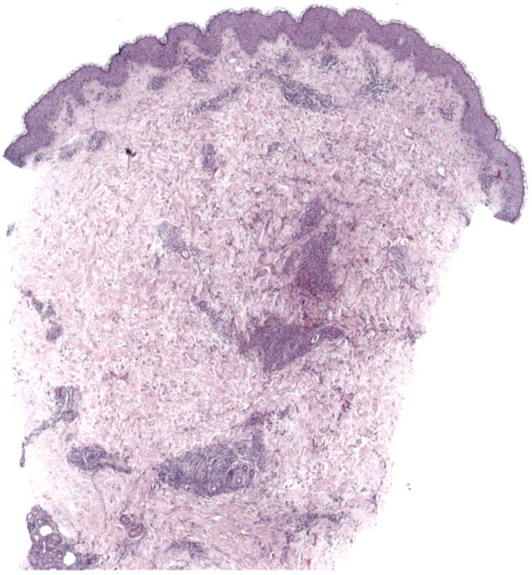

Fig. 21.8 Histopathology of pathergy test: Neutrophil-predominating infiltrate around the vessels (H&Ex100)

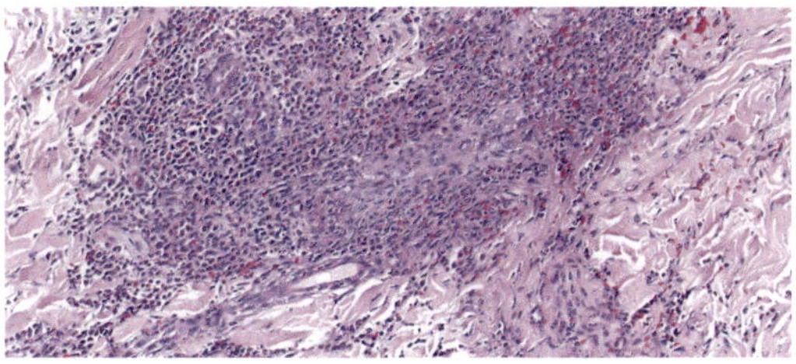

Fig. 21.9 Leukocytoclastic vasculitis, accompanying the dermal infiltration (H&Ex400)

Controversial results were reported in direct immunflourescence evaluation in pathergy test. Some authors showed depositions with IgM, IgG and complement 3, in the pathergy test sites in almost all patients [28, 29], while others could not demonstrated any accumulation [30].

21.8 Sweet Syndrome-Like Skin Manifestations

There is dense, diffuse, or patchy neutrophilic infiltration within the dermis, sometimes extending to the subcutaneous fat tissue. [Fig. 21.10]. There is usually prominent edema in the papillary dermis. Leukocytoclasis and extravasated erythrocytes are present together with the neutrophilic infiltration. Endothelial swelling is prominent in the vessels. Sometimes, fibrinoid material is evident in the vessel walls. In later stages, this neutrophilic infiltration can be replaced by a lymphohistiocytic infiltration. The Sweet syndrome-like neutrophilic dermatosis is considered a neutrophilic vascular reaction not infrequently encountered in patients with BD [31, 32].

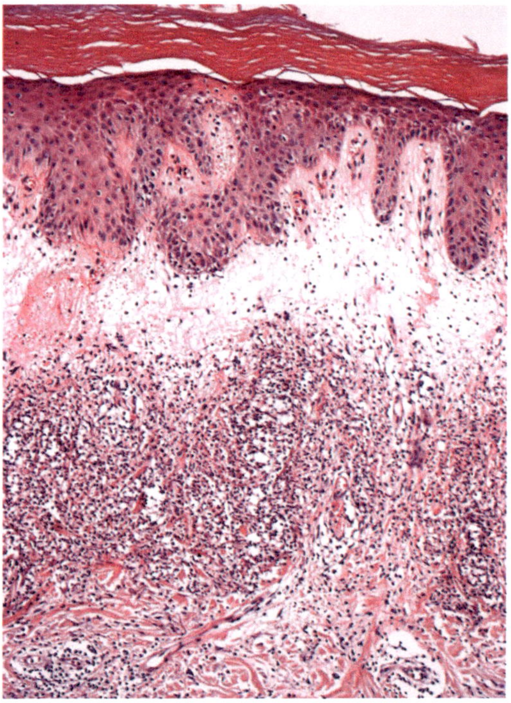

Fig. 21.10 Sweet syndrome: Prominent edema in the papillary dermis, with diffuse infiltration of neutrophils (H&Ex200)

21.9 Other Reported Associations

Pyoderma gangrenosum-like lesions, erythema multiforme-like lesions, pernio-like lesions, neutrophilic eccrine hidradenitis, bullous lesions due to necrotizing vasculitis, and palpable purpura may be seen in patients with BD [1–4, 33–35].

The earliest presentation of pyoderma gangrenosum is follicular/perifollicular neutrophil-rich inflammation with abscess formation. In later stages, there is ulceration, and diffuse neutrophilic infiltration resembling Sweet syndrome. Abscess and leukocytoclastic vasculitis accompany.

Erythema multiforme is characterized by interphase dermatitis. Hydropic degeneration in the basal cell layer of the epidermis, with many colloid bodies are present together with many lymphoctes, forming satellite cell necrosis.

In pernio-like lesions, papillary dermal edema, lymphocytic vasculitis, thickenning of the vessel walls, and endothelial swelling are documented.

Neutrophilic eccrine hidradenitis can be seen as result of a neutrophilic vascular reaction in BD [33, 34]. There is an infiltrate of neutrophils around the eccrine glands, involving the secretory coil epithelium and sometimes destroying the gland. Necrosis of the secretory coil epithelium may be present.

In conclusion, BD is an inflammatory disease of unknown origin. Cutaneous lesions may be the first manifestation of the disease. Pathergy test caused by external stimulus is often recognizable. However, it should be kept in mind that BD has no pathognomonic features on histopathology, although it is possible to see wide range of microscopic changes in various systems. Vascular changes, such as vasculitis or occlusive vasculopathy play role in most cutaneous lesions. Neutrophil-rich infiltration is evident in early, active stages of the lesions. It seems that the research topics dealing with interactions between T cells, neutrophils, cytokines and antigen presenting cells would contribute to better understanding of pathogenesis of BD.

References

1. Chun SI, Su WP, Lee S. Histopathologic study of cutaneous lesions in Behcet's syndrome. J Dermatol. 1990;17:333–41.
2. Alpsoy E, Zouboulis CC, Ehrlich GE. Mucocutaneous lesions of Behcet's disease. Yonsei Med J. 2007 Aug 31;48(4):573–85. https://doi.org/10.3349/ymj.2007.48.4.573.
3. Lee ES, Bang D, Lee S. Dermatologic manifestation of Behcet's disease. Yonsei Med J. 1997;38:380–9.
4. Cantini F, Salvarani C, Niccoli L, et al. Behcet's disease with unusual cutaneous lesions. J Rheumatol. 1998;25:2469–72.
5. Gao C. Clinical pathological analysis of recurrent oral ulcer and Behcet's syndrome. Zhonghua Kou Qiang Yi Xue Za Zhi. 1990;25(82–5):125.
6. Kose O, Stewart J, Waseem A, et al. Expression of cytokeratins, adhesion and activation molecules in oral ulcers of Behcet's disease. Clin Exp Dermatol. 2008;33:62–9.
7. Luderschmidt C, Wolff HH, Scherer R. Apthae: histologic, immunofluorescent and immuno--electron microscopy study of their pathogenesis. Hautarzt. 1981;32:364–9.
8. Reimer G, Luckner L, Hornstein OP. Direct immunofluorescence in recurrent aphthous ulcers and Behçet's disease. Dermatologica. 1983;167:293–8.

9. Boyvat A, Heper AO, Kocyigit P, et al. Can specific vessel-based papulopustular lesions of Behcet's disease be differentiated from nonspecific follicular-based lesions clinically? Int J Dermatol. 2006;45:814–8.
10. Alpsoy E, Uzun S, Akman A, et al. Histological and immunofluorescence findings of non-follicular papulopustular lesions in patients with Behcet's disease. J Eur Acad Dermatol Venereol. 2003;17:521–4.
11. Demirkesen C, Tuzuner N, Mat C, et al. Clinicopathologic evaluation of nodular cutaneous lesions of Behcet syndrome. Am J Clin Pathol. 2001;116:341–6.
12. Kim B, LeBoit PE. Histopathologic features of erythema nodosum-like lesions in Behcet disease: a comparison with erythema nodosum focusing on the role of vasculitis. Am J Dermatopathol. 2000;22:379–90.
13. Chun SI, Su WP, Lee S, et al. Erythema nodosum-like lesions in Behcet's syndrome: a histopathologic study of 30 cases. J Cutan Pathol. 1989;16:259–65.
14. Misago N, Tada Y, Koarada S, Narisawa Y. Erythema nodosum-like lesions in Behçet's disease: a clinicopathological study of 26 cases. Acta Derm Venereol. 2012;92:681–6.
15. Mat C, Demirkesen C, Melikoğlu M, Yazıcı H. Behçet's Syndrome. In: Sarzi-Puttini P, Doria A, Girolomoni G, Kuhn A, editors. The skin in systemic autoimmune diseases. Handbook of systemic autoimmune diseases, vol. 5. Amsterdam/Boston/London/New York/Oxford/Paris/Tokyo: Elsevier; 2006. p. pg: 186-205.
16. Senturk T, Aydintug O, Kuzu I, et al. Adhesion molecule expression in erythema nodosum-like lesions in Behcet's disease. A histopathological and immunohistochemical study. Rheumatol Int. 1998;18:51–7.
17. Uchio E, Matsumoto T, Tanaka SI, et al. Soluble intercellular adhesion molecule-1 (ICAM-1), CD4, CD8 and interleukin-2 receptor in patients with Behcet's disease and Vogt-Koyanagi-Harada's disease. Clin Exp Rheumatol. 1999;17:179–84.
18. Verity DH, Vaughan RW, Kondeatis E, et al. Intercellular adhesion molecule-1 gene polymorphisms in Behcet's disease. Eur J Immunogenet. 2000;27:73–6.
19. Triolo G, Accardo-Palumbo A, Carbone MC, et al. Enhancement of endothelial cell E-selectin expression by sera from patients with active Behcet's disease: moderate correlation with anti-endothelial cell antibodies and serum myeloperoxidase levels. Clin Immunol. 1999;91:330–7.
20. Demirkesen C, Tüzüner N, Senocak M, Türkmen I, Aki H, Kepil N, Mat C, Yazici H. Comparative study of adhesion molecule expression in nodular lesions of Behçet syndrome and other forms of panniculitis. Am J Clin Pathol. 2008;130:28–33.
21. Ergun T, Gurbuz O, Harvell J, et al. The histopathology of pathergy: a chronologic study of skin hyperreactivity in Behcet's disease. Int J Dermatol. 1998;37:929–33.
22. Kutlubay Z, Tüzün Y, Wolf R. The pathergy test as a diagnostic tool. Skinmed. 2017;15(2):97–104. eCollection 2017
23. Alibaz-Oner F, Direskeneli H. Update on the diagnosis of Behçet's disease. Diagnostics (Basel). 2022 Dec 23;13(1):41. https://doi.org/10.3390/diagnostics13010041.
24. Sobel JD, Haim S, Shafrir A, Gellei B. Cutaneous hyperreactivity in Behcet's disease. Dermatologica. 1973;146:350–6.
25. Jorizzo JL, Solomon AR, Cavallo T. Behcet's syndrome-immunopathologic and histopathologic assessment of pathergy lesions is useful in diagnosis and follow up. Arch Pathol Lab Med. 1985;109:747–51.
26. Akmaz O, Erel A, Gürer MA. Comparison of histopathologic and clinical evaluations of pathergy test in Behçet's disease. Int J Dermatol. 2000;39:121–5.
27. Ozluk E, Balta I, Akoğuz O, et al. Histopathologic study of Pathergy test in Behçet's disease. Indian J Dermatol. 2014;59:630.
28. Azizlerli G, Saylan T, Cologlu AS, Bozan G, Urgancioglu M. Major immunoglobulins in Behçet's disease and a study with direct and indirect immunoflourescent methods. Excepta Medica. Int Congr Ser. 1977:232–5.
29. Kose AA. Direct immunofluorescence in Behçet's disease: a controlled study with 108 cases. Yonsei Med J. 2009;50:505–11.
30. Haim S, Sobel JD, Friedman-Birnbaum R, et al. Histological and direct immunofluorescence study of cutaneous hyperreactivity in Behcet's disease. Br J Dermatol. 1976;95:631–6.
31. Magro CM, Crowson AN. Cutaneous manifestations of Behcet's disease. Int J Dermatol. 1995;34:159–65.
32. Nelson CA, Stephen S, Ashchyan HJ, James WD, Micheletti RG, Rosenbach M. Neutrophilic dermatoses: pathogenesis, sweet syndrome, neutrophilic eccrine hidradenitis, and Behçet disease. J Am Acad Dermatol. 2018;79:987–1006.
33. Bilic M, Mutasim DF. Neutrophilic eccrine hidradenitis in a patient with Behcet's disease. Cutis. 2001;68:107–11.
34. Mercader-Garcia P, Vilata-Corell JJ, Pardo-Sanchez J, et al. Neutrophilic eccrine hidradenitis in a patient with Behcet's disease. Acta Derm Venereol. 2003;83:395–6.

Activity Scales Used in Behçet's Disease

22

Filiz Canpolat and Ümit Türsen

Contents

22.1 Introduction

Behçet's disease (BD) is a rare and chronic autoimmune disorder characterized by inflammation in blood vessels. Symptoms include recurring mouth and genital ulcers, ocular inflammation, as well as involvement of joints, gastrointestinal tract, and the central nervous system [1–3]. The International Study Group diagnostic criteria, published in 1990, are the most widely used and recognized, but to enhance sensitivity, the International Criteria for Behçet's Disease was developed in 2014 [4, 5]. Due to the inadequacy of basic biochemical and laboratory analyses in understanding disease activity, clinical scoring systems have become crucial for diagnosis, treatment evaluation, and monitoring. Consequently, there is a need for measures assessing severity of organ involvement, patients' quality of life, and guiding physicians in management. Evaluating disease activity in BD is pivotal for treatment selection and monitoring. As a result, various activity measures have been developed. One well-established scoring method is the simplified Behçet's Disease Current Activity Form (BDCAF) and its 2006 version [6, 7] Subsequently, several other activity tools have been proposed and utilized for research purposes. This chapter aims to summarize these tools and their clinical significance.

F. Canpolat (✉)
Department of Dermatology, Ankara Etlik City Hospital, Ankara, Türkiye

Ü. Türsen
Department of Dermatology, Mersin University, Mersin, Türkiye
e-mail: utursen@mersin.edu.tr

E. Alpsoy et al. (eds.), *Behçet's Disease: An Integrated Approach*,
https://doi.org/10.1007/978-3-031-77251-1_22

22.2 Disease Activity Indexes

The presence of recurring acute inflammation attacks that affect various organs in BD makes it challenging to assess disease activity. Main problems in the assessment of disease activity are as follows;

1. The disease exhibits a fluctuating course, complicating assessment.
2. There are no laboratory tests that reliably reflect and correlate with disease manifestations.
3. There is no standardized tool for estimating the severity of disease symptoms.
4. The lack of consensus on diagnostic criteria, and the emergence of new ones leads to difficulties in assessing disease severity. Despite these challenges, disease activity indexes have been developed, primarily based on clinical history [8, 9].

22.3 Activity Index Studies

First, Yazıcı et al. developed the Turkish Behçet's Disease Activity Index [9], followed by the development of Iranian Behçet's Disease Dynamic Activity Measure (IBDDAM) [10] and the European Disease Activity Index [6, 11]. Turkish Behçet's Disease Activity Index, published in 1984, is outlined in Table 22.1 [12]. These scales were later amalgamated, and the Behçet's Disease Current Activity Form (BDCAF) index was redefined and evaluated by Bhakta, at a Behçet's disease meeting held in Leeds, England in 1994 [6]. Subsequently, Bhakta, Baltacı, Hamuryudan, Lawton, Monastero, Bodur et al. tested BDCAF's performance in various clinical studies [13, 14]. All of the aforementioned activity indexes are primarily based on clinical findings. In the Turkish version, clinical findings were evaluated only during visits, whereas in the European form, the findings of the last month were considered, and in the Iranian form, findings of the last 12 months were evaluated.

In the IBDDAM form developed in 1991 by Davatchi et al., 18 clinical symptoms related to BD and pathergy testing are assessed. Oral ulcers, genital ulcers, pustular lesions, erythema nodosum, and the presence and number of superficial thrombophlebitis have been queried for the past 4 weeks. Additionally, epididymitis, the presence of monoarthritis, oligoarthritis, or arthralgia regardless of symptom duration are evaluated during this period (Table 22.2). If lesions do not resolve, the same score is assigned during monthly evaluations. Notably, the assessment of

Table 22.1 Turkish Behçet's Disease activity index [9]

Involevement	Evaluation
Eye	0: Normal 1: Only in vitreous and/or anterior chamber cells 2: 50% vision 3: 30% vision loss, 4: Seeing in a few steps 5: Blindness
Skin	1: Oral aphthous 1: Erythema nodosum 1: Genital ulcer
Vascular involvement	5: Throma in the superior and inferior vena cava gray and/or arterial occlusion 4: Vena cava superior or inferior thrombosis 3: Thrombosis and/or bedsores in calf veins Superficial thrombophlebitis requiring rest 2: Thrombosis in bilateral calf veins and/or superficial thrombophlebitis 1: Thrombosis in unilateral calf veins and/or superficial thrombophlebitis
Arthritis	1: Each joint
Neurological involvement	2: Intracranial hypertension 3: Multiple sclerosis-like syndrome 5: Pyramidal and/or cerebellar involvement

Table 22.2 Iranian *Behçet's disease* dynamic activity measure [IBDDAM] [10]

Oral ulcer	1 point for every 5 ulcer
Genital ulcer	1 point for each lesion
Skin lesions	1 point for every 10 papulopustular eruptions and 1 point for every 5 erythema nodosum
Eye lesion	1–4 points for depending on the presence of activation of anterior uveitis, hypopyon, cell, and keratic precipitate, 1–4 points for the presence of posterior uveitis cell, snowball, snow bank, 1–4 points depending on the presence of the disc of retinal vasculitis, retinal and macular edema, periphlebitis, periarteritis, papillitis
Joint	It is evaluated as 1 points for arthralgia regardless of the number of joints, 2 points for monoarthritis, 3 points for polyarthritis
Central nervous system	Isolated lesion 1, mild involvement 3, moderate and severe involvement 6 points
Vascular thrombosis	Superficial phlebitis 1, deep venous thrombosis for each vein 2, large vessel involvement for each vein 6 points
Gastrointestinal system	Mild symptoms such as chronic diarrhea, rectal bleeding, abdominal pain 3 points, moderate and severe symptoms 6 points
Epididymitis	2 points
Positive pathergy	1 point

pathergy test, eye involvement, and major vascular involvement in this form relies on objective examination findings rather than history [10].

The European Behçet's Disease Activation Index was initially published in 1993. It assesses the presence of oral ulcers, genital ulcers, skin findings, and joint symptoms occurring within the past month. Furthermore, it evaluates the severity and localization of vascular disease, eye findings and degree of vision loss, gastrointestinal system involvement and symptom severity, and central nervous system involvement based on functional defects [meningeal, parenchymal, vascular]. Each extraocular organ involvement is scored between 0 and 5 points, and each eye is scored between 0 and 47 points. Oro-genital ulcerations and skin lesion size and numbers are not considered [6].

In 1999, the BDCAF index was defined by Bhakta et al., evaluating 10 common clinical symptoms of BD (Table 22.3). These include fatigue, headache, oral ulcers, genital ulcers, erythema nodosum, superficial thrombophlebitis, papulopustular eruption, arthralgia, arthritis, nausea, vomiting or abdominal pain, and bloody diarrhea. Manifestations are scored between 0 and 4 points based on their occurrence over the previous 4 weeks. In addition, three organ systems including eye, large vessels, and central nervous system are assessed using two different variables. Patients indicate their feelings over the last 4 weeks using a visual Likert scale with seven different facial expressions, while clinicians evaluate similar visual scores according to physician-assessed disease activity. In evaluating the effectiveness of BDCAF, Bhakta et al. observed its strength in assessing oral ulcers, genital ulcers, skin manifestations, arthritis, headache, large vessels, central nervous system, and eye involvement but noted weakness in evaluating bloody diarrhea and fatigue [7].

Hamuryudan et al. assessed the effectiveness of the BDCAF form in Turkish Behçet's patients, finding it useful for evaluating oro-genital ulcers and ocular involvement but not for erythema nodosum, vascular involvement, central nervous system, and gastrointestinal involvement [11].

Şimşek et al. compared BDCAF and IBDDAM forms in 2008. They found BDCAF useful for evaluating oro-genital ulcers, skin lesions, arthralgia, arthritis, and eye involvement but unsuitable for evaluating gastrointestinal symptoms and headaches. Both forms were deemed useful for retrospectively assessing daily disease activity despite some differences, relying almost exclusively on clinical symptom history [15].

Neves et al. observed BDCAF's effectiveness for oro-genital ulcers, skin symptoms, articular symptoms, with a high kappa score (>0.6) for general symptoms of patients with BD. However, its utility was moderate for evaluating ocular activity (kappa score: 0.483), gastrointestinal tract, and low for evaluating the central nervous system and large vessel involvement (kappa

Table 22.3 Behçet's disease Current Activity Form 2006

BEHÇET'S DISEASE INSTANT ACTIVITY FORM-2006

Date: Name: Gender: M/F

Center: Telephone: Date of birth:

Country: Address:

Clinician:

ASSESSMENT OF THE PATIENT'S ACTIVITY

Question: With which facial expression could you describe your illness in the last 4 weeks [Choose a face]

HEAD PAIN, ORAL ULCERS, GENITAL ULCERS, SKIN LESIONS, JOINT INVOLVEMENT AND GASTROINTESTINAL SYMPTOMS

Question: If you have had any of the following symptoms for the last 4 weeks, fill in the associated box.

Manifestation	No symptoms	Present in the last 4 weeks
Headache		
Oral ulceration		
Genital ulceration		
Erythema		
Skin pustules		
Joints-arthralgia		
Joints-arthritis		
Nausea/vomiting/ abdominal pain		
Diarrhea/significant bleeding from therectum		

EYE INVOLVEMENT

[ask the questions below.]

Have you had the following symptoms in the last 4 weeks?

	Right eye		Left eye	
Red eye	Yes	No	Yes	No
Painful eye	Yes	No	Yes	No
Blurred and decreased vision	Yes	No	Yes	No
Are any of the above symptoms new?	Yes		No	

NERVOUS SYSTEM INVOLVEMENT [involving intracranial vascular disease]

[in the form of a new symptom related to the nervous system and major intracranial vessels that have not been previously reported or noted by the patient, ask the questions below]

Have you had any of the following symptoms in the last 4 weeks?

Symptom	Yes	No	Check if new
Fainting and blackening			
Hard of hearing			
Speech difficulty			
Blurred or double vision			
Loss of sensation and weakness in the face			
Loss of sensation and weakness in the arm			
Loss of sensation and weakness in the leg			
Memory loss			
Loss of balance			

(continued)

Table 22.3 (continued)

Is there new evidence of active nervous system involvement? Yes No			
LARGE VESSEL INVOLVEMENT [except for intracranial vascular disease]			
Have you had any of the following symptoms in the last 4 weeks?			
Symptom	Yes	No	Check if new
Chest pain			
Breathlessness			
Cough with blood			
Facial pain/swelling/ discoloration			
Pain/swelling/ discoloration in the arm			
Pain/swelling/ discoloration in the leg			
Is there new evidence of active great vasculitis? Yes no			
CLINICIAN'S OBSERVATION ABOUT DISEASE ACTIVITY			
Choose a face from which you can describe your illness in the last 4 weeks.			

BEHÇET'S DISEASE ACTIVITY INDEX			
Add up all the scores in the black-colored areas. An initial yes score becomes 1, while a final yes score on other symptoms is calculated as 1, and the total disease activity index score is evaluated out of 12.			
Patient's index score 0 1 2 3 4 5 6 7 8 9 10 11 12			
Transformed index score 0 3 5 7 8 9 10 11 12 13 15 17 20			

score: 0.322). Consequently, it was useful for assessing classic mucocutaneous, articular, and general symptoms but weak for evaluating visceral involvement in disease activity, suggesting the need for additional and complementary criteria [16].

22.4 Other Activation Index Studies

Various groups developed tools for assessing the disease activity. Japanese Behçet's Disease Research Committee developed an activity phase classification in 2003 [17]. Accordingly, the presence of the following disease features and laboratory parameters are evaluated;

1. Active phase: Presence of one of the following symptoms
   - Uveitis
   - Subcutaneous venous thrombosis
   - Skin symptoms such as erythema nodosum, genital ulcers (cases related to menstruation will be excluded)
   - Arthralgia
   - Gastrointestinal ulceration
   - Progressive central nervous system lesions
   - Progressive vasculitis
   - Epididymitis
2. Presence of clinical findings, including ophthalmological examination and/or serum CRP, cerebrospinal fluid, colonoscopy, and other laboratory findings.

In this evaluation, a score of 2 or more for oral aphthae, genital ulcers, skin and eye symptoms are interpreted as the active phase. If defined symptoms of the active phase are excluded, the patients with BD are stated as non-active.

In addition, the authors concluded that the following issues to be taken into consideration for the activation phase:

1. In the presence of active phase findings, increasing the dosage of current treatment, drug change, or combination therapies can be considered.
2. Since there are no good criteria for disease activity, other symptoms and findings should be taken into account in patients with the presence of oral aphtha and papulopustular eruption only, such as number, width, variability in frequency, and length of recovery period.
3. In cases with uveitis activation, the active phase usually regresses within 2 weeks. If significant inflammatory findings persist for more than 2 weeks, it is assumed that the active phase continues.
4. Cases in the inactive phase may suddenly develop exacerbation.
5. Patients having inactive phase for more than 1 year are considered as having stable phase (remission) with an index of 0 [17].

The activity index proposed by the Japanese Behçet's Disease Research Committee is shown in Table 22.4.

In another study, Japanese Behçet's Disease Research Committee Disease Severity Criteria, which classifies disease severity in six stages, was published. Accordingly, the severity is stated as follows;

Stage 1: The presence of main symptoms such as oral ulcer, genital ulcer, and skin lesions other than ocular lesions.
Stage 2: Addition to stage 1 symptom, iridocyclitis as an ocular symptom or the addition of arthritis and/or epididymitis.
Stage 3: Retinochondritis cases.
Stage 4: Presence of retinochondritis causing vision loss in the other eye or possible vision loss.
Stage 5: Special BD involvement with risky prognosis and moderate neuro-Behçet's disease affecting intelligence to a greater degree or more severely.
Stage 6: Death (caused by the symptom of BD or complication needs to be explained) [17].

In another study, Yossipovitch et al. developed a scale by classifying the severity of the disease into four categories: mild, moderate, very active, and severe. [Table 22.5] [18].

In their research, Krause et al., evaluated Behçet's disease severity index as shown in the Table 22.6 [19]. Krause et al. observed that it had a higher activity index and more severe course in their patients of North African origin [20].

Table 22.4 Japanese Behçet's Disease Research Committee Disease Activity Index [17]

Oral aphthous ulcers	0: No aphthous ulcer 1: Lasting less than 2 weeks in the last 4 weeks 2: Lasting more than 2 weeks or in the last 4 lasting more than 2 weeks per week 3: Aphthous ulcers that have persisted mostly for the last 4 weeks
Skin symptoms like erythema nodosum	0: No lesion 1: Less than 2 weeks in the last 4 weeks 2: Lasting more than 2 weeks or in the last 4 for more than 2 weeks 3: The lesion that has usually been present for the last 4 weeks
Eye symptoms	0: No uveitis 1: Only 1 ocular attack in the last 4 weeks [also in the opposite eye in a few days] 2: Attack twice in the last 4 weeks 3: Attacks occurring 3 times in the last 4 weeks
Arthritis	Arthralgia, swelling, difficulty walking, deformity, and other symptoms
Gastrointestinal	Acute/chronic abdominal pain, melena, or occult symptoms blood
Epididymitis	Pain, swelling
Vascular lesions	Cardiac/aortic diseases, moderate or minor vascular occlusion, thrombophlebitis, and other symptoms
Central nerve	Headache, dizziness, paralysis, mental system lesions symptoms, and others

In addition to measures focusing on overall disease activity, several organ-specific scales have also been developed. BenEzra et al. constructed an eye specific tool, Behçet's Oculopathy Index, at which, both activity and damage are evaluated with a score between 0 and 4 points for each eye. Parameters such as anterior cell inflammation, synechiae, posterior vitreous retinal infiltrate, dissociation, branch vein or central vein occlusion, new vascularization, hemorrhage, presence of detachment, neuro-ophthalmic pupillary defect, disc swelling, optic atrophy, visual acuity, intraocular pressure, and lymph opacity (aphakia/pseudoaphakia) are assessed [21].

Table 22.5 Yossipovitch's activity classification of Behçet's disease [18]

Mild activity	Minor oral aphtha and genital ulcers Skin symptoms Arthritis in less than two joints
Moderate	Arthritis of fewer than three joints Recurrent genital ulcer Mild anterior uveitis
Very active	Major oral aphthous ulcers and genital ulcers Arthritis in two or more joints Eye symptoms Neurological symptoms Large vessel involvement
Severe	Anterior and posterior uveitis Large vessel involvement Arterial aneurysm Recurrent arthritis in more than three joints

In 1998, Kaklamani et al. published an easier BD severity scoring system, assigning 1 point for oral aphthae, skin lesions, epididymoorchitis, pleurisy, and pericarditis; 2 points for genital ulcer, gastrointestinal involvement, and arthritis; and 3 points for eye, central nervous system, and vascular involvement [22].

In another study, Chang et al. reported Behçet's disease clinical activity scoring with mucocutaneous findings scoring 1 each and organ involvements scoring 2 or three according to severity (Table 22.7) [23].

The Korean Behçet's Disease Activity Form was developed in 2003, incorporating the patient's self-evaluation. Points were assigned as follows: 20 points for oral aphthous ulcers, genital ulcers, skin lesions, and eye involvement; 2 points for vascular involvement, central nervous system involvement, epididymitis, and other involvements; 7 points for joint involvement; and 5 points for gastrointestinal system involvement. The authors concluded that this index was weak

Table 22.6 Krause's the evaluation of Behçet's disease activity index [20]

Mild [1 point for each findings]	Oral aphthosis Genital ulcer Typical skin lesions [Erythema nodosum, papulopustular eruption, folliculitis, leukocytoclastic vasculitis] Arthralgia Recurrent headache Epididymitis Mild gastrointestinal symptoms [chronic diarrhea, chronic recurrent colicky abdominal pain] Pleuritic pains Superficial vein thrombosis
Moderate [2 points for each findings]	Arthritis Deep vein thrombosis in the leg Anterior uveitis Gastrointestinal bleeding
Severe [3 points for each findings]	Posterior/pan uveitis, retinal vasculitis Arterial thrombosis or aneurysm Large vein [vena cava, hepatic] thrombosis Neuro-Behçet's Bowel perforation

Table 22.7 Chang's Behçet's disease clinical activity scoring [23]

1 point	Oral ulcer genital ulcer Skin lesions: Erythema nodosum-like lesions/Papulopustular eruption Superficial thrombophlebitis
2 points	Arthritis in two or more joints Complicated gastrointestinal ulcer Small or medium-sized vascular involvement unrelated to vital organ
3 points	Uveitis Gastrointestinal ulcer causing bleeding or perforation Large vessel involvement Large organ involvement, such as the brain, lungs, or heart

for evaluating vascular, gastrointestinal, and central nervous system involvements but strong for assessing other symptoms [24].

22.5 Scales for Assessment of Quality of Life

Several tools have been devised to evaluate the quality of life of patients with BD. Bodur et al. utilized the BDCAF scoring index in a study and identified articular involvement, fatigue, and genital ulcerations as the primary factors affecting the quality of life of these patients. Articular involvement and disease activity were particularly detrimental to pleasure and overall well-being [14]. In a study by Tanriverdi et al. in 2003, ocular involvement was identified as the main factor affecting the quality of life index, leading to increased tendencies toward anxiety and depression [25]. In addition, Blackford et al. in 1997 demonstrated that painful oral and genital ulcers significantly impacted the dermatological quality of life index [26]. Mumcu et al. investigated the quality of life of patients with BD using tools for both oral and general quality of life indexes [27]. In 1993, Davis et al. reported that patients with BD primarily complained about oral ulcer pain, fatigue, arthralgia, weight gain, swelling, difficulty in moving arms and legs, and loss of vision as major health issues [28].

In their study, Prokaeva et al. found that fatigue was frequently observed in patients with BD and was associated with disease activity and severity of depression [29].

In summary, although various general and organ-specific measures have been developed for the evaluation of disease severity and quality of life in patients with BD, there is no single scale that has achieved consensus for clinical and research purposes.

22.6 Conclusion

Behçet's disease lacks any laboratory markers directly relevant to clinical activity. A thorough history, meticulous clinical assessment, and tools such as BDCAF can aid in daily clinical practice. BDCAF is easy to use and typically takes a relatively short time to complete. The current version is readily available and is also used for research.

References

1. Kurokawa MS, Suzuki N. Behçet's disease. Clin Exp Med. 2004;3:10–20.
2. Lee S, Lee ES, Bang D, Jun JB. Clinical manifestations of late-onset Behçet's disease. In: Bang D, Lee ES, Lee S, editors. Behçet's disease. International conference on Behçet's disease, 9th, Seoul, Korea, 2000, p. 946–8.
3. Tursen U, Gurler A, Boyvat A. Evaluation of clinical findings according to sex in 2313 Turkish patients with Behçet's disease. Int J Dermatol. 2003;42:346–51.
4. International Study Group for Behcet's Disease. Criteria for diagnosis of Behcet's disease. Lancet. 1990;335(8697):1078–80.
5. International Team for the Revision of the International Criteria for Behçet's Disease (ITR-ICBD). The International Criteria for Behcet's Disease (ICBD): a collaborative study of 27 countries on the sensitivity and specificity of the new criteria. J Eur Acad Dermatol Venereol. 2014;28(3):338–47.
6. Bhakta BB, Brennan P, James TE, Chamberlain MA, Noble BA, Silman AJ. Behçet's disease: evaluation of a new instrument to measure clinical activity. Rheumatology. 1999;38:728–33.
7. https://behcetdiseasesociety.org/behcetwsData/Uploads/files/BehcetsDiseaseActivityForm.pdf
8. Alpsoy E, Donmez L, Onder M, Gunasti S, Usta A, Karincaoglu Y, et al. Clinical features and natural

course of Behçet's disease in 661 cases: a multicentre study. Br J Dermatol. 2007;157:901–6.
9. Yazici H, Tuzun Y, Pazarli H, Yurdakul S, Ozyazgan Y, Ozdoğan H, et al. Influence of age of onset and patient's sex on the prevalence and severity of manifestations of Behçet's syndrome. Ann Rheum Dis. 1984;43:783–9.
10. Davatchi F, Akbaran M, Shahram F, Jamshidi A, Gharibdoost F, Chams C. Iran Behçet's disease dynamic activity measure. Abstracts of the XIIth European Congress of Rheumatology. Hung Rheumatol Suppl. 1991;32:10–100.
11. Hamuryudan V, Fresko I, Direskeneli H, Tenant MJ, Yurdakul S, Akoglu T, et al. Evaluation of the Turkish translation of a disease activity form for Behçet's syndrome. Rheumatology (Oxford). 1999;38:734–6.
12. Lawton G, Bhakta BB, Chamberlain MA, Tennant A. The Behçet's disease activity index. Rheumatology. 2004;43:73–8.
13. Baltaci M. A review on disease activity scores in Behçet's disease. Arthritis Res Ther. 2005;5:7.
14. Bodur H, Borman P, Ozdemir Y, Atan C, Kural G. Quality of life and life satisfaction in patients with Behçet's disease: relationship with disease activity. Clin Rheumatol. 2006;25:329–33.
15. Simsek I, Meric C, Erdem H, Pay S, Kilic S, Dinc A. Accuracy of recall of the items included in disease activity forms of Behçet's disease: comparison of retrospective questionnaires with a daily telephone interview. Clin Rheumatol. 2008;27:1255–60.
16. Neves FS, Moraes JC, Kowalski SC, Goldenstein-Schainberg C, Lage LV, Goncalves CR. Cross-cultural adaptation of the Behçet's Disease Current Activity Form [BDCAF] to Brazilian Portuguese language. Clin Rheumatol. 2007;26:1263–7.
17. Suzuki KM, Suzuki N. Behçet's disease. Clin Exp Med. 2004;4:10–20.
18. Yosipovitch G, Shohat B, Bshara J, Wysenbeek A, Weinberger A. Elevated serum interleukin 1 receptors and interleukin 1B in patients with Behçet's disease: correlations with disease activity and severity. Isr J Med Sci. 1995;31:345–8.
19. Krause I, Rosen Y, Kaplan I, Milo G, Guedj D, Molad Y, Weinberger A. Recurrent aphthous stomatitis in Behçet's disease: clinical features and correlation with systemic disease expression and severity. J Oral Pathol Med. 1999;28:193–6.
20. Krause I, Mader R, Sulkes J, Paul M, Uziel Y, Molad Y, Weinberger A. The expression of Behçet's disease in Israeli ethnic groups. In: Bang D, Lee ES, Lee S, editors. Behçet' s disease. International conference on Behçet's disease. 9th, Seoul, Korea, 2000, p. 73–6.
21. Benezra D, Cohen E. Treatment and visual prognosis in Behcet's disease. Br J Ophthalmol. 1986;70:589–92.
22. Kaklamani VG, Vaipoulos G, Markomichelakis N, Palimeris G, Markaki J, Kaklamanis PH. Correlation of the severity of Adamantiades-Behçet's disease with clinical and demographic parameters. In: Bang D, Lee ES, Lee S, editors. Behçet' s disease. International conference on Behçet's disease. 9th, Seoul, Korea 2000, p. 902.
23. Chang HK, Cheon KS. The clinical significance of a pathergy reaction in patients with Behçet's disease. J Korean Med Sci. 2002;17:371–4.
24. Lee ES, Kim HS, Bang D, Yu HG, Chung H, Shin DH, et al. Development of clinical activity form for Korean patients with Behçet's disease. Adv Exp Med Biol. 2003;528:153–6.
25. Tanriverdi N, Taskintuna DC, Ozdal P, Ortac S, Firat E. Healthrelated quality of life in Behçet patients with ocular involvement. Jpn J Ophthalmol. 2003;47:85–92.
26. Blackford S, Finlay AY, Roberts DL. Quality of life in Behçet's syndrome: 335 patients surveyed. Br J Dermatol. 1997;136:293.
27. Mumcu G, Niazi S, Stewart J, Hagi-Pavli E, Gokani B, Seoudi N, et al. Oral health and related quality of life status in patients from UK and Turkey: a comparative study in Behçet's disease. J Oral Pathol Med. 2009;38:406–9.
28. Davis GL, Brissett D. Experiencing Behçet's disease: a view from 245 patients. In: Godeau P, Wechsler B, editors. Behçet's disease. Amsterdam: Elsevier; 1993. p. 211–4.
29. Prokaeva T, Alekberova Z, Nassonova V. Fatigue in Behçet's disease. In: Bang D, Lee ES, Lee S, editors. International conference on Behçet's disease. 9th, Seoul, Korea, 2000, p. 974–981.

23 Quality of Life and Scales Used in Behçet's Disease

Ahmet Metin and Aylin Türel Ermertcan

Contents

23.1 Introduction

QoL is an individual's perception of their position in life in the context of the culture and value systems in which they live and about their goals, expectations, standards, and concerns. BD can significantly impact the QoL of affected individuals [1]. Therefore, assessing and improving the QoL of people with BD is an important goal of clinical care and research. This chapter aims to review the current literature on the effects of BD on QoL and to identify the factors that influence QoL in BD patients.

23.2 The Impact of Behçet's Disease on Quality of Life

BD is a complex, chronic, and rare condition that leads to inflammation in multiple areas of the body. This inflammation has the potential to impact various organs beyond the mucocutaneous

A. Metin (✉)
Dermatology and Venereology, Pamukkale University, Denizli, Türkiye

A. T. Ermertcan
Dermatology and Venereology, Manisa Celal Bayar University, Manisa, Türkiye

E. Alpsoy et al. (eds.), *Behçet's Disease: An Integrated Approach*,
https://doi.org/10.1007/978-3-031-77251-1_23

region. The exact cause of the disease is unknown, but genetic and environmental factors are thought to play a role [2]. The disease is particularly prevalent in regions along the Silk Road and treatment options focus on reducing the frequency and severity of attacks and preventing or treating complications [3].

Patients may experience symptoms such as recurrent oral and genital ulcers, uveitis, vision loss, neurological, vascular complications, and arthritis. These conditions can lead to chronic pain, functional impairment, and psychological distress, which negatively affects quality of life [4]. The physical health of patients with BD is often limited by pain and general health perception. Psychological health is associated with emotional well-being and cognitive functioning.

The BH-QoL Scale has been used to evaluate the quality of life of patients with BD, and the results indicate a low quality of life. This scale covers aspects such as mood, social interaction, sexual activity, work and leisure time activities, and concerns about the disease [5].

The disease activity and severity of BD negatively correlate with the QoL of patients. The disease activity can be measured by tools such as the Behçet's Syndrome Activity Scale (BSAS), the Behçet's Disease Current Activity Form (BDCAF), or the oral ulcer activity index. The disease severity can be assessed by the number and type of organ involvement, such as mucosal, ocular, neurological, musculoskeletal, or vascular manifestations [6].

The oral ulcers of BD are one of the main factors that affect the QoL of patients. The oral ulcers can cause pain, discomfort, difficulty in eating and speaking, and social embarrassment. The painful ulcers of oral mucosa heal within 10–14 days. Oral ulcers can also affect the oral health-related QoL (OHRQoL) of patients, which is a specific aspect of QoL that reflects the impact of oral conditions on functional and psychosocial well-being. The OHRQoL can be measured by tools such as the Oral Health Impact Profile-14 (OHIP-14) or the composite index [7–11].

The ocular involvement of BD is another major factor that affects the QoL of patients. The ocular involvement can cause uveitis, which is an inflammation of the eye that can lead to vision loss or blindness. The ocular involvement can also affect the visual function and visual acuity of patients, which are important indicators of QoL. The visual function and visual acuity can be measured by tools such as the National Eye Institute Visual Functioning Questionnaire-25 (VFQ-25) or the best-corrected visual acuity (BCVA) [12].

Gender and age are important factors affecting the QoL of BD patients. Female patients often report a lower QoL compared to their male counterparts, particularly in areas such as psychological health, social relationships, sexual activity, and mood [4]. This disparity may be attributed to the higher incidence and severity of genital ulcers and depression among female patients. Similarly, age plays a pivotal role in determining the QoL of BD patients; older individuals tend to report diminished QoL in domains like physical health, social relationships, and vitality [13, 14]. The decline in these areas can be associated with the prolonged duration and progression of the disease along with its complications that are more prevalent among older patients.

23.2.1 The Physical Impact

BD is a condition that causes inflammation in various organs of the body, with different levels of severity and impact. The type and severity of the organ involvement determine the physical impact, which can range from mild to life-threatening. The common physical manifestations of BD include oral and genital ulcers, skin lesions, eye inflammation, and joint inflammation. Other possible complications include vascular inflammation, which can affect any organ and cause life-threatening events, nervous system inflammation, which can affect the brain and spinal cord functions, and digestive tract inflammation, which can cause bleeding and perforation [15, 16].

According to several studies, BD patients have a lower QoL than healthy individuals in most domains of QoL, especially in physical health and psychological health [17–20]. The physical impact of BD on QoL is influenced by several factors, such as:

- The type and number of symptoms: BD patients with more severe and frequent symptoms, such as oral ulcers, genital ulcers, joint problems, neurological problems, and eye problems, have a lower QoL than those with less severe and frequent symptoms. The number of symptoms is inversely correlated with the QoL scores in both specific and general instruments [7, 20–22].
- The disease activity: BD patients with active disease have a lower QoL than those with inactive disease. The disease activity is positively correlated with the pain and functional disability scores and negatively correlated with the QoL scores in both specific and general instruments [23–27].
- The gender: Female BD patients have a lower QoL than male BD patients in some domains of QoL, such as psychological health and social relationships. This may be due to the higher prevalence of genital ulcers, skin lesions, and fatigue among female patients, as well as the social stigma and emotional distress associated with these manifestations [20].
- The age: Older BD patients have a lower QoL than younger BD patients in some domains of QoL, such as physical health and social relationships. This may be due to the cumulative effect of chronic inflammation, organ damage, and disability over time [28].
- The education level: BD patients with higher education levels have a higher QoL than those with lower education levels in some domains of QoL, such as environment. This may be due to better access to health care, information, and social support among educated patients [29].

The physical impact of BD varies among individuals and over time. Some people may have mild symptoms that do not affect their daily activities, while others may have severe and disabling symptoms that require intensive treatment and hospitalization. The disease course is unpredictable and may alternate between remission (when symptoms improve or disappear) and relapse (when symptoms worsen or reappear).

23.2.2 Psychological Impact

BD affects various organ systems and impairs the QoL and life satisfaction of patients, caregivers, and families. The reduced QoL in BD patients may be attributed to several factors, such as disease activity and severity, psychological distress, social and occupational impairment, and treatment side effects. These factors can interfere with the physical, mental, and social well-being of patients and limit their coping abilities [20, 30, 31].

Patients with BD often experience depression and anxiety. These problems are worse than in healthy controls and relate to the disease activity, severity, duration, and symptoms [32]. Depression and anxiety impair the patients' coping, treatment adherence, stress management, and social relationships. They also raise the risk of suicide [33].

Other psychological problems include somatic symptoms (fatigue, pain, insomnia, and sexual dysfunction), psychotic symptoms (hallucinations and delusions), and cognitive impairment (memory loss, attention deficit, and executive dysfunction) [34].

The psychological impact varies by demographic (age, gender, education, and marital status), clinical (symptoms, organ involvement, and treatment), and psychosocial (social support, coping strategies, illness perception, and stigma) factors [35, 36]. It should be assessed and managed routinely. Validated instruments (e.g., the Leeds BD-QoL or the WHOQOL-BREF questionnaires) can measure the QoL and identify the needs of the patients [37]. Narrative medicine (e.g., collecting and analyzing illness stories) can explore the patients' perspectives and experiences [38].

Psychological well-being can be improved by pharmacological treatments (antidepressants or antipsychotics), psychological treatments (cognitive-behavioral therapy or mindfulness-based therapy), psychosocial support (peer support groups or online communities), and educational programs (self-management or health literacy) [39].

23.2.3 Social Impact

BD has negative effects on the QoL, well-being, self-esteem, social relationships, work productivity and daily functioning of patients, caregivers, and families. Several factors influence the QoL of BD patients, such as disease activity, severity, duration, organ involvement, treatment side effects, pain, disability, depression, anxiety, and stigma. BD patients have lower QoL than healthy individuals, especially in physical and psychological domains. They experience pain, eating difficulties, tension, irritability, depression, and dissatisfaction with life [40]. The QoL of BD patients can be improved by early diagnosis, effective treatment, multidisciplinary care, patient education, psychological support, and social integration. BD patients face many social challenges, such as stigma, discrimination, isolation, rejection, misunderstanding, and lack of support. They may have problems fulfilling their social roles as spouses, parents, friends, students, or workers due to the unpredictable and disabling nature of the disease [17]. They may also suffer from reduced work productivity and increased absenteeism, presenteeism, and unemployment, leading to financial difficulties and lower socioeconomic status [41, 42]. Moreover, BD patients may have impaired sexual and reproductive health due to genital ulcers, pain, dyspareunia, infertility, pregnancy complications, and sexual dysfunction. BD patients need *more social support and understanding from their family, friends, health professionals, and* society to cope with the disease and its consequences. BD can also cause social and economic burdens [43]. Some of the social effects on patients are:

Reduced QoL Patients with BD report lower levels of physical and mental well-being and social functioning than healthy individuals or patients with other chronic diseases. The disease impairs their ability to perform daily activities, work, study, or enjoy leisure time. They also face stigma, isolation, or discrimination due to their visible symptoms or disability [44].

Psychological distress Patients with BD suffer from various psychological problems such as depression, anxiety, anger, frustration, fear, guilt, or low self-esteem. These problems are related to the uncertainty of the disease course, the lack of effective treatments, the impact of symptoms on appearance and function, the loss of control over their life, or the lack of social support [40, 45].

Social support Patients with BD benefit from adequate and appropriate social support from their family, friends, health care providers, or peer groups. Social support helps them cope with the emotional and practical challenges of living with a rare and chronic disease. However, some patients have difficulties accessing or maintaining social support due to geographical distance, cultural differences, communication barriers, or lack of awareness or understanding of the disease [6, 46].

Economic impact Patients with BD incur substantial direct and indirect costs associated with their disease management and care. Direct costs include medical expenses for diagnosis, treatment, hospitalization, or rehabilitation. Indirect costs include productivity losses due to absenteeism, presenteeism (reduced performance at work), unemployment, disability, or premature mortality. The economic impact of BD varies depending on the country, health care system, insurance coverage, and severity of the disease [41].

As a challenging condition, BD can affect many aspects of a person's life. However, with proper diagnosis, treatment, and follow-up, most people with BD can manage their symptoms and lead a fulfilling life.

23.3 Quality of Life Scales in BD

QoL is an important outcome measure for patients with BD and can be influenced by a range of factors, including disease activity, psychological distress, sleep quality, and social functioning [20]. Many scales have been used to assess.

QoL in BD patients can be broadly classified into two categories: generic and specific [47]. Specific scales were adapted to capture the impact of BD on QoL [Table 23.1], while generic scales were adapted to measure QoL in general populations or in different diseases, including BD [Table 23.2].

23.3.1 Specific Scales for BD Patients

Behçet's disease quality of life (BD-QoL) A 30-item questionnaire that measures the impact of BD on the QoL of patients. It covers the physical, psychological, social, and environmental aspects of QoL. Higher scores indicate lower QoL. It has been validated and translated into different languages, such as Persian, Arabic, and Korean [5, 32, 48–53].

Behçet's Disease Current Activity Form (BDCAF) A tool to assess the disease activity and severity of BD. It consists of a visual analogue scale (VAS) for patients and clinicians to rate the overall perceived QoL and a patient index score that sums up the number and severity of symptoms in different organ systems. The patient index score can be transformed into a 0–20 scale. Higher scores indicate higher disease activity [26, 28, 32, 34, 43, 49, 50, 52, 54–60].

Behçet's Syndrome Activity Scale (BSAS) A composite index that combines clinical and laboratory parameters to measure the disease activity of BD. It includes oral ulcers, genital ulcers, skin lesions, eye lesions, joint involvement, vascular involvement, neurological involvement, gastrointestinal involvement, and erythrocyte sedimentation rate. Each parameter is assigned a weight according to its severity and frequency. The total score ranges from 0 to 284, with higher scores indicating higher disease activity [40, 50, 59, 61].

Behçet's Disease-Checklist 92 This is a tool for assessing the physical and psychosocial problems of patients with BD based on the International Classification of Functioning, Disability and Health (ICF). It consists of 92 items that cover three domains: body functions and structures, activities and participation, and environmental factors. The items are rated on a scale of 0–4, indicating the severity of the problem. The BD-checklist 92 has been shown to have good validity and reliability for measuring the functioning and quality of life of patients with BD [62–64].

Table 23.1 Specific quality of life scales used in Behçet's disease

	Total items	Total score	Aspects of QoL	Developed by	References
BD-QoL	30	0–30	Physical, psychological, social, and environmental factors	Gilworth et al. 2004 [5]	[5, 32, 48–53]
BDCAF	6	0–20	Assessment of disease activity	Bhakta et al. 1999 [54]	[26, 28, 32, 34, 43, 49, 50, 52, 54–60]
BSAS	10	0–100	Combines clinical symptoms and laboratory parameters	Forbess et al. 2008 [59]	[40, 50, 59, 61]
BD-checklist 92	92	0–4	Functions, structures, activities participation, and environmental factors.	Tsutsui et al. 2022 [63]	[62–64]

Abbreviations: *BD* Behçet's disease, *BDCAF* Behçet's disease current activity form, *BSAS* Behçet's syndrome activity scale

Table 23.2 Generic quality of life scales used in Behçet's disease

Scales, questionnaires, indexes	Items	Descriptions	Domains	References
Beck anxiety inventory (BAI)	21	Covers cognitive, somatic, affective, and behavioral aspects of anxiety	Psy	[65, 66]
Beck inventory scale or Beck Depression Inventory (BDI)	21	Covers four domains of depression: Cognitive, affective, somatic, and behavioral	Psy	[67, 68]
Brief Disability Questionnaire (BDQ)	11	Physical disability (6 items) and social disability (5 items). The total score reflects the severity of disability	Phy	[69]
Brief symptoms inventory (BSI)	53	Somatization, depression, anxiety, hostility, and psychoticism	Psy	[70]
Central Sensitization Inventory (CSI)	25	CSI is a 25-item questionnaire that measures the symptoms and severity of central sensitization syndrome, which is a condition characterized by hypersensitivity to pain and other stimuli due to increased excitability of the central nervous system.	Phy	[60, 71]
Composite index	3	The composite index is a scoring system between 0 and 10 consisting of the sum of three domains: Presence of oral ulcer, pain, and functional effect.	Phy	[8]
Dermatology Life Quality Index (DLQI)	10	Symptoms, emotions, daily activities, leisure, work or school, personal relationships, and treatment	Phy, Psy, social	[72]
Epworth Sleepiness Scale (ESS)	8	It is used for measuring the general level of daytime sleepiness in adults and adolescents	Phy	[73, 74]
Euro Quality of life 5D (EQ-5D)	5	Mobility, self-care, usual activities, pain/discomfort, and anxiety/depression	Phy, Psy, social	[75, 76]
Extended Disability Status Scale (EDSS)	19	Pyramidal, cerebellar, brainstem, sensory, bowel and bladder, visual, mental functions ambulation score	Phy	[77, 78]
Fatigue Severity Scale (FSS)	9	Assesses physical functioning and disability, psychological Well-being and mood, social and occupational performance, general health and satisfaction with life	Phy	[79]
Generalized Anxiety Disorder-7 (GAD-7)	7	Assesses the frequency of anxiety symptoms over the previous 2 weeks	Psy	[80, 81]
General Well-Being Index (GWBI)	18	Measures severity, distress, degree of interference in activities of daily living, and timing of fatigue	Psy	[17, 82]
Genital Ulcer Severity Score (GUSS)	N/A	It consists of six domains: Average number, average size, duration, ulcer-free period, pain and site of ulcers.	Phy	[34]
Global Fatigue Index (GFI)	16	Four aspects of fatigue: Severity, distress, degree of interference in activities of daily living, and timing	Phy	[40, 81]
Health Assessment Questionnaire (HAQ)	20	It's eight domains are; dressing and grooming, arising, eating, walking, hygiene, reach, grip, and activities	Phy	[84]
Hospital Anxiety and Depression Scale (HADS)	14	Measures the levels of anxiety and depression	Psy	[85–87]

(continued)

Table 23.2 (continued)

Scales, questionnaires, indexes	Items	Descriptions	Domains	References
Inflammatory Bowel Disease Questionnaire (IBDQ)	32	Bowel symptoms, systemic symptoms, emotional function, and social function	Phy, Psy, social	[19, 84]
Leeds Assessment of Neuropathic Symptoms and Signs (LANSS)	7	Global fatigue index, fatigue severity, distress caused by fatigue, and interference of fatigue with daily activities	Phy	[17, 88]
Multidimensional Assessment of Fatigue (MAF)	16	Assess four dimensions of fatigue (severity, distress, degree of interference in activities of daily living, and timing)	Phy	[40, 52]
Multidimensional Health Assessment Questionnaire (MD-HAQ)	10	It covers physical and psychological aspects, as well as scales and indices to measure pain, fatigue, helplessness, joint count, symptoms, and clinical severity.	Phy	[89]
National Eye Institute Visual Function Questionnaire-25 (NEI-VFQ-25)	25	Measures the impact of visual impairment on health-related QoL. It covers domains such as general health, vision-specific mental health, social functioning, role difficulties, dependency, driving, color vision, peripheral vision, and ocular pain	Phy, Psy, social	[22, 90–92]
Nottingham Health Profile (NHP)	38	It covers domains such as energy, pain, emotional reactions, sleep, social isolation, and physical mobility	Phy, Psy, social	[25, 60, 93–96]
Oral Health Impact Profile-14 (OHIP-14)	14	Covers seven domains of oral health-related quality of life: Functional limitation, physical pain, psychological discomfort, physical disability, psychological disability, social disability, and handicap	Phy, Psy, social	[7, 11, 96]
General Oral health assessment index (GOHAI)	12	Covers three domains: Physical function, psychosocial function, and pain and discomfort. The items are scored on a Likert-type scale and summed up to give a total score ranging from 12 to 60. Higher scores indicating better OHRQoL	Phy, Psy, social	[97–100]
Oral ulcer severity score (OUSS)	N/A	It covers four domains: Number, size, pain, and functional limitation of oral ulcers. Higher scores indicating more severe ulcers	Phy	[55, 56]
Patient Global Impression of Change (PGIC)	1	A single-item questionnaire that measures the patient's perception of improvement or worsening of their condition after treatment	Psy	[17, 96]
Patient Health Questionnaire-9 (PHQ-9)	9	A questionnaire that measures the severity of depressive symptoms in the past two weeks.	Psy	[56, 80, 81]
Pittsburgh Sleep Quality Index (PSQI)	19	A self-report questionnaire assessing sleep quality over a 1-month period. It consists of 7 sleep components that produce a single global score	Phy	[18, 83, 86, 101]
Psychological General Well-Being (PGWB)	22	A questionnaire that measures the psychological Well-being and distress of patients with chronic diseases. It covers physical and social functioning, role limitations due to physical and emotional problems, bodily pain, general health, vitality, social functioning, and mental health	Psy	[17]

(continued)

Table 23.2 (continued)

Scales, questionnaires, indexes	Items	Descriptions	Domains	References
Short Form-36 (SF-36)	36	It covers eight domains: Physical functioning, role limitations due to physical problems, bodily pain, general health perceptions, vitality, social functioning, role limitations due to emotional problems, and mental health	Phy, Psy, social	[30, 102, 103]
Social Economic Status (SES)	10	A multifactorial questionnaire that measures the social and economic status of an individual or a household within a community. It's score ranges from 0 to 100, with higher scores indicating higher SES	Social	[17, 43, 51]
Standard Gamble (SG)	N/A	The SG scale is applied by asking individuals to choose between a gamble of living in perfect health or dying, and living in a certain health state for the rest of their lives, and then calculating their utility by subtracting the percentage risk of death from	Psy	[17, 81]
State Trait Anxiety Inventory (STAI-T)	20	Asses the affective, cognitive, and physiological aspects of trait anxiety, such as nervousness, worry, tension, calmness, confidence, and relaxation	Psy	[21, 104]
Structured Clinical Interview for Diagnostic and Statistical Manual of Mental Disorders (SCID-CV)	10	Covers major categories of DSM such as mood disorders, psychotic disorders, anxiety disorders, substance use disorders, eating disorders, somatoform disorders, adjustment disorders, and personality disorders	Psy	[17, 44]
Temperament and Character Inventory (TCI)	240	It measures four temperament dimensions and three-character dimensions of personality	Psy	[104–107]
Time Trade Off (TTO)	2	Can measure the utility of different health states, and it can cover various domains of health	Psy	[17, 81]
Venous insufficiency epidemiological and Economic Study Quality of Life/Symptoms (VEINES-QoL/Sym)	26	A QoL and symptoms related to chronic venous disorders. It covers four domains: physical, physical, pain, and social	Phy, Psy, social	[17, 108]
Visual analogue scale (VAS)	N/A	This is a psychometric response scale that can be used in questionnaires to measure subjective characteristics or attitudes that cannot be directly measured, such as pain intensity, mood, or quality of life	Phy, Psy	[17, 88, 109]
Warwick-Edinburgh Mental Well-being Scale (WEMWBS)	14	A scale that measures positive mental Well-being. It covers affective, cognitive, and physical aspects	Psy	[17, 34, 80, 110]
Work and Social Adjustment Scale (WSAS)	5	A self-report measure of functional impairment due to a specific problem or disorder. It measures the impact of the problem on the following domains: Work, home management, social leisure, private leisure, and personal or family relationships.	Social	[17, 56, 80, 110, 111]
World Health Organization Quality of Life scales (WHOQOL)		These are instruments that measure different aspects of QoL in various populations and settings. They include the WHOQOL-100, a comprehensive questionnaire, the WHOQOL-BREF a shorter version, and the WHODAS 2.0, a tool that measures disability [112]		

(continued)

Table 23.2 (continued)

Scales, questionnaires, indexes	Items	Descriptions	Domains	References
WHOQOL-100	100	Physical health, psychological health, level of Independence, social relationships, environment, and spirituality/religion/personal beliefs	Phy, Psy, social	[12, 17, 18, 24, 32, 33, 37, 38, 49, 82, 113, 114]
WHOQOL-BREF	26	Physical health, psychological health, social relationships, and environment		[12, 20, 33, 35, 37, 53, 112–115]
WHO disability assessment schedule 2.0 (WHODAS 2.0)	36	This is a generic instrument that measures health and disability that covers six domains: Cognition, mobility, self-care, getting along, life activities, and participation		[116]

Abbreviations: *Psy* physical, *Psy* psychological

23.3.2 Generic scales for BD Patients

These tools play an important role in determining the diagnosis, treatment, and prognosis of the BD. Additionally, this can be used to understand the epidemiological, clinical, and pathophysiological features of the disease. The development and standardization of these tools are a challenge for researchers in the field of BD. BD is a rare disease that affects multiple organ systems and has a heterogeneous course. Therefore, the psychometric properties of these instruments, such as validity, reliability, and sensitivity, should be continually evaluated and improved.

23.4 Factors Influencing Quality of Life in Behçet's Disease

Some factors that have been found to influence the QoL of BD patients are gender, age, marital status, education level, medication use, lifestyle habits, employment status, and benefit claims. For example, female gender, older age, lower education level, unemployment, and receiving benefits have been associated with poorer QoL in BD patients. On the other hand, using immunosuppressants, doing regular exercise, and continuing employment have been associated with better QoL in BD patients [117].

The most common symptoms that have a negative impact on the QoL of BD patients are joint and neurological problems, followed by mucosal, ocular, skin, and gastrointestinal manifestations. These symptoms can cause pain, disability, emotional distress, social isolation, and reduced self-esteem in BD patients. For ocular disease, the visual acuity and the type of uveitis can also affect the QoL of BD patients [57, 99].

23.5 Improving Quality of Life in BD

BD can have a negative impact on the QoL of the affected patients, especially in terms of physical and psychological health [118]. Therefore, improving QoL is an important goal in the management of BD. To improve QoL in BD, several strategies can be considered:

Early diagnosis and treatment of BD can prevent or reduce the severity of organ damage and complications, which can impair QoL. The International Criteria for BD may help to identify the patients based on clinical manifestations and exclude other differential diagnoses [119].

Effective control of disease activity and symptoms can improve QoL by reducing pain, disability, and psychological distress. Various medications can be used to treat BD, such as corticosteroids, immunosuppressants, biologics, and colchicine. The choice of treatment depends on the type and severity of organ involvement, as well as the patient's preferences and comorbidities [50, 115].

Regular monitoring and follow-up of BD patients can help to assess the response to treatment, detect any adverse effects or new manifestations, and adjust the treatment regimen accordingly. The BD BDCAF is a validated tool that can measure the disease activity and its impact on QoL [58, 59, 120].

Multidisciplinary care and collaboration among different specialists can provide comprehensive and holistic care for BD patients, addressing their physical, psychological, social, and emotional needs. For example, rheumatologists, ophthalmologists, neurologists, dermatologists, gastroenterologists, dentists, psychiatrists, nurses, physiotherapists, and social workers can work together to provide optimal care for BD patients [6].

Patient education and empowerment can enhance QoL by increasing the patient's knowledge, awareness, self-management skills, coping strategies, and treatment adherence. Patients can benefit from reliable sources of information about BD, such as websites, books, or leaflets. They can also join support groups or networks to share their experiences and receive emotional support from other BD patients or caregivers [121, 122].

Lifestyle modifications and complementary therapies can improve QoL by promoting general health and well-being, reducing stress, and alleviating symptoms. For example, patients can adopt a healthy diet, exercise regularly, quit smoking, practice relaxation techniques, or use herbal remedies. However, these interventions should be used with caution and under medical supervision, as they may have potential interactions or side effects [1, 29].

In conclusion, QoL in BD can be improved by early diagnosis and treatment, effective control of disease activity and symptoms, regular monitoring and follow-up, multidisciplinary care and collaboration, patient education and empowerment, lifestyle modifications, and complementary therapies. These strategies can help BD patients achieve a better physical and psychological health status, reduce their suffering and disability, and enhance their social functioning and satisfaction with life.

23.6 Future Directions in Research

QoL is a complex and multidimensional concept that reflects the subjective perception of individuals about their well-being and satisfaction in various domains of life. QoL is influenced by both personal and environmental factors and can vary significantly among individuals and groups. BD can cause various symptoms and complications that impair the physical, psychological, social, and sexual functioning of patients, and consequently reduce their QoL. Therefore, assessing and improving QoL is an important goal in the management of BD [1, 17].

However, there are still many gaps and challenges in the research on QoL in BD patients [14]. Some of the future directions that could advance the knowledge and practice in this field are:

Developing and validating more comprehensive and specific QoL measures that capture the multidimensional and dynamic aspects of BD: Existing QoL instruments may not adequately reflect the impact of BD on different domains of life, such as oral ulcers, ocular involvement, neurological complications, and sexual and reproductive health. Moreover, QoL may change over time depending on the course and severity of the disease, the response to treatment, and the adaptation to the illness. Therefore, there is a need for more sensitive and reliable QoL measures that can assess the specific needs and preferences of BD patients and monitor their QoL changes over time [5, 17].

Conducting longitudinal studies that follow BD patients over time and examine the changes in QoL and its determinants: Most of the previous studies on QoL in BD patients were cross-sectional [123], which limits the ability to infer causal relationships and temporal patterns. Longitudinal studies can provide more insight into the natural history of QoL in BD patients and identify the factors that influence QoL positively or negatively over time [46]. Some of the potential determinants of QoL in BD patients are disease activity, severity, duration, organ involvement, treatment response, psychological distress, sleep quality, social support, coping strategies, illness perception, and stigma [1].

Comparing the QoL of BD patients with other chronic inflammatory diseases or rare diseases to identify the similarities and differences in QoL domains and influencing factors: BD is often considered as a model disease for studying the impact of inflammation on QoL. However, BD is also a heterogeneous and complex disorder that has unique features and challenges. Comparing the QoL of BD patients with other patient groups can help to understand the common and specific aspects of QoL in BD, and to develop more tailored interventions for improving QoL in different populations [47].

Exploring the relationship between QoL and clinical outcomes, such as disease progression, complications, disability, mortality, and health care utilization in BD patients: QoL is not only an outcome measure but also a predictor of clinical outcomes in chronic diseases. There is evidence that lower QoL is associated with a worse prognosis and higher health care costs in various conditions [124]. However, there is limited research on how QoL affects or is affected by clinical outcomes in BD patients. Understanding this relationship can help to optimize the management of BD patients by addressing both their medical and psychosocial needs.

Evaluating the effectiveness of interventions that aim to improve QoL in BD patients, such as pharmacological treatments, psychological treatments, psychosocial support, educational programs, lifestyle modifications, and complementary therapies: Although there are several treatment options for controlling the symptoms and preventing the complications of BD, there is a lack of evidence-based interventions that specifically target QoL improvement in BD patients. Moreover, there may be individual differences in the response to different interventions depending on various factors [43, 125]. Therefore, there is a need for a more rigorous and comprehensive evaluation of the efficacy and cost-effectiveness of various interventions for enhancing QoL in BD patients.

Investigating the role of genetic and environmental factors in QoL variation among BD patients across different populations and regions: BD has a strong genetic component that involves several genes related to immune regulation [126]. However, environmental factors, such as infections, stress, diet, climate, and culture, may also modulate the expression and severity of BD. These factors may also affect QoL directly or indirectly through their impact on disease manifestations or coping mechanisms [127]. Therefore, there is a need for more research on how genetic and environmental factors interact to influence QoL among BD patients from different backgrounds.

23.7 Conclusion

To conclude, the QoL of BD patients is influenced in multiple areas, including physical, psychological, social, and environmental aspects. In this section, the general and specific scales used to assess the quality of life for patients with BD were discussed, emphasizing their strengths and weaknesses. Similar to many other chronic and systemic diseases, evaluating, improving, and enhancing the QoL is a crucial objective in the clinical care and research of patients with BD.

References

1. Senusi AA, Mather J, Ola D, Bergmeier LA, Gokani B, Fortune F. The impact of multifactorial factors on the quality of life of Behcet's patients over 10 years. Front Med (Lausanne). 2022;9:996571. https://doi.org/10.3389/fmed.2022.996571.
2. Zeidan MJ, Saadoun D, Garrido M, Klatzmann D, Six A, Cacoub P. Behçet's disease physiopathology: a contemporary review. Autoimmun Highlights. 2016;7(1):4. https://doi.org/10.1007/s13317-016-0074-1.
3. Alpsoy E. Behçet's disease: a comprehensive review with a focus on epidemiology, etiology and clinical features, and management of mucocutaneous lesions. J Dermatol. 2016;43(6):620–32. https://doi.org/10.1111/1346-8138.13381.
4. Ali S, Nagieb CS, Fayed HL. Effect of Behcet's disease-associated oral ulcers on oral health related quality of life. Spec Care Dentist. 2023;43(4):435–42. https://doi.org/10.1111/scd.12782.

5. Gilworth G, Chamberlain MA, Bhakta B, Haskard D, Silman A, Tennant A. Development of the BD-QoL: a quality of life measure specific to Behcet's disease. J Rheumatol. 2004;31(5):931–7.
6. Bernabe E, Marcenes W, Mather J, Phillips C, Fortune F. Impact of Behcet's syndrome on health-related quality of life: influence of the type and number of symptoms. Rheumatology. 2010;49(11):2165–71. https://doi.org/10.1093/rheumatology/keq251.
7. Mumcu G, Inanc N, Ergun T, Ikiz K, Gunes M, Islek U, et al. Oral health related quality of life is affected by disease activity in Behcet's disease. Oral Dis. 2006;12(2):145–51. https://doi.org/10.1111/j.1601-0825.2005.01173.x.
8. Mumcu G, Karacayli U, Yay M, Aksoy A, Tas MN, Armagan B, et al. Oral ulcer activity assessment with the composite index according to different treatment modalities in Behcet's syndrome: a multicentre study. Clin Exp Rheumatol. 2019;37 Suppl 121(6):98–104.
9. Mumcu G, Niazi S, Stewart J, Hagi-Pavli E, Gokani B, Seoudi N, et al. Oral health and related quality of life status in patients from UK and Turkey: a comparative study in Behcet's disease. J Oral Pathol Med. 2009;38(5):406–9. https://doi.org/10.1111/j.1600-0714.2009.00752.x.
10. Sogur E, Onem E, Kalfa M, Emmungil H, Bostanci N, Aksu K, et al. Oral health and oral quality of life in inactive patients with familial Mediterranean fever without amyloidosis. Clin Exp Rheumatol. 2013;31(3 Suppl 77):15–9.
11. Mumcu G, Hayran O, Ozalp DO, Inanc N, Yavuz S, Ergun T, Direskeneli H. The assessment of oral health-related quality of life by factor analysis in patients with Behcet's disease and recurrent aphthous stomatitis. J Oral Pathol Med. 2007;36(3):147–52. https://doi.org/10.1111/j.1600-0714.2007.00514.x.
12. Oklar M, Zorlutuna Kaymak N, Tanyildiz B, Tezcan ME, Şimşek Ş. Treatment adherence effect on the visual acuity of Behçet's uveitis patients. Ocul Immunol Inflamm 2023:1–9. doi: https://doi.org/10.1080/09273948.2023.2288905, 32, 1698.
13. Floris A, Piga M, Laconi R, Espinosa G, Lopalco G, Serpa Pinto L, et al. Accrual of organ damage in Behçet's syndrome: trajectory, associated factors, and impact on patients' quality of life over a 2-year prospective follow-up study. Arthritis Res Ther. 2022;24(1):253. https://doi.org/10.1186/s13075-022-02947-y.
14. Masoumi M, Sharifi A, Rezaei S, Rafiei S, Hosseinifard H, Khani S, et al. Global systematic review and meta-analysis of health-related quality of life in Behcet's patients. Caspian J Intern Med. 2022;13(3):447–57. https://doi.org/10.22088/cjim.13.3.447.
15. Behçet H. Uber rezidivierende aphthouse durch ein virüs verursachte Geschwuere am Mund, am Auge und an den Genitalien. Dermatol Monatsschr. 1937;105:1152–7.
16. Tursen U, Gurler A, Boyvat A. Evaluation of clinical findings according to sex in 2313 Turkish patients with Behçet's disease. Int J Dermatol. 2003;42(5):346–51. https://doi.org/10.1046/j.1365-4362.2003.01741.x.
17. Mastrolia MV, Marinello D, Di Cianni F, Talarico R, Simonini G. Assessing quality of life in Behçet's disease: a systematic review. Clin Exp Rheumatol. 2022;40:1560. https://doi.org/10.55563/clinexprheumatol/sian1b.
18. Shaddad AM, Hussein AARM, Safwat SM, Talaat EA, Farrag S, Gamal NM, Khaleel WGE. Assessment of sleep quality, anxiety, depression, and quality of life in Behçet's disease. The Egyptian Journal of Bronchology. 2023;17(1) https://doi.org/10.1186/s43168-023-00200-x.
19. Kim WH, Cho YS, Yoo HM, Park IS, Park EC, Lim JG. Quality of life in Korean patients with inflammatory bowel diseases: ulcerative colitis, Crohn's disease and intestinal Behçet's disease. Int J Color Dis. 1999;14(1):52–7. https://doi.org/10.1007/s003840050183.
20. Canpolat O, Yurtsever S. The quality of life in patients with Behcet's disease. Asian Nurs Res (Korean Soc Nurs Sci). 2011;5(4):229–35. https://doi.org/10.1016/j.anr.2011.12.003.
21. Gur A, Sarac AJ, Burkan YK, Nas K, Cevik R. Arthropathy, quality of life, depression, and anxiety in Behcet's disease: relationship between arthritis and these factors. Clin Rheumatol. 2006;25(4):524–31. https://doi.org/10.1007/s10067-005-0100-6.
22. Onal S, Savar F, Akman M, Kazokoglu H. Vision- and health-related quality of life in patients with Behcet uveitis. Arch Ophthalmol. 2010;128(10):1265–71. https://doi.org/10.1001/archophthalmol.2010.209.
23. Khabbazi A, Ebrahimzadeh Attari V, Asghari Jafarabadi M, Malek MA. Quality of life in patients with Behcet disease and its relation with clinical symptoms and disease activity. Reumatol Clin (Engl Ed). 2021;17(1):1–6. https://doi.org/10.1016/j.reuma.2019.03.002.
24. Fabiani C, Vitale A, Orlando I, Sota J, Capozzoli M, Franceschini R, et al. Quality of life impairment in Behçet's disease and relationship with disease activity: a prospective study. Intern Emerg Med. 2017;12(7):947–55. https://doi.org/10.1007/s11739-017-1691-z.
25. Bodur H, Borman P, Özdemir Y, Atan Ç, Kural G. Quality of life and life satisfaction in patients with Behçet's disease: relationship with disease activity. Clin Rheumatol. 2006;25(3):329–33. https://doi.org/10.1007/s10067-005-0046-8.
26. Oktayoglu P, Mete N, Caglayan M, Bozkurt M, Bozan T, Em S, Nas K. Elevated serum levels of calprotectin (MRP8/MRP14) in patients with Behcet's disease and its association with disease activity and quality of life. Scand J Clin Lab Invest. 2015;75(2):106–12. https://doi.org/10.3109/00365513.2014.984319.

27. Gorial FI, Jabbar MA. Impact of disease activity on health related quality of life in patients with Behçet's disease: a cross-sectional study. Ann Med Surg. 2020;54:43–6. https://doi.org/10.1016/j.amsu.2020.03.010.
28. Floris A, Laconi R, Espinosa G, Lopalco G, Serpa Pinto L, Kougkas N, et al. AB0636 relationship between organ damage and impairment of health-related quality of life in patients with Behçet's syndrome: results from a longitudinal extension of the BODI project. Ann Rheum Dis. 2022;81(Suppl 1):1445.1. https://doi.org/10.1136/annrheumdis-2022-eular.4060.
29. Senusi AA, Ola D, Mather J, Mather J, Fortune F. Behcet's syndrome and health-related quality of life: influence of symptoms, lifestyle and employment status. Clin Exp Rheumatol. 2017;35 Suppl 108(6):43–50.
30. Santos-Faria D, Silva J, Cerqueira M, Rodrigues J, Sousa-Neves J, Teixeira F, et al. FRI0318 Quality of life in patients with Behcet's disease. Annual European Congress of Rheumatology, 14–17 June, 2017: BMJ Publishing Group Ltd and European League Against Rheumatism; 2017. p. 607.2-.
31. Yi SW, Kim J-H, Lim K-Y, Bang D, Lee S, Lee E-S. The Behçet's disease quality of life: reliability and validity of the Korean version. Yonsei Med J. 2008;49(5):698. https://doi.org/10.3349/ymj.2008.49.5.698.
32. Lee J, Kim S-S, Jeong H-J, Son C-N, Kim J-M, Cho Y-W, Kim S-H. Association of sleep quality in Behcet disease with disease activity, depression, and quality of life in Korean population. Korean J Intern Med. 2017;32(2):352–9. https://doi.org/10.3904/kjim.2016.367.
33. Uğuz F, Dursun R, Kaya N, Savas CA. Quality of life in patients with Behçet's disease: the impact of major depression. Gen Hosp Psychiatry. 2007;29(1):21–4. https://doi.org/10.1016/j.genhosppsych.2006.10.001.
34. Senusi A, Seoudi N, Bergmeier LA, Fortune F. Genital ulcer severity score and genital health quality of life in Behcet's disease. Orphanet J Rare Dis. 2015;10:117. https://doi.org/10.1186/s13023-015-0341-7.
35. Melikoglu M, Melikoglu MA. What affects the quality of life in patients with Behcet's disease? Acta Reumatol Port. 2014;39(1):46–53.
36. Çakir EN, Yenisoy Y, Kapusuz A, Abacar K, Alibaz-Oner F, Yay M, et al. AB0895 a moderated mediation analysis for poor oral health-related quality of life in patients with Behçet's disease. Ann Rheum Dis. 2021;80(Suppl 1):1471.1. https://doi.org/10.1136/annrheumdis-2021-eular.3043.
37. Fidaner H. Measuring quality of life WHOQOL-100 and WHOQOL-bref. J Psychiatr Psychol Psychopharmacol. 1999;7:23–41.
38. Uğuz F, Dursun R, Kaya N, Çilli AS. Psychiatric symptoms and quality of life in Behçet patients. Anadolu Psikiyatri Dergisi. 2006;7:133–9.
39. Izuno T, Miyakawa M, Sugimori H, Takahashi E, Yoshida K, Hoshi K. The effect of quality of life in Behcet disease patients on subjective life satisfaction. Nihon Koshu Eisei Zasshi. 1998;45(10):979–87.
40. Ilhan B, Can M, Alibaz-Oner F, Yilmaz-Oner S, Polat-Korkmaz O, Ozen G, et al. Fatigue in patients with Behçet's syndrome: relationship with quality of life, depression, anxiety, disability and disease activity. Int J Rheum Dis. 2018;21(12):2139–45. https://doi.org/10.1111/1756-185X.12839.
41. Mumcu G, Lehimci F, FiDan Ö, Gük H, Alpar U, Ünal AU, et al. The assessment of work productivity and activity impairment in Behçet's disease. Turk J Med Sci. 2017;47:535–41. https://doi.org/10.3906/sag-1603-161.
42. Serin N, Ozguler Y, Esatoglu SN, Hamuryudan V, Hatemi G. FRI0519 Work productivity is impaired in patients with behÇet's syndrome. Annual European Congress of Rheumatology, EULAR 2018, Amsterdam, 13–16 June 2018: BMJ Publishing Group Ltd and European League Against Rheumatism; 2018. p. 786.1-.
43. Zayed HS, Medhat BM, Seif EM. Evaluation of treatment adherence in patients with Behçet's disease: its relation to disease manifestations, patients' beliefs about medications, and quality of life. Clin Rheumatol. 2019;38(3):761–8. https://doi.org/10.1007/s10067-018-4344-3.
44. Atay IM, Erturan I, Demirdas A, Yaman GB, Yürekli VA. The impact of personality on quality of life and disease activity in patients with Behcet's disease: a pilot study. Compr Psychiatry. 2014;55(3):511–7. https://doi.org/10.1016/j.comppsych.2013.11.008.
45. Talarico R, Parma A, Zera E, Calabresi E, Tani C, Baldini C, Mosca M. AB0618A snapshot of disease activity in patients with behcet's syndrome: predictive factors and relationship with quality of life. Annual European Congress of Rheumatology, EULAR 2019, Madrid, 12–15 June 2019: BMJ Publishing Group Ltd and European League Against Rheumatism; 2019. p. 1769.2–70.
46. Bullinger M. Measuring health related quality of life. An international perspective. Adv Exp Med Biol. 2003;528:113–22. https://doi.org/10.1007/0-306-48382-3_23.
47. Hatemi G, Merkel PA, Hamuryudan V, Boers M, Direskeneli H, Aydin SZ, Yazici H. Outcome measures used in clinical trials for Behçet syndrome: a systematic review. J Rheumatol. 2014;41(3):599–612. https://doi.org/10.3899/jrheum.131249.
48. Touma Z, Ghandour L, Sibai A, Puzantian H, Hamdan A, Hamdan O, et al. Cross-cultural adaptation and validation of Behcet's disease quality of life questionnaire. BMC Med Res Methodol. 2011;11:52. https://doi.org/10.1186/1471-2288-11-52.
49. Vojdanian M, Faezi ST, Tennant A, Morgan AW, Paragomi P, Qorbani M, et al. Validity and reliability of the Persian version of Behcet's disease quality-of-life (BD-QoL) questionnaire: a cross-cultural adap-

tation. Rheumatol Int. 2015;35(4):677–84. https://doi.org/10.1007/s00296-014-3128-6.
50. Hatemi G, Mahr A, Takeno M, Kim D, Melikoglu M, Cheng S, et al. Impact of apremilast on quality of life in Behcet's syndrome: analysis of the phase 3 RELIEF study. RMD Open. 2022;8(2):e002235. https://doi.org/10.1136/rmdopen-2022-002235.
51. Gaggiano C, Del Bianco A, Sota J, Gentileschi S, Ruscitti P, Giacomelli R, et al. A patient-driven registry on Behcet's disease: the AIDA for patients pilot project. Front Med (Lausanne). 2023;10:1188021. https://doi.org/10.3389/fmed.2023.1188021.
52. Sandikci CS, Colak S, Omma A, Enecik ME. An evaluation of depression, anxiety and fatigue in patients with Behcet's disease. Int J Rheum Dis. 2019;22(6):974–9. https://doi.org/10.1111/1756-185X.13411.
53. Aflaki E, Farahangiz S, Salehi A. Quality of life assessment in patients with Behcet's disease using the Persian Version of the leeds BD-QoL questionnaire. Iran J Med Sci. 2020;45(5):352–8. https://doi.org/10.30476/ijms.2020.72634.0.
54. Bhakta BB, Brennan P, James TE, Chamberlain MA, Noble BA, Silman AJ. Behçet's disease: evaluation of a new instrument to measure clinical activity. Rheumatology. 1999;38(8):728–33. https://doi.org/10.1093/rheumatology/38.8.728.
55. Senusi A, Kang A, Buchanan JAG, Adesanya A, Aloraini G, Stanford M, Fortune F. New mouthwash: an efficacious intervention for oral ulceration associated with Behcet's disease. Br J Oral Maxillofac Surg. 2020;58(8):1034–9. https://doi.org/10.1016/j.bjoms.2020.07.027.
56. Senusi A, Higgins S, Fortune F. The influence of oral health and psycho-social Well-being on clinical outcomes in Behcet's disease. Rheumatol Int. 2018;38(10):1873–83. https://doi.org/10.1007/s00296-018-4117-y.
57. Sakai T, Watanabe H, Kuroyanagi K, Akiyama G, Okano K, Kohno H, Tsuneoka H. Health- and vision-related quality of life in patients receiving infliximab therapy for Behcet uveitis. Br J Ophthalmol. 2013;97(3):338–42. https://doi.org/10.1136/bjophthalmol-2012-302515.
58. Neves FS, Moraes JCB, Kowalski SC, Goldenstein-Schainberg C, Lage LV, Gonçalves CR. Cross-cultural adaptation of the Behçet's Disease Current Activity Form (BDCAF) to Brazilian Portuguese language. Clin Rheumatol. 2007;26(8):1263–7. https://doi.org/10.1007/s10067-006-0484-y.
59. Forbess C, Swearingen C, Yazici Y. Behcet's Syndrome Activity Score (BSAS): a new disease activity assesment tool, composed of patient-derived measures, only, is strongly correlated with The Behcet's Disease Current Activity Form (BDCAF). Clinical and Experimental Rheumatology: Clinical & Experimental Rheumatology via Santa Maria 31, 56126 Pisa, İtaly; 2008. p. S28-S.
60. Ayar K, Okmen BM, Altan L, Ozturk EK. Central sensitization and its relationship with health profile in Behcet's disease. Mod Rheumatol. 2021;31(2):474–80. https://doi.org/10.1080/14397595.2020.1780076.
61. Alibaz-Oner F, Aldag B, Aldag M, Unal AU, Mutis A, Toptas T, et al. Post-thrombotic syndrome and venous disease-specific quality of life in patients with vascular Behcet's disease. J Vasc Surg Venous Lymphat Disord. 2016;4(3):301–6. https://doi.org/10.1016/j.jvsv.2016.01.003.
62. Tsutsui H, Kikuchi H, Oguchi H, Nomura K, Ohkubo T. Identification of physical and psychosocial problems based on symptoms in patients with Behçet's disease. Rheumatol Int. 2019;40(1):81–9. https://doi.org/10.1007/s00296-019-04488-1.
63. Tsutsui H, Kikuchi H, Oguchi H, Kono H, Ohkubo T. Validity and reliability of a checklist for patients with Behcet's disease based on the International Classification of Functioning, Disability and Health. Rheumatol Int. 2022;42(1):159–65. https://doi.org/10.1007/s00296-021-05001-3.
64. Üsküdar Cansu D, Korkmaz C. Seasonal variations and Behçet's disease activity. Cent Asian J Med Hypotheses Ethics. 2022;3(1):21–6. https://doi.org/10.47316/cajmhe.2022.3.1.02.
65. Beck A, Steer R. Beck anxiety inventory manual. 2nd ed. San Antonio: Psychological Corporation; 1993.
66. Ulusoy M, Sahin NH, Erkmen H. Turkish version of the Beck anxiety inventory: psychometric properties. J Cogn Psychother. 1998;12(2):163.
67. Beck AT. An inventory for measuring depression. Arch Gen Psychiatry. 1961;4(6):561. https://doi.org/10.1001/archpsyc.1961.01710120031004.
68. Hisli N. Beck depresyon envanterinin universite ogrencileri icin gecerliligi, guvenilirligi. (A reliability and validity study of Beck depression inventory in a university student sample). J Psychol. 1989;7:3–13.
69. Eren I, Şahin M, Tunc SE, Cure E, Civi İİ. Psychiatric symptoms and quality of life in patients with Behçet's disease. Neurol Psychiatry Brain Res. 2006;13(4):169–74.
70. Wood WD. An attempt to validate the psychoticism scale of the brief symptom inventory. Br J Med Psychol. 1982;55(4):367–73. https://doi.org/10.1111/j.2044-8341.1982.tb01521.x.
71. Mayer TG, Neblett R, Cohen H, Howard KJ, Choi YH, Williams MJ, et al. The development and psychometric validation of the central sensitization inventory. Pain Pract. 2012;12(4):276–85. https://doi.org/10.1111/j.1533-2500.2011.00493.x.
72. Finlay AY, Khan GK. Dermatology Life Quality Index (DLQI)-a simple practical measure for routine clinical use. Clin Exp Dermatol. 1994;19(3):210–6. https://doi.org/10.1111/j.1365-2230.1994.tb01167.x.
73. Johns MW. A new method for measuring daytime sleepiness: the Epworth sleepiness scale. Sleep. 1991;14(6):540–5. https://doi.org/10.1093/sleep/14.6.540.

74. Ahmed AE, Fatani A, Al-Harbi A, Al-Shimemeri A, Ali YZ, Baharoon S, Al-Jahdali H. Validation of the Arabic version of the Epworth sleepiness scale. J Epidemiol Glob Health. 2014;4(4):297. https://doi.org/10.1016/j.jegh.2014.04.004.
75. Euro-Qol Group. EuroQol—a new facility for the measurement of health-related quality of life. Health Policy. 1990;16(3):199–208. https://doi.org/10.1016/0168-8510(90)90421-9.
76. Brooks R. EuroQol: the current state of play. Health Policy. 1996;37(1):53–72. https://doi.org/10.1016/0168-8510(96)00822-6.
77. Siva A, Kantarci OH, Saip S, Altintas A, Hamuryudan V, Islak C, et al. Behçet's disease: diagnostic and prognostic aspects of neurological involvement. J Neurol. 2001;248(2):95–103. https://doi.org/10.1007/s004150170242.
78. Gündüz T, Emir Ö, Kürtüncü M, Mutlu M, Tumaç A, Akca Ş, et al. Cognitive impairment in Neuro-Behcet's disease and multiple sclerosis: a comparative study. Int J Neurosci. 2012;122(11):650–6. https://doi.org/10.3109/00207454.2012.704454.
79. Krupp LB. The fatigue severity scale: application to patients with multiple sclerosis and systemic lupus erythematosus. Arch Neurol. 1989;46(10):1121. https://doi.org/10.1001/archneur.1989.00520460115022.
80. Zulfiqar MH, Shamdas M, Bashir A, Douglas S, Murray PI. Longitudinal study investigating the relationship between disease activity and psychological status of patients with Behcet's disease. Ocul Immunol Inflamm. 2020;28(4):613–21. https://doi.org/10.1080/09273948.2019.1616770.
81. Murray PI, Sekaran A, Javidi H, Situnayake D. Interrelationships between heath utility measurements, disease activity and psychological factors in Behçet's disease. Gen Hosp Psychiatry. 2021;70:103–8. https://doi.org/10.1016/j.genhosppsych.2021.03.001.
82. Senthil MP, Simon S, Constable PA. A review of patient-reported outcome measures used in uveitis. Surv Ophthalmol. 2023;68(2):225–40. https://doi.org/10.1016/j.survophthal.2022.11.004.
83. Senusi AA, Liu J, Bevec D, Bergmeier LA, Stanford M, Kidd D, et al. Why are Behçet's disease patients always exhausted? Clin Exp Rheumatol. 2018;36(6):53–62.
84. Alder NM, Fisher M, Yazici Y. Behçet's syndrome patients have high levels of functional disability, fatigue and pain as measured by a Multi-dimensional Health Assessment Questionnaire (MDHAQ). Clin Exp Rheumatol. 2008;26(Suppl 50):S110–3.
85. Herrmann C. International experiences with the hospital anxiety and depression scale-a review of validation data and clinical results. J Psychosom Res. 1997;42(1):17–41. https://doi.org/10.1016/S0022-3999(96)00216-4.
86. Yazmalar L, Batmaz İ, Sarıyıldız MA, Yıldız M, Uçmak D, Türkçü F, et al. Sleep quality in patients with Behçet's disease. Int J Rheum Dis. 2017;20(12):2062–9. https://doi.org/10.1111/1756-185X.12459.
87. AL-Omiri MK, Karasneh J, Lynch E. Psychological profiles in patients with recurrent aphthous ulcers. Int J Oral Maxillofac Surg. 2012;41(3):384–8. https://doi.org/10.1016/j.ijom.2011.12.024.
88. Evcik D, Dogan SK, Ay S, Cuzdan N, Guven M, Gurler A, Boyvat A. Does Behcet's disease associate with neuropathic pain syndrome and impaired Well-being? Clin Rheumatol. 2012;32(1):33–6. https://doi.org/10.1007/s10067-012-2086-1.
89. Gibson KA, Pincus T. A self-report Multidimensional Health Assessment Questionnaire (MDHAQ) for Face-To-Face or Telemedicine Encounters to Assess Clinical Severity (RAPID3) and Screen for Fibromyalgia (FAST) and Depression (DEP). Curr Treat Options Rheumatol. 2021;7(3):161–81. https://doi.org/10.1007/s40674-021-00175-0.
90. Mangione CM. Development of the 25-list-item National Eye Institute Visual Function Questionnaire. Arch Ophthalmol. 2001;119(7):1050. https://doi.org/10.1001/archopht.119.7.1050.
91. Toprak AB, Eser E, Guler C, Baser FE, Mayali H. Cross-validation of the Turkish version of the 25-item National Eye Institute Visual Functioning Questionnaire (NEI-VFQ 25). Ophthalmic Epidemiol. 2005;12(4):259–69. https://doi.org/10.1080/09286580590967763.
92. Fitzpatrick R. The measurement of health status and quality of life in rheumatological disorders. Baillieres Clin Rheumatol. 1993;7(2):297–317. https://doi.org/10.1016/S0950-3579(05)80091-3.
93. Coons SJ, Rao S, Keininger DL, Hays RD. A Comparative Review of Generic Quality-of-Life Instruments:. PharmacoEconomics. 2000;17(1):13–35. doi: https://doi.org/10.2165/00019053-200017010-00002.
94. Guillemin F. Functional disability and quality-of-life assessment in clinical practice. Rheumatology. 2000;39(suppl_1):17–23. https://doi.org/10.1093/oxfordjournals.rheumatology.a031489.
95. Hunt SM, McEwen J, McKenna SP. Measuring health status: a new tool for clinicians and epidemiologists. J R Coll Gen Pract. 1985;35(273):185–8.
96. Hayran O, Mumcu G, Inanc N, Ergun T, Direskeneli H. Assessment of minimal clinically important improvement by using Oral Health Impact Profile-14 in Behcet's disease. Clin Exp Rheumatol. 2009;27(2 Suppl 53):S79–84.
97. Atchison K, Dolan T. Development of the Geriatric Oral Health Assessment Index. J Dent Educ. 1990;54(11):680–7. https://doi.org/10.1002/j.0022-0337.1990.54.11.tb02481.x.
98. Naito M, Suzukamo Y, Nakayama T, Hamajima N, Fukuhara S. Linguistic adaptation and validation of the General Oral Health Assessment Index (GOHAI) in an elderly Japanese population. J Public Health Dent. 2006;66(4):273–5. https://doi.org/10.1111/j.1752-7325.2006.tb04081.x.

99. Naito M, Suzukamo Y, Wakai K, Azechi M, Kaneko F, Nakayama T, et al. One-year period prevalence of oral aphthous ulcers and oral health-related quality of life in patients with Behcet's disease. Genet Res Int. 2014;2014:930348. https://doi.org/10.1155/2014/930348.
100. Schmalz G, Patschan S, Patschan D, Ziebolz D. Oral-health-related quality of life in adult patients with rheumatic diseases-a systematic review. J Clin Med. 2020;9(4) https://doi.org/10.3390/jcm9041172.
101. Italiano N, Di Cianni F, Marinello D, Elefante E, Mosca M, Talarico R. Sleep quality in Behcet's disease: a systematic literature review. Rheumatol Int. 2023;43(1):1–19. https://doi.org/10.1007/s00296-022-05218-w.
102. Mchorney CA, Johne W, Anastasiae R. The MOS 36-item short-form health survey (SF-36): II. Psychometric and clinical tests of validity in measuring physical and mental health constructs. Med Care. 1993;31(3):247–63. https://doi.org/10.1097/00005650-199303000-00006.
103. Demiral Y, Ergor G, Unal B, Semin S, Akvardar Y, Kıvırcık B, Alptekin K. Normative data and discriminative properties of short form 36 (SF-36) in Turkish urban population. BMC Public Health. 2006;6(1) https://doi.org/10.1186/1471-2458-6-247.
104. Ucar D, Yıldırım Y, Gultekin G, Ozyazgan Y, Emul M. Temperament and character traits in patients with Behçet's disease with/without eye involvement. Semin Ophthalmol. 2015;32(2):210–5. https://doi.org/10.3109/08820538.2015.1053624.
105. Cloninger CR, Przybeck T, Svrakic DM, Wetzel R. Temperam Charac Invent. 2011; https://doi.org/10.1037/t03902-000.
106. Köse S, Sayar K, Kalelioglu Ü, Aydin N, Ak I, Kirpinar I, et al. Turkish version of the Temperament and Character Inventory (TCI): reliability, validity, and factorial structure. Bull Clin Psychopharmacol. 2004;14(3):107–13.
107. Arkar H, Sorias O, Tunca Z, Safak C, Alkin T, Akdede BB, et al. Factorial structure, validity, and reliability of the Turkish temperament and character inventory. Turk Psikiyatri Dergisi. 2005;16(3):190.
108. Dumantepe M, Aydin S, Ökten M, Karabulut H. Endophlebectomy of the common femoral vein and endovascular iliac vein recanalization for chronic iliofemoral venous occlusion. J Vasc Surg Venous Lymphat Disord. 2020;8(4):572–82. https://doi.org/10.1016/j.jvsv.2019.11.008.
109. Baglan Yentur S, Bilek F, Koca SS. Physical activity and psychosomatic status in patients with Behcet's disease during coronavirus disease pandem. Eur J Rheumatol. 2022;9(3):144–7. https://doi.org/10.5152/eurjrheum.2021.20166.
110. Ogunkolade W, Senusi AA, Desai P, Sacoor S, Bibi A, Gokani B, et al. Profiling the microbiome of oral and genital mucosal surfaces in Behçet's disease. Clin Immunol. 2023;253:253. https://doi.org/10.1016/j.clim.2023.109654.
111. Mundt JC, Marks IM, Shear MK, Greist JM. The work and social adjustment scale: a simple measure of impairment in functioning. Br J Psychiatry. 2018;180(5):461–4. https://doi.org/10.1192/bjp.180.5.461.
112. Organization WH. WHOQOL-BREF: introduction, administration, scoring and generic version of the assessment: field trial version, December 1996. World Health Organization; 1996.
113. Nejat S, Montazeri A, Holakouie Naieni K, Mohammad K, Majdzadeh S. The World Health Organization quality of life (WHOQOL-BREF) questionnaire: translation and validation study of the Iranian version. J School Public Health Ins Public Health Res. 2006;4(4):1–12.
114. Harputluoglu N, Alkan Ozdemir S, Yilmaz U, Celik T. Evaluation of primary caregiver parents' quality of life in pediatric palliative care with the WHOQOL-Bref (TR). Turk Arch Pediatr. 2021;56(5):429–39. https://doi.org/10.5152/TurkArchPediatr.2021.20262.
115. Ertam I, Kitapcioglu G, Aksu K, Keser G, Ozaksar A, Elbi H, et al. Quality of life and its relation with disease severity in Behcet's disease. Clin Exp Rheumatol. 2009;27(2 Suppl 53):S18–22.
116. Meesters JJL, Verhoef J, Liem ISL, Putter H, Vliet Vlieland TPM. Validity and responsiveness of the World Health Organization disability assessment schedule II to assess disability in rheumatoid arthritis patients. Rheumatology. 2009;49(2):326–33. https://doi.org/10.1093/rheumatology/kep369.
117. Tuğrul Ayanoğlu B, Gürler A, Erdoğan FG, Gündüz Ö, Alhan A. Quality of life in patients with Behcet's disease and recurrent aphthous stomatitis. Turkderm. 2015;49(4):276–84. https://doi.org/10.4274/turkderm.00868.
118. Tascilar NF, Tekin NS, Ankarali H, Sezer T, Atik L, Emre U, et al. Sleep disorders in Behçet's disease, and their relationship with fatigue and quality of life. J Sleep Res. 2011;21(3):281–8. https://doi.org/10.1111/j.1365-2869.2011.00976.x.
119. Mumcu G, Yazici Y, Hatemi G. Disease assessment in Behçet syndrome. Behçet Syndrome. 2020:261–78.
120. Hamuryudan V, Fresko İ, Direskeneli H, Tenant MJ, Yurdakul S, Akoglu T, Yazıcı H. Evaluation of the Turkish translation of a disease activity form for Behçet's syndrome. Rheumatology. 1999;38(8):734–6. https://doi.org/10.1093/rheumatology/38.8.734.
121. Lee JS, Cinanni N, Di Cristofaro N, Lee S, Dillenburg R, Adamo KB, et al. Parents of very young children with congenital heart defects report good quality of life for their children and families regardless of defect severity. Pediatr Cardiol. 2020;41(1):46–53. https://doi.org/10.1007/s00246-019-02220-1.
122. Oymak Y, Kaygusuz A, Turedi A, Yaman Y, Eser E, Cubukcu D, Vergin C. Comparing the quality of life of patients with hemophilia and juvenile idiopathic arthritis in which chronic Arthropathy

is a common complication. J Pediatr Hematol Oncol. 2015;37(8):600–4. https://doi.org/10.1097/MPH.0000000000000429.
123. Aloyouny AY, Almufarji F, Almutairi GG, Alkait S, Al-Mohaya MA, Alserwi R. Impact of rheumatic diseases on oral health-related quality of life. Cureus. 2022;14(12):e32268. https://doi.org/10.7759/cureus.32268.
124. Lorenzoni V, Marinello D, Palla I, Mosca M, Turchetti G, Talarico R. A cost-of-illness study of Behçet syndrome in Italy. Eur J Health Econ. 2023;25:411. https://doi.org/10.1007/s10198-023-01593-8.
125. Ozguler Y, Ozdede A, Hatemi G. Recent insights into the management of Behcet syndrome. J Inflamm Res. 2021;14:3429–41. https://doi.org/10.2147/JIR.S285400.
126. Alpsoy E, Bozca BC, Bilgic A. Behçet disease: an update for dermatologists. Am J Clin Dermatol. 2021;22(4):477–502. https://doi.org/10.1007/s40257-021-00609-4.
127. Kirino Y, Nakajima H. Clinical and genetic aspects of Behcet's disease in Japan. Intern Med. 2019;58(9):1199–207. https://doi.org/10.2169/internalmedicine.2035-18.

Clinical Features and Differential Diagnosis in Pediatric Behçet's Disease

24

Müzeyyen Gönül and Hayriye Sarıcaoğlu

Contents

Behçet's disease (BD) is a type of vasculitis that affects vessels of all types and sizes. It was first described by the Turkish dermatologist Hulusi Behçet as a clinical triad consisting of recurrent oral and genital ulcers (GU) and uveitis [1–9]. The complete understanding of the etiopathogenesis of BD remains elusive, but the leading hypothesis suggests that the disease is a result of a complex interplay between autoimmunity and autoinflammation. The human leukocyte antigen (HLA)-B51 allele is the major genetic predisposing factor to BD. In this genetically susceptible group, it has been hypothesized that various infectious agents could act as triggers [5].

Pediatric (juvenile) BD is defined as a fully manifested disease that occurs before the age of 16 years and it should be distinguished from the juvenile-onset BD in which symptoms first appear in childhood but disease manifestation is complete thereafter [3, 4, 9–12]. Although today the pediatric age group is considered to be 18 years or less [13], it would be appropriate to

M. Gönül (✉)
Clinic of Dermatology, University of Health Sciences, Ankara Etlik City Hospital, Ankara, Türkiye

H. Sarıcaoğlu
Department of Dermatology, Uludağ University Faculty of Medicine, Bursa, Türkiye
e-mail: hayriye@uludag.edu.tr

E. Alpsoy et al. (eds.), *Behçet's Disease: An Integrated Approach*,
https://doi.org/10.1007/978-3-031-77251-1_24

use the term pediatric BD for those fulfilling the diagnostic criteria of the disease until 16 years of age in order to set standards in studies and ensure objective evaluation of the results. It is regrettable that not all published studies include pediatric patients diagnosed before the age of 16. Furthermore, the inclusion criteria employed in different studies differ, making it challenging to conduct studies on pediatric BD.

Diagnosing BD in children is challenging because of its rarity [12]. The Pediatric Behçet's Disease (PEDBD) study is a prospective cohort study with the aim of describing the main features of the disease and proposing a classification of pediatric BD. This study highlighted the limitations of the adult criteria for the pediatric population and defined the diagnostic criteria for pediatric BD. The pediatric classification consists of six categories, and at least three criteria are required to diagnose pediatric BD and recurrent oral ulcer (ROU) is not mandatory criterion (Table 24.1) [12]. Kurt et al. retrospectively compared 67 patients diagnosed with pediatric BD to the control group which included 31 patients with periodic fever, aphthous stomatitis, pharyngitis, and adenitis (PFAPA) syndrome and 37 systemic lupus erythematosus patients. They showed that the sensitivity of the PEDBD criteria was lower than the International Criteria for BD (ICBD) and the International Study Group (ISG) criteria. They reported that the limitations of the PEDBD criteria included not testing for pathergy, and that all symptoms were considered to be of equal importance. Moreover, GU were defined as being "typically with scars" in PEDBD criteria but, nearly, one-third of BD GU heal without scars. This study also showed that pathergy testing might be useful in the diagnosis of pediatric BD in some patients [14]. As a result, the literature suggests that current criteria have some limitations and the gold standard for diagnosis is still the expert opinion and patient-based evaluation [3, 14]. This chapter offers an overview of the epidemiology, clinical features, and differential diagnosis of pediatric BD.

Three of six items are required to classify a patient as having pediatric BD.

24.1 Epidemiological and Demographic Features

Pediatric cases are rare and there is still a limited amount of research on BD in children. It has been shown that 4–26% of BD patients experienced their first symptoms in childhood before the age of 16 years [8]. Recent studies have reported that BD is completed before 16 years old aproximately 2.5–14% of all cases [5, 6, 9, 10]. The prevalence of BD in children <15 years is estimated to be 1 in 600.000 according to a French nationwide survey but the exact incidence/prevalence is still unknown [1, 3, 11]. The male-female ratio varies between 0.6 and 1.6 [2, 9, 12].

An international collaborative study showed that male patients had a more severe course (uveitis and/or retinal vasculitis) than females. Risk of vascular complications including arterial aneurysms and deep vein thrombosis was higher in male patients. The disease pattern in females

Table 24.1 Consensus classification of pediatric BD in PEDBD study [12]

Item	Description	Value/item
ROU	At least three attacks/year	1
GU	Typically with scar	1
Skin involvement	Acneiform lesions, erythema nodosum	1
Ocular involvement	Anterior uveitis, posterior uveitis, retinal vasculitis	1
Neurological signs	With the exception of isolated headaches	1
Vascular signs	Venous thrombosis, arterial thrombosis, arterial aneurysm	1

was more benign and characterized with isolated mucosal lesions and arthritis [1]. Similarly, the PEDBD study also showed that males had more often cutaneous, ocular, and vascular symptoms than females, whereas females had more GU than males [12].

The studies have demonstrated that the systemic involvement and the severity of BD may vary according to the different population groups. In France and Saudi Arabia, pediatric population with BD experienced higher rates of neurological and gastrointestinal complications compared to their Turkish counterparts, who had a higher incidence of mucocutaneous findings. In this study, 86 cases were reviewed retrospectively via a questionnaire consisting of 286 items, including family history, mucocutaneous, neurologic, psychiatric, ocular, digestive, pulmonary, cardiac, and nephrologic features which was completed by five BD specialists from Türkiye, France, Iran, or Saudi Arabia [1]. A study including pediatric BD patients from Türkiye and Israel showed that Turkish BD patients had more frequent neurologic involvement [6]. In PEDBD study, vascular involvements were less frequent in European BD children than non-European children [12]. Shahram et al. reported that GU, skin manifestations (especially erythema nodosum), and gastrointestinal involvement were less frequent, while ocular lesions were more frequent and severe in the Iranian population compared to other cohorts [10].

The studies of pediatric BD patients found that they had a higher frequency of family history (9.9–47%) than adult BD patients [3, 4, 7, 15, 16]. The results of studies on pediatric BD throughout the previous 25 years are summarized in Table 24.2. Although these studies have been published in the field of pediatric BD, there is a lack of uniformity in the inclusion criteria of the patients, with varying age restrictions. These studies revealed that mucocutaneous lesions were the most common manifestations in both pediatric and adult BD. The initial presentation was ROU in all pediatric BD patients [1–4, 6, 9, 10, 12, 15, 17–26] (Table 24.2). However, GU, ocular, and articular involvements were less common in children than in adult BD patients. Neurological involvement was the highest in Krause et al. cohort and the authors reported that neuro-Behçet's disease was more frequent among children rather than adults. They also reported that pediatric patients had more frequent gastrointestinal system (GIS) involvement and suggested that this may be related to more common occurrence of abdominal pain and diarrhea in children [15]. Reports by Fujikawa et al. (54.8%) and Nanthapisal et al. (56.5%) showed a higher frequency of GIS involvement than other studies [18, 19]. Zou et al. found that follicular manifestations and GIS involvement were more common in children but ocular and cardiac involvement were more common in adults [7, 22]. It has been reported that uveitis in children progresses with acute exacerbations causing severe visual loss therefore early diagnosis and treatment are important [27]. Unlike previous studies, a recent study from Türkiye comparing the pediatric and adult BD revealed that there was no statistical difference between the rates of mucocutaneous and systemic involvement among pediatric and adult BD patients, and the pediatric and adult BD patients had a similar clinical course with a similar frequency of clinical manifestations [26]. In summary, the discrepancies observed between the current studies may be due to differences in the number of patients recruited, the duration of follow-up, and the ethnic background.

There are only a few case reports of neonatal BD in which symptoms occurred at or shortly after birth. The role of maternal autoantibody transfer in these cases was uncertain, as some of the mothers in these cases had no symptoms of BD [7, 28].

Table 24.2 Studies about the paediatric BD from different countries

Studies	Number M/F	Age at diagnosis	Family history BD	Oral ulcer %	Genital ulcers %	Skin lesions %	Joint involvement %	Ocular involvement %	Neurological involvement %	Vascular involvement %	GIS involvement %	Patergy test %
Fujikawa [19][a] 1997	31 0.82	NA	1/31	100	58	55	54.8	25	16.1	6.5	54.8	59.1
Koné-Paut [1][a] 1998	65 1.03	13	10/86	96	70	92	46	61	21.5	15	13.8	80
Krause [15][a] 1999	19 1.3	NA	36.8 % for ROU	100	31.6	89.5	78.9	47.4	63.2	10.5	36.8	41.2
Koné-Paut [21][a] 2002	55 0.89	11.6	9%	100	79	NA	17	NA	NA	21	40	NA
Borlu [4][a] 2006	17 2.4	12	47%	100	94	NA	76	24	12	6.25	12	76
Karıncaoğlu [24][b] 2008	83 1.25	12.3±3.5	19%	100	81.9	51.8	39.8	34.9	7.2	7.2	4.8	50
Atmaca [9][a] 2011	110 0.59	14.15 ± 2.13	12.3%	100	82.7	76	22.7	30.9	3.6	3.6	NA	45.5
Koné-Paut [12][a] 2015 PED-BD	156 1.01	13.9±3.8	24.4%	100	58.3	66.6	41	46.7	46.1	17.3	29.4	NA
Nanthapisal [18][c] 2016	46 1.09	3.7	17%	97.8	73.9	23.9	30.4	8.7	28.3	6.5	56.5	60 [d]
Gallizzi [25] [e] 2017	110 0.77	11.3±3.9	12/110	94.5	33.6	NA	42.7	43.6	30.9	10	42.7	14.5
Shahram [10][a] 2018	204 0.98	NA	9.9%	91.7	42.2	51.5	30.9	66.2	4.9	6.4	5.9	57
Çirkinoğlu [17][f] 2018	34 0.88	16.5±4.1	15%	97	62	82	38	35	17.6	32	5.8	50
Aviel 2020 [6] [f] Turkish Israeli	165 0.92 40 0.7	12.7 13	Total 26.3% 29.1% 15%	100 97.5	64.8 67.5	55.2 22.5	44.8 35	13.3 17.5	15.8 10	11.5 7.5	12.1 17.5	27.3 23.1
Ekinci [2][f] 2020	16 1.66	13.3	31.2%	93.8	50	NA	75	37.5	6.3	6.3	NA	31.2

Gezgin [23][a] 2020	57 1.37	12	31%	100	56	46	63	47	9	17	9	19
Zou 2021 [22][a]	69 0.86	NA	15/69 for ROU	100	79.7	58	13	8.7	4.3	14.5	29	NA
Tekin [29][a] 2022	72 1.25	14	41.7%	100	68.1	34.7	20.3	36.1	15.3	18.1	NA	27.8
Açarı [20] [f] 2023	34 0.7	12.5±3.0	26.4%	97.1	47	32.3	26.4	44.1	17.6	17.6	NA	58.8
Boyvat [26][a] 2023	101 0.44	14.1±1.7	13.6%	100	90.1	PPL 45.5 EN 40.6	42.6	26.7	4	12.9	4	43.2

GIS gastrointestinal system, *NA* not available
[a]Patients who met the diagnostic criteria before the age of 16 were included
[b]Juvenil-onset BD
[c]Patients under 18 years of age were included
[d]Patergy test was done only,in five patients
[e]Patients whose symptoms started after the age of 16 were excluded
[f]Age of inclusion not specified

24.2 Clinical Findings

24.2.1 Mucocutaneous Manifestations

The mean age at diagnosis of pediatric disease varies from 3,74 to 16,5 years old in investigations of different populations [17, 18]. Diagnosing pediatric BD can be challenging because of the significant time gap between the first symptom and diagnosis in children [3, 5, 9, 25]. Delay from first symptoms to diagnosis varies from 2.5 to 5 years [4, 9, 21]. The initial manifestation of pediatric BD is most commonly (63.8–98.2%) ROU [5, 6, 8, 9, 20, 21, 23, 29]. ROU are seen in almost all patients with BD (96–100%) and are a major clue for the diagnosis of BD although they are not rare in the pediatric population [5, 30]. These lesions do not differ from ROU in adult BD. They are painful, round, or oval ulcers with a yellow-grey pseudomembranous base with an erythematous halo. They are localised on the tongue, lips, cheeks, and palate. ROU may be minor, major, or herpetiform [7, 8, 30] and usually heal within 3–10 days without scarring. But, some lesions may persist for weeks [7]. Simultaneous observation of multiple oral ulcers of different sizes with diffuse erythematous surroundings located in the soft palate and oropharynx was emphasized as a clue for the recognition of BH [5].

Although GU is the second most common finding, it has been reported to occur less frequently in children than in adults in most studies [4, 6, 9, 33] and their frequency varies between 33.16% and 94% of pediatric patients in different populations [4, 25]. In contrast to these data, Çirkinoğlu et al. reported that the second most common presentation in pediatric patients was other cutaneous lesions (82%) [17]. GU of BD are similar to oral ulcers, although larger and deeper and are more commonly seen in girls than in boys [8]. Atmaca et al. found that GU were observed in 61% of male patients and in 95.7% of female patients [9]. GU usually heal with scarring differently from ROU, but scarring is less common in pediatric BD than in the adult population [7]. GU are usually localized on the vulva and the scrotum, but may also be observed in the perianal region (7–30%) and perianal ulceration appears to be a specific feature of pediatric BD [3, 8, 9]. However, differentiation of inflammatory bowel disease (IBD) is very important in this localization [3, 8].

Skin manifestations of BD are erythema nodosum-like lesions, papulopustular lesions (follicular or non-follicular) superficial thrombophlebitis, and cutaneous vasculitic lesions. It has been documented that cutaneous manifestations are observed in between 38% and 99% of adults diagnosed with BD and in between 22.5% and 92% of pediatric BD patients [1, 6]. A study investigating the characteristics of pediatric BD in Turkey and Israel showed that Turkish patients had a higher incidence of skin involvement than Israeli patients (55.2% vs 22.5%, respectively). The lowest reported rate was 22.5% (from the Israeli population) [6]. Pseudofolliculitis was more often seen in males, and erythema nodosum-like lesions were more common in females. Erythema nodosum-like lesions are primarily localized on the lower limbs, especially on the anterior and lateral surfaces of the legs. Dermal nodules may also indicate superficial thrombosis. Other neutrophilic lesions may also be seen in BD [8].

BD patients may exhibit a skin hypersensitivity known as Pathergy phenomenon [8]. The pathergy test may show a positivity rate of 37–80% in pediatric cases due to geographical and population variations, but it is not regularly performed in all BD patients [6–9]. Aviel et al. found that patients from Turkey underwent more pathergy tests compared to those from Israel (93.3% vs. 32.5%), with similar positivity rates in both groups [6]. Pathergy test can be used as a diagnostic tool though it is not specific for BD [7].

24.2.2 Musculoskeletal Involvement

Articular symptoms are seen in 13–78.9% of children [15, 22]. A study noted that the most commonly affected joints were the knees, ankles, elbows, and wrists [1]. The course of BD arthritis in children is recurrent, but overall favorable, the disease is nonerosive and mostly does not cause any deformity but rarely can lead to joint destruction or functional disability [5, 7, 31]. Sacroiliac involvement is not common, and there is a low correlation with HLA-B27 (2%) [5]. Gaggiano et al. reviewed musculoskeletal manifestations of pediatric BD. They found that 26.2% of patients had musculoskeletal symptoms at disease onset. Recurrent oral and GU and pseudofolliculitis were the most common symptoms associated with musculoskeletal manifestations. Arthralgia was seen in 89.2% and arthritis in 83.8% of patients with musculoskeletal manifestations. The most common arthritis was oligoarthritis, followed by monoarthritis and polyarthritis, but sacroiliitis was not uncommon in children. The median follow-up duration was 21.8 years in this study. In a study, it was found that arthritis became chronic-recurrent in 67.7% of cases, and joint erosions developed in 22.6% of patients during the follow-up period. The authors emphasize the importance of a high index of clinical suspicion, particularly for sacroiliitis, and note that early diagnosis is crucial [31]. Krause et al. found joint involvement in 78.9% of their cohort, which was the highest rate in the literature [15].

24.2.3 Ocular Involvement

There are controversial results about the ocular involvement in BD in children compared to adults [1, 5]. A study found that ocular disease was more common as the initial presenting sign in children than in adults [32]. Gallizzi et al. found that 43.6% of the patients had ocular involvement and it was the second most common manifestation of BD after ROU [25]. The frequency of ocular involvement (62%) and its severity in Iranian children with BD were found to be notably higher than what has been reported previously [10]. However, a British study showed that ocular involvement was seen in 8.7% of pediatric BD patients [18]. Symptoms of ocular involvement include redness, blurred vision, photophobia, epiphora, and periorbital pain [5]. Chronic relapsing posterior and anterior uveitis with necrotizing retinal vasculitis are characteristic findings. There is mostly bilateral involvement but sometimes unilateral involvement can be seen [7]. Other ocular manifestations are iridocyclitis, optic neuritis, keratitis, episcleritis, scleritis, vitritis, vitreous hemorrhage, cataract, glaucoma, and retinal detachment [5]. Sungur et al. noted that anterior uveitis was the most common ocular finding in patients younger than 10 years, panuveitis was the most frequent finding in patients older than 10 years. They suggested that family screening for BD may be crucial for early and accurate diagnosis of BD because the patients younger than 10 years had a higher family history of BD [16]. Kramer et al. found that 70% of pediatric BD patients with ocular involvement had recurrent attacks and the mean number of acute exacerbations was 4.1 ± 2.7. They reported that most of the exacerbations were severe and although a decrease of visual acuity during exacerbations may be observed in 68% of pediatric cases, 80% of the affected eyes improved after therapy [27].

24.2.4 Neurological Involvement

The frequency of neurological involvement in pediatric patients varies from 3.6% to 63.2% [9, 15]. Headaches can be the presenting symptom of BD in up to 25% of patients [7, 8]. Manifestations usually occur during puberty and are more common in males [33]. Neurological involvement in BD presents mainly in two major forms: parenchymal and cerebral venous sinus thrombosis. The main neurological manifestations in pediatric BD patients are cerebral venous thrombosis and cranial nerve palsy (especially nerve VI), in contrast to the more common parenchymal lesions in adults [5, 33]. Cerebral venous thrombosis has a better prognosis [33]. However, different outcomes have been reported in different populations [15]. According to a study, neurological complications can affect up to 75% of children, resulting in long-term consequences for their schooling. Half of the children with neurological involvement could not follow a normal curriculum [8, 34, 35]. Other neurological findings include optic atrophy-related visual disturbances, personality changes, and motor and sensory sequelae. Imaging studies such as cranial computed tomography, especially magnetic resonance imaging (MRI) and the cerebrospinal fluid (CSF) examination can be helpful in the diagnosis in childhood [7, 36]. CSF examination may reveal elevated protein levels, polymorphonuclear cells and lymphocytes, and elevated interleukin-6 levels [7].

24.2.5 Vascular Involvement

All types and sizes of vessels are affected by BD, especially the venous system. Vascular involvement is now integrated into the classification criteria for both adult and pediatric BD [7, 8, 12].

Vascular involvement is less commonly seen in children compared to adults [36]. The percentage of adults with vascular involvement can vary between 5% and 40%, while in children, it can range from 1.8% to 21% [5, 7, 20]. Vascular symptoms are more commonly observed in male patients. The results of a study indicated that there was a male/female ratio of 6 to 1 among children with thrombosis. Furthermore, it was found that male patients presented with a more severe form of BD [37]. The most common type of vascular involvement is superficial or deep venous thrombosis of the lower extremities. Deep vein thrombosis can also be seen in large vessels like iliofemoral artery (with pulmonary artery aneurysms, known as Hughes-Stovin syndrome), superior or inferior vena cava and hepatic veins (Budd-Chiari syndrome) [7, 30, 36]. Arterial involvement is most commonly seen in the pulmonary arteries and presents as an aneurysm, pseudoaneurysm, thrombosis, and stenosis. Chest radiography is the imaging modality of first choice in a child to detect aneurysms of the thoracic aorta or pulmonary arteries. Chest CT, CT-angiography, and cardiac MRI can be used as imaging modalities for cardiovascular symptoms [34]. Although there is a lack of data in pediatric patients with BD, recurrent vascular events have been documented to be in the range of 0–21%, in contrast to the high relapse rate in adult patients. Pulmonary arterial involvement and Budd-Chiari syndrome are associated with high morbidity and mortality in BD patients [7].

Thrombophilic factors such as anticardiolipin antibodies and protein C deficiency may be risk factors for vascular manifestations [7, 37]. The thrombus in BD does not cause a secondary embolism due to its adherence to the vessel wall [8].

24.2.6 Gastrointestinal System Involvement

Gastrointestinal system involvement differs between different populations and ranges from 4% to 56.5% in pediatric cohorts [18, 26]. Intestinal involvement has been reported to be more frequent in pediatric patients than in adults. The whole gastrointestinal tract from the mouth to the anus, particularly the ileum and the colon, can be affected by the lesions of the BD. Various symptoms, such as abdominal pain, nausea, diarrhea, melena, or hematochezia can be signs of gastrointestinal involvement [5, 7, 15]. Deep aphthous and necrotic ulcerations leading to abscesses and perforation may be seen more rarely [7, 8]. Another form is intestinal ischemia and infarction stemming from mesenteric artery involvement [5]. Endoscopy and biopsy, computed tomography, and magnetic resonance enterography might be needed for the diagnosis of GIS involvement in BD and to make a differential diagnosis with inflammatory bowel disease (IBH), particularly Crohn's Disease (CD). IBD and BD share many manifestations including abdominal symptoms [5, 7]. A study of CD and intestinal BD showed that the most predictive symptoms of BD on colonoscopy were round ulcers, focal single/focal multiple distribution of ulceration, fewer than six ulcers, absence of cobblestone appearance, or aphthous lesions [38]. Also, anal complications such as stricture, fistula, and abscess formation, that may be seen in CD, are rare in BD [7].

24.2.7 Miscellaneous Involvement

Glomerulonephritis, orchitis, epididymitis, urethritis, and sterile cystitis are rarely seen in pediatric BD. The frequency of AA amyloidosis has decreased with better management of BD [8].

24.3 Differential Diagnosis

24.3.1 Differential Diagnosis of Mucocutaneous Findings

Given the absence of a pathognomonic test that definitively identifies BD, it is vital to adhere to the diagnostic criteria based on clinical findings for confirming the disease and ruling out other conditions that present similar symptoms [28]. The manifestations of BD show a wide range, so there are many diseases included in the differential diagnosis. ROU is the most frequent finding in BD may be seen in many conditions such as viral infections *herpes simplex virus* (HSV), human immunodeficiency virus (HIV), nutritional deficiencies (vitamins B1, B2, B6, B12 folate, iron, zinc), cyclic neutropenia, erythema multiforme, IBD, Celiac disease, systemic lupus erythematosus, reactive arthritis and autoinflammatory diseases (PFAPA), familial Mediterranean fever (FMF), and hyperimmunoglobulinemia D (HID) syndrome. GU caused by HSV infection, erythema multiforme, fixed drug eruption, syphilis, and HIV infection should be distinguished from GU of BD [30].

Complex aphthosis is one of the most important differential diagnoses. It is an uncommon, persistent, chronic type of ROU and may be associated with anogenital ulcers [39, 40]. Bipolar aphthosis is considered a forme fruste of BD by some authors, and a different disease entity by others [40]. Although it fulfills the ICBD criteria, the association of oral ulcers and GU can also be seen in gluten-sensitive enteropathy, IBD, ulcus vulva acutum, MAGIC syndrome (mouth and GU with inflamed cartilage), PFAPA syndrome, cyclic neutropenia, and HIV infection [39].

The papulopustular lesions must be differentiated from acne vulgaris, especially during childhood. The fact that papulopustular lesions are not only located in typical areas (face and upper part of the trunk) for acne vulgaris but also on the lower limbs may be helpful in differential diagnosis [40]. Patergy test positivity is not specific for BD and may also be seen in pyoderma gangrenosum and acute febrile neutrophilic dermatosis (Sweet's syndrome) [34].

We will not discuss the differential diagnosis of other manifestations of BD in detail here, as it is covered in the relevant chapters of this book. BD can be misdiagnosed as acute rheumatic fever, Still's disease, and other autoimmune connective tissue disorders in children. The most important group of diseases that should be considered in the differential diagnosis of childhood BD, unlike adults, are autoinflammatory syndromes that can mimic BD.

24.4 Mimickers of BD

An increasing number of autoinflammatory diseases have been identified in recent years, some of which have clinical manifestations similar to BD. Autoinflammatory diseases are characterized by unprovoked episodes of sterile inflammation, fever, and cytokine amplification due to disorders of innate immunity [41, 42]. Monogenic autoinflammatory disorders can have clinical manifestations overlapping with BD [42]. One of these is haploinsufficiency 20 (HA20) which has a heterozygous mutation of the TNFAIP3 gene. It is an early-onset autoinflammatory disease presenting with BD-like features such as ROU, GU, and gastrointestinal symptoms. ROU are the most common symptoms and they may be scarring. The disease course ranges from mild disease to severe or fatal multisystemic inflammation. Patients with HA20 can also present with autoimmune and/or immunodeficiency symptoms, fluctuating autoantibodies, and can show a treatment-refractory disease course [43, 44]. Other clinical manifestations include recurrent fever, ocular disease, skin lesions, vasculitis, gastrointestinal ulcers, musculoskeletal disease, autoimmune thyroid disease, renal and hepatic injury, recurrent respiratory disease, interstitial lung disease, and dental abnormalities. Symptoms of HA20 are early onset compared to BD and it has autosomal dominant inheritance. BD is a polygenic disease and has a complex inheritance pattern. Fever is not a usual symptom in BD [43]. HA20 can present with variable vasculitis similar to BD [45].

Other autoinflammatory disorders with ROU/GU are mevalonate kinase deficiency, cryopyrin-associated periodic syndrome (CAPS), tumor necrosis factor receptor-associated periodic syndrome (TRAPS); NFKB1-associated Behçet-like disease (NFKB1-BLD); C/EBPε-associated autoinflammation and immune impairment of neutrophils (CAIN); chronic granulomatous disease (CGD); periodic fevers with immunodeficiency and thrombocytopenia (PFIT) (early-onset fevers, recurrent perianal ulceration, ROU causing scarring and microstomia); trisomi 8; relative v-rel reticuloendotheliosis viral oncogene homolog A (RELA); and NF-κB essential modulator (NEMO) deficiency (arthritis, colitis, and dermatitis) [33, 42, 44].

RELA haploinsufficiency is a recently described autoinflammatory condition and leads to decreased NF-kB signalling promoting TNF-driven mucosal apoptosis with impaired epithelial recovery. Clinical features include BD-like mucocutaneous ulcerations, rash, joint inflammation, fever, conjunctivitis, recurrent infections, and neuromyelitis optica [33, 42, 44, 46].

Ocular manifestations similar to BD are observed in Blau syndrome, CAPS, TRAPS, NEMO, and Fabry disease (fever of unknown origin, ROU, myalgia, colitis, and a skin rash reminiscent of panniculitis) [33, 34, 44]. Acne-like skin lesions may also be observed in deficiency of interleukin-1 receptor antagonist (DIRA), pyogenic arthritis, pyoderma gangrenosum and acne syndrome (PAPA) chronic recurrent multifocal osteomyelitis, and congenital dyserythropoietic anemia and pyrin-associated autoinflammation with neutrophilic dermatosis (PAAND). The pathergy reaction may also be positive in some autoinflammatory syndromes such as PAPA syndrome, HA20, and NFKB1-BLD [42].

Vasculitis has been defined in many autoinflammatory syndromes such as FMF, CAPS, MKD, TRAPS, HIDS, STING-associated vasculopathy with onset in infancy (SAVI), deficiency of adenosine deaminase-2 (DADA2), and HA20 [45].

Otulipenia is characterized by loss-of-function mutations in OTULIN that is a protein playing a role in the regulation of innate immune signalling complexes. Clinical findings are neonatal-onset fever, neutrophilic dermatosis/panniculitis, and failure to thrive in the absence of primary immunodeficiency [34, 45].

DADA-2 is an early-onset vasculopathy due to the *ADA2* mutation. Lacunar strokes, livedoid rash, and other neurovascular manifestations are clinical findings of DADA2. Hematological involvement and immunodeficiency may be observed. Cases with GU, recurrent fever, arthralgia, ROU, vertigo, and erythema nodosum have also been reported [34].

Differential diagnosis is very important as the management of monogenic BD mimics may differ significantly from standard BD management. In cases of early-onset pediatric BD, genetic evaluation should be conducted to differentiate this condition from autoinflammatory diseases [40].

Other differential diagnoses of BD include immunodeficiency syndromes such as DNA ligase 4 deficiency, RELA haplodeficiency, NFKB1 deficiency, X-linked anhidrotic ectodermal dysplasia with immunodeficiency, NEMO deleted exon5-autoinflammatory syndrome, incontinentia pigmenti, congenital defects in phagocyte number or function (CGD, PFIT), and defects in intrinsic and innate immunity (ID 31A, ID 31B, ID 31C) [47].

Non-monogenic periodic fever syndromes like PFAPA can be misdiagnosed as BD in infancy and early childhood. Conversely, patients initially diagnosed with PFAPA may be found to actually have BD later in life [34]. PFAPA syndrome, the most common periodic fever syndrome in children, is characterized by recurrent, regular attacks of high fever associated with pharyngeal inflammation, aphthous stomatitis, and/or cervical lymphadenopathy, the frequency of which decreases with age. Some authors have suggested that BD and PFAPA syndrome may be two different disorders within the same spectrum [48]. Neutrophilic dermatoses, like pyoderma gangrenosum and Sweet's syndrome, as well as IBD, other vasculitis conditions, and seronegative spondyloarthropathies, can also imitate BD [34].

In conclusion, BD, which is a diverse illness, presents a challenging differential diagnosis, particularly during childhood. Because the diagnosis relies on clinical symptoms, the full clinical picture may not be available yet, and it may take some time to establish a definitive diagnosis [30]. Moreover, there is insufficient information in the literature on the clinical characteristics and differential diagnosis of pediatric BD due to its rarity. New multicenter and multinational studies with larger case series should be done in the future to better define the characteristics of pediatric BD. Additionally, these studies will generate reliable information on pediatric BD by excluding recently identified autoinflammatory disorders that may have been mistakenly diagnosed as BD before.

References

1. Kone-Paut I, Yurdakul S, Bahabri SA, Shafae N, Ozen S, Ozdogan H, et al. Clinical features of Behcet's disease in children: an international collaborative study of 86 cases. J Pediatr. 1998;132(4):721–5.
2. Kisla Ekinci RM, Esen E, Erol AH, Sızmaz S, Karagoz D, Altintas D, Balcı S. Evaluation of different classification criteria in children with Behcet disease: results from a single referral center. Expert Rev Clin Immunol. 2020;16(11):1093–7.
3. Batu ED. Diagnostic/classification criteria in paediatric Behçet's disease. Rheumatol Int. 2019;39:37–46.
4. Borlu M, Ukşal Ü, Ferahbaş A, Evereklioglu C. Clinical features of Behçet's disease in children. Int J Dermatol. 2006;45:713–6.
5. Yıldız M, Köker O, Adroviç A, Şahin S, Barut K, Kasapçopur Ö. Paediatric Behçet's disease—clinical aspects and current concepts. Eur J Rheumatol. 2020;7(Suppl1):S38–47.
6. Butbul Aviel Y, Batu ED, Sözeri B, Aktay Ayaz N, Baba L, Amarilyo G, et al. Characteristics of paediatric Behçet's disease in Turkey and Israel: a cross-sectional cohort comparison. Semin Arthritis Rheum. 2020;50:515–20.
7. Ya-Chiao Hu YC, Chiang BL, Yang YH. Clinical manifestations and management of paediatric Behçet's disease. Clin Rev Allergy Immunol. 2021;61(2):171–80.
8. Koné-Paut I. Behçet's disease in children, an overview. Paediatric Rheumatology. 2016;14:10.
9. Atmaca L, Boyvat A, Yalcindag FN, Atmaca-Sonmez P, Gurler A. Behcet disease in children. Ocul Immunol Inflamm. 2011;19(2):103–7.
10. Shahram F, Nadji A, Akhlaghi M, Faezi ST, Chams Davatchi C, Shams H, et al. Paediatric Behçet's disease in Iran: report of 204 cases. Clin Exp Rheumatol. 2018;36(6 Suppl 115):135–40.
11. Seyahi E, Özdoğan H. Juvenile Behçet's syndrome. In: Yazıcı Y, Yazıcı H, editors. Behçet's Syndrome. New York: Springer; 2010. p. 205–14.
12. Koné-Paut I, Shahram F, Darce-Bello M, Cantarini L, Cimaz R, Gattorno M, et al. Consensus classification criteria for paediatric Behçet's disease from a prospective observational cohort: PEDBD. Ann Rheum Dis. 2016;75:958–64.
13. Lansdown G, Vaghri Z. Article 1: definition of a child. In: Vaghri Z, Zermatten J, Lansdown G, Ruggiero R, editors. Monitoring state compliance with the UN convention on the rights of the child. An analysis of attributes. Springer; 2022. p. 407–12.
14. Kurt T, Aydın F, Sezer M, Tekgöz PN, Tekin ZE, Çelikel E, et al. Performance of diagnostic criteria in paediatric Behçet's disease. Rheumatol Int. 2022;42(1):127–32.
15. Krause I, Uziel Y, Guedj D, Mukamel M, Harel L, Molad Y, et al. Childhood Behçet's disease: clinical features and comparison with adult-onset disease. Rheumatology. 1999;38:457–62.
16. Sungur GK, Hazirolan D, Yalvac I, Ozer PA, Yuksel D, Vural ET, et al. Clinical and demographic evaluation of Behcet disease among different paediatric age groups. Br J Ophthalmol. 2009;93(1):83–7.
17. Çirkinoğlu MS, Demir S, Bilginer Y, Özen S. Behçet's disease in children: single-center experience. Turk Pediatri Ars. 2019;54:179–84.
18. Nanthapisal S, Klein NJ, Ambrose N, Eleftheriou D, Brogan PA. Paediatric Behçet's disease: a UK tertiary centre experience. Clin Rheumatol. 2016;35:2509–16.
19. Fujikawa S, Suemitsu T. Behcet disease in children: a nationwide retrospective survey in Japan. Acta Paediatr Jpn. 1997;39:285–9.
20. Açarı C, İşgüder R, Torun R, Makay B, Ünsal ŞE. Paediatric Behçet's disease: experience of a single tertiary center. Arch Rheumatol. 2022;38(2):282–90.
21. Kone-Paut I, Gorchakoff-Molınas A, Weschler B, Touıtou I. Paediatric Behçet's disease in France. Ann Rheum Dis. 2002;61:655–6.
22. Zou J, Luo JF, Shen Y, Guan JL. Distinct clinical characteristics of paediatric Behçet's syndrome: a study from a referral center in China. Mod Rheumatol. 2021 Nov;31(6):1158–63.
23. Gezgin Yıldırım D, Bakkaloğlu SA, Hasanreisoglu M, Buyan N. Disease activity and outcomes in juvenile Behçet's disease: 10 years' experience of a single centre. Clin Exp Rheumatol. 2020;38(Suppl 127):105–11.
24. Karıncaoglu Y, Borlu M, Toker SC, Akman A, Onder M, Gunasti S, et al. Demographic and clinical properties of juvenile-onset Behçet's disease: a controlled multicenter study. J Am Acad Dermatol. 2008;58:579–84.
25. Gallizzi R, Pidone C, Cantarini L, Finetti M, Cattalini M, Filocamo G, et al. A national cohort study on paediatric Behçet's disease: cross-sectional data from an Italian registry. Pediatr Rheumatol Online J. 2017 Dec;21;15(1):84:1–7.
26. Boyvat A, Oktem A, Kalay Yildizhan I, Ates A, Yalcindag N, Koksoy C, et al. A comparison of adult and juvenile Behcet's patients and a look at clinical trends: retrospective data from a Turkish follow-up cohort study. Dermatology. 2023;239(6):958–65.

27. Kramer M, Amer R, Mukamel M, Snir M, Jaouni T, Friling R. Uveitis in juvenile Behcet's disease: clinical course and visual outcome compared with adult patients. Eye (Lond). 2009;23(11):2034–41.
28. Clarke K, Shastry D, Chetcuti P, Wood M, Morgan A. Neonatal Behçet's disease. Arch Dis Child. 2017 Nov;102(11):1062.
29. Ekici Tekin Z, Çelikel E, Aydin F, Kurt T, Sezer M, Tekgöz N, et al. Juvenile Behçet's disease: a tertiary center experience. Clin Rheumatol. 2022;41:187–94.
30. Costagliola G, Cappelli S, Consolini R. Behçet's disease in children: diagnostic and management challenges. Ther Clin Risk Manag. 2020;16:495–507.
31. Gaggiano C, Maselli A, Sfikakis PP, Laskari K, Ragab G, Hegazy MT, et al. AIDA network musculoskeletal manifestations in children with Behçet's syndrome: data from the AIDA network Behçet's syndrome registry. Intern Emerg Med. 2023 Apr;18(3):743–54.
32. Pivetti-Pezzi P, Accortini M, Abdulaziz MA, La Cava M, Torella M, Riso D, et al. Behçet's disease in children. Jpn J Ophthalmol. 1995;39:309–14.
33. Uluduz D, Kürtüncü M, Yapıcı Z, Seyahi E, Kasapçopur Ö, Özdoğan H, et al. Clinical characteristics of paediatric-onset neuro-Behcet disease. Neurology. 2011;77(21):1900–5.
34. Kul Cinar O, Romano M, Guzel F, Brogan PA, Demirkaya E. Paediatric Behçet's disease: a comprehensive review with an emphasis on monogenic mimics. J Clin Med. 2022;11(5):1278:1–23.
35. Metreau-Vastel J, Mikaeloff Y, Tardieu M, Koné-Paut I, Tran TA. Neurological involvement in paediatric Behçet's disease. Neuropaediatrics. 2010;41(5):228–34.
36. Topcuoglu OM, Topcuoglu ED, Altay CM, Genc S. Imaging pearls of paediatric Behcet's disease. Eur J Radiol. 2017;94:115–24.
37. Krupa B, Cimaz R, Ozen S, Fischbach M, Cochat P, Koné-Paut I. Paediatric Behçet's disease and thromboses. J Rheumatol. 2011;38(2):387–90.
38. Lee SK, Kim BK, Kim TI, Kim WH. Differential diagnosis of intestinal Behcet's disease and Crohn's disease by colonoscopic findings. Endoscopy. 2009;41:9–16.
39. Rogers RS 3rd. Complex aphthosis. Adv Exp Med Biol. 2003;528:311–6.
40. Boyvat A, Ekmekçi P, Gürgey E. Bipolar aphthosis. A forme fruste of Behçet's disease. Adv Exp Med Biol. 2003;528:321–2.
41. Miller JJ, Venna N, Siva A. Neuro-Behcet disease and autoinflammatory disorders. Semin Neurol. 2014;34(4):437–43.
42. Perazzio SF, Allenspach EJ, Eklund KK, Varjosalo M, Shinohara MM, Torgerson TR, et al. Behçet disease (BD) and BD-like clinical phenotypes: NF-κB pathway in mucosal ulcerating diseases. Scand J Immunol. 2020;92(5):e12973.
43. Aeschlimann FA, Batu ED, Canna SW, Go E, Gül A, Hoffmann P, et al. A20 haploinsufficiency (HA20): clinical phenotypes and disease course of patients with a newly recognised NF-kB-mediated autoinflammatory disease. Ann Rheum Dis. 2018;77(5):728–35. p. 1–14
44. Chen Y, Ye Z, Chen L, Qin T, Seidler U, Tian D, et al. Association of Clinical Phenotypes in Haploinsufficiency A20 (HA20) with disrupted domains of A20. Front Immunol. 2020;11:s38–47.
45. Demir S, Sag E, Dedeoglu F, Ozen S. Vasculitis in systemic autoinflammatory diseases. Front Pediatr. 2018;6(377):1–10.
46. An JW, Pimpale-Chavan P, Stone DL, Bandeira M, Dedeoglu F, Lo J, et al. Case report: novel variants in RELA associated with familial Behcet's-like disease. Front Immunol. 2023;14(1127085):1–7.
47. Shiraki M, Kadowaki S, Kadowaki T, Kawamoto N, Ohnishi H. Primary immunodeficiency disease mimicking paediatric Bechet's disease. Children (Basel). 2021;8(2):75:1–11.
48. Cantarini L, Vitale A, Bersani G, Nieves LM, Cattalini M, Lopalco G, et al. PFAPA syndrome and Behçet's disease: a comparison of two medical entities based on the clinical interviews performed by three different specialists. Clin Rheumatol. 2016;35(2):501–5.

Treatment and Prognosis of Pediatric Behçet's Disease

25

Mehmet Yıldız, Elif Kiliç Könte, and Özgür Kasapçopur

Contents

25.1 Introduction

Behcet's disease is a multisystemic vasculitis that can involve vessels of all types and size [1–4]. The disease was first described by Dr. Hulusi Behçet in 1937 as a combination of recurrent oral and genital ulcer and uveitis [1]. The prevalence of it varies significantly across the world. Although Behçet's disease is most common in communities living along the historic Silk Road, it is not limited to the countries along the Silk Road [5, 6]. The disease is generally considered an affliction of adult individuals and is diagnosed between the ages of 20 and 40; however, approximately one-fourth of cases have pediatric onset [7–9]. Although various studies have demonstrated a similar clinical spectrum of the disease in both adult-onset and pediatric-onset cases, many studies report a milder clinical severity in pediatric-onset cohorts [10, 11]. The treatment of Behçet's disease generally takes a long time and varies depending on the affected organ systems. While there are evidence-based treatment guidelines for adult Behçet's disease, there is no specific treatment guide for pediatric cases due to a lack of an adequate number of studies on the treatment of pediatric cases [12]. Therefore, the treatment of pediatric cases is carried out in accordance with adult guidelines and in parallel with the practices of our colleagues from adult department, as there is no specific treatment guide for pediatric cases.

M. Yıldız · E. K. Könte · Ö. Kasapçopur (✉)
Pediatric Rheumatology Department, Istanbul University-Cerrahpaşa, Istanbul, Türkiye
e-mail: yildizmehmet@istanbul.edu.tr; ozgurkc@istanbul.edu.tr

E. Alpsoy et al. (eds.), *Behçet's Disease: An Integrated Approach*,
https://doi.org/10.1007/978-3-031-77251-1_25

The main objective of this chapter is to furnish a comprehensive and critical assessment of the existing knowledge on the management and prognosis of pediatric Behçet's disease. Behçet's disease is a rare, chronic, and debilitating autoimmune disorder that affects both children and adults. Despite its impact on the quality of life of affected children and their families, there is no consensus on the optimal treatment approach for pediatric Behçet's disease, and additional research is needed in this area. This literature review aims to address this gap by summarizing the current literature on the treatment and prognosis of pediatric Behçet's disease and identifying areas for further research. By offering a synthesis of current knowledge and a critical evaluation of its limitations, this literature review aims to contribute to a better understanding of pediatric Behçet's disease and inform the development of evidence-based treatment guidelines and quality improvement initiatives.

25.2 Treatment of Pediatric Behçet's Disease

Behçet's disease is an illness that can involve blood vessels of any type and size, affecting various organ systems and leading to a range of clinical presentations with different severity levels. Therefore, making treatment decisions for individuals diagnosed with Behçet's disease requires personalized decisions, taking into consideration the affected organ systems and the severity of involvement (personalized treatment). Additionally, a multidisciplinary approach involving experts in pediatric rheumatology, neurology, gastroenterology, pulmonology, ophthalmology, dermatology, and cardiovascular surgery is crucial for the optimal management of this multisystemic condition. The primary goals of treatment are the rapid suppression of disease flares, prevention of subsequent flares, and the prevention of irreversible organ damage [12–14].

It is important to provide lifestyle recommendations, promote a healthy and balanced diet, encourage physical activity, and offer appropriate vaccination advice in the follow-up and management of children and adolescents diagnosed with Behçet's disease [14]. It is crucial to take into account the issue of childhood immunizations when dealing with Behçet's disease in pediatric patients. Given that immunosuppressive medications are often necessary for treating the disease, it is important to assess the patient's immunization history as soon as possible and to administer any missing vaccinations. The medications that are commonly administered to pediatric patients with Behçet's disease, along with their respective dosages and possible adverse effects, are systematically presented in Table 25.1.

Table 25.1 Pediatric doses and possible side effects of medications commonly used in the treatment of pediatric Behçet's disease

	Mechanism of action	Pediatric dose	Doses per day	Side effects
NSAIDs[a]				
Ibuprofen	Inhibition[c] of COX 1 and 2 enzymes	30–40 mg/kg/day (max. 2400 mg)	3–4 doses	Gastrointestinal discomfort, ulcers, hepatitis, cutaneous reactions (pruritus, urticaria, rashes, erythema multiforme), renal toxicity (reversible acute renal failure, acute interstitial nephritis, nephrotic syndrome, papillary necrosis, water retention), hematologic toxicity (macrocytic anemia, leukopenia, thrombocytopenia)
Indomethacin	Inhibition[c] of COX 1 and 2 enzymes	1.5–3 mg/kg/day (max. 150 mg)	3 doses	
Diclofenac	Inhibition[c] of COX 1 and 2 enzymes	2–3 mg/kg/day (max. 150 mg)	3 doses	
Acetylsalicylic acid	Inhibition[c] of COX 1 and 2 enzymes	5 mg/kg/day (4900 mg/day)	2–4 doses	
Celecoxib	[c]Inhibition of COX 2 enzyme	100 mg/day (>2 years old, 10–25 kg); 200 mg/day (>2 years old, 25–50 kg);	2–4 doses	

(continued)

Table 25.1 (continued)

	Mechanism of action	Pediatric dose	Doses per day	Side effects
Conventional DMARDs[b]				
Methotrexate	Inhibition of dihydrofolate reductase enzyme	10–15 mg/m²/week	1 dose/week	Gastrointestinal discomfort, nausea, mucositis, transaminase elevation, liver fibrosis, (folic aside replacement may be effective in reducing gastrointestinal side effects)
Sulfasalazine	Analog of 5-aminosalicylic acid	Start with 10–15 mg/kg/day and gradually increase over a period of 4 weeks to 30–50 mg/kg/day (max 2 g/day).	2–3 doses	Maculopapular rash, oral ulcer, Stevens Johnson syndrome, cytopenia, drug-induced lupus erythematosus, hepatitis, Raynaud phenomenon, pulmonary fibrosis, alveolitis, reversible decrease in sperm count
Cytotoxic, antimetabolic, and immunomodulatory drugs				
Azathioprine	Inhibition of purine synthesis	Start with 1–1.5 mg/kg/day; gradually increase 2–2.5 mg/kg/day (max 150 mg/day)	1 dose	Gastrointestinal discomfort, nausea, vomiting, diarrhea, oral ulcers, maculopapular rash, bone marrow suppression, hepatitis, pancreatitis,
Mycophenolate Mofetil	Inhibitor of inosine monophosphate dehydrogenase	Start with 300 mg/m²/dose twice daily; increase over a period of 2 weeks to 600 mg/m²/dose twice daily (max 2–3 g/day)	2–4 doses	Gastrointestinal discomfort and toxicity, bone marrow suppression
Cyclophosphamide	Binds guanine in DNA and disrupts DNA replication	Oral/IV: 0.5–2 mg/kg/day Iv pulse: 500–1000 g/m²/2–4 weeks	Oral: 1–2 doses	Cytopenias, bladder toxicity (hemorrhagic cystitis, carcinoma, fibrosis), nausea, vomiting, alopecia, infections, pubertal development problems and infertility (risk increases prepubertal individuals), myeloproliferative disease, and malignity (bladder, skin) (Mesna is recommended for preventing hemorrhagic cystitis and, gonadotropin-releasing hormone agonist/luteinizing hormone–releasing hormone agonists may decrease ovarian toxicity)
Cyclosporine	Calcineurin inhibitor	3–5 mg/kg/day	2 doses	Renal toxicity, hypertension, hepatic toxicity, tremor, nausea, vomiting

(continued)

Table 25.1 (continued)

	Mechanism of action	Pediatric dose	Doses per day	Side effects
Biologic DMARDs[b]				
Etanercept	Dimeric fusion protein comprises the human TNF-α receptor p75 linked to the fc region of immunoglobulin G1.	0.8 mg/kg/week (max 50 mg/week)	1 dose/week	Increased risk of opportunistic infections (tuberculosis, fungal, etc.), possible increased risk of malignancy (leukemia, lymphoma, melanoma, solid organ cancers), demyelinating events of central nervous system
Adalimumab	Recombinant human IgG1 monoclonal antibody	24 m^2/2 weeks or 10 mg/2 weeks (10–15 kg) 20 mg/2 weeks (15–30 kg) 40 mg/2 weeks (30–45 kg)	1 dose/2 weeks	
Infliximab	Chimeric monoclonal antibody to the human IgG1	6–10 mg/kg/dose	Single dose administered in weeks 0, 2, and 6, followed by doses every 4–8 weeks thereafter	
Tocilizumab	Humanized monoclonal antibody the soluble IL-6 receptor	10–12 mg/kg (<30 kg) 8–10 mg/kg (>30 kg)	2–4 weeks	Infections, hematologic toxicity (leukopenia, thrombocytopenia), hyperlipidemia, gastrointestinal toxicity (intestinal ulceration, diverticulitis, peritonitis, perforation, fistulae, abscesses)
Other				
Colchicine	Inhibition of microtubule formation	0.5–2 mg/day	2–3 doses	Diarrhea, gastrointestinal discomfort, myelosuppression

The table has been created based on the data from [46]
[a]Non-steroidal anti-inflammatory Drugs
[b]Disease modifying drugs
[c]Cyclooxygenase

25.2.1 Mucocutaneous Involvement

Oral and genital ulcerations, although they are the mildest symptoms of the disease, significantly impact the quality of life of patients due to the associated pain. Painful oral lesions can lead to disruptions in routine oral care procedures, compromised oral hygiene, triggering infections and inflammation, and even exacerbation of systemic disease activity. Additionally, mucosal lesions can disrupt the patient's nutrition by affecting the intake of vitamins and minerals essential for mucosal and epithelial integrity, potentially increasing the frequency and severity of mucosal lesions. Therefore, as a general preventive approach, it is crucial to provide oral hygiene education and encouragement to patients [14]. In this context, the use of oral chlorhexidine-containing antiseptic mouthwashes or gels may be considered in selected cases [14].

Oral ulcers can be managed using various topical agents aimed at reducing pain and shortening the healing time. Analgesic/anesthetic sprays and gels containing lidocaine are effective in pain control. Hyaluronic acid in local preparations has been shown to shorten the healing time of oral ulcers [14, 15]. Similarly, the application of topical sucralfate has been demonstrated to be effective in reducing pain and shortening the healing time of oral and genital ulcers in Behçet's patients [16].

In addition to the preparations mentioned above, there are also topically used nonsteroidal anti-inflammatory drugs (such as diclofenac and choline salicylate) and steroids (triamcinolone acetonide, dexamethasone, hydrocortisone) [14]. The use of topical steroids is recommended for the treatment of oral and genital ulcers in the EULAR guideline [12].

Mucocutaneous lesions are treated and prevented primarily with systemic therapy, and colchicine is the first choice in treatment [12–14]. Colchicine has been shown to be effective in the treatment of genital ulcers and erythema nodosum in numerous studies; however, there are controversial reports regarding its efficacy in the treatment of oral ulcers [12, 14]. Similarly, the efficacy of colchicine treatment is considered low in papulopustular lesions. Topical and systemic treatments used for acne vulgaris may be beneficial for mild papulopustular lesions or lesions resembling acne [12]. It is recommended to try an appropriate dose of colchicine for at least 3–6 months in patients before considering them as nonresponsive, taking into account their age and weight [13]. Topical or systemic steroids (only in severe cases) can be used to control flares in mucocutaneous manifestations [13, 14].

In cases with recurrent mucocutaneous lesions despite colchicine treatment, alternatives such as azathioprine, thalidomide, dapsone, interferon alpha, anti-TNF agents, or apremilast can be considered [12–14]. The choice of which alternative to use should be determined based on the patient's characteristics, disease severity, involvement of other areas, treatment cost, potential side effects, patient preferences, and accessibility.

Azathioprine treatment has been shown to be effective in Behçet's disease-associated oral and genital ulcers, arthritis and prevention of new eye disease [17]. The oral phosphodiesterase 4 inhibitor, apremilast, has been demonstrated to be effective in the treatment of oral ulcers in adult Behçet's patients, and it is listed as an alternative treatment for mucocutaneous involvement in EULAR recommendations [12, 18]. Apremilast treatment has also been shown to be effective in the treatment of genital ulcers, skin lesions, and arthritis, in addition to oral ulcers. Its oral administration, safety profile, and compatibility with other disease-modifying agents are its most significant positive features [14]. Clinical studies investigating the effectiveness of apremilast treatment in pediatric cases are still ongoing. Ustekinumab, a monoclonal antibody targeting interleukin-12 and interleukin-23, has been shown to be effective in the treatment of colchicine-resistant oral ulcers [19]. Similarly, secukinumab, a monoclonal antibody targeting interleukin-17A, has been shown to be effective in Behçet's disease-associated mucocutaneous manifestations and articular involvement [20]. Interestingly, there are reported cases in the literature of the development of Behçet's syndrome after the use of secukinumab [14, 21]. Publications in the literature suggest that anti-IL-1 agents are effective in the mucocutaneous manifestations of the disease [12, 14]. The use of tocilizumab, a monoclonal antibody to the IL-6 receptor, has been shown to be ineffective for mucocutaneous manifestations and can even lead to disease activation [12].

25.2.2 Eye Involvement

Behçet's disease with ocular involvement should be managed in collaboration with ophthalmologists experienced in chronic inflammatory eye diseases. For uncomplicated isolated anterior segment inflammation (anterior uveitis), local agents such as steroid-containing eye drops (e.g., prednisolone acetate 1%, dexamethasone 0.1%, prednisolone sodium phosphate 1%, difluprednate 0.05%, etc.) should be tried [12, 14]. In addition to local steroids, mydriatic and cycloplegic agents (e.g., tropicamide 1%, atropine 0.01%, cyclopentolate 1%, phenylephrine 2.5%, etc.) are often added to the treatment to reduce pain caused by ciliary muscle spasm and prevent adhesions [13, 14].

Posterior uveitis, panuveitis, and relapsed/refractory disease require systemic treatment. Similarly, hypopyon uveitis is often associated with the need for systemic steroid use [13]. Studies in adult patients suggest that early disease onset and male gender are poor risk factors for ocular involvement. Therefore, it is recommended to keep the threshold low for starting systemic treatment in these patients [12–14].

Systemic steroids can be used as a bridging therapy in acute flares and until the effectiveness of systemic immunosuppressants becomes apparent, due to their rapid and effective anti-inflammatory activity [12–14]. However, treating posterior uveitis with systemic steroids alone is not recommended [12].

Behçet's disease-associated uveitis is treated with various systemic immunosuppressive/immunomodulatory therapies, including azathioprine, cyclosporin-A, interferon-alpha, and anti-TNF agents [12–14]. Azathioprine (2 mg/kg/day) or cyclosporin-A (3 mg/kg/day) treatments have been shown to be effective in preventing relapses and improving visual acuity [13, 14, 17]. The combination of azathioprine and interferon-alpha should be avoided due to an increased risk of myelosuppression [14]. Cyclosporin-A, a selective calcineurin inhibitor, has been shown in numerous studies to be effective in preserving visual acuity and preventing uveitis attacks [12–14, 22]. When using cyclosporin-A and azathioprine in combination, it should be kept in mind that cyclosporin-A serum levels may decrease [12, 23]. In cases unresponsive to cyclosporin-A and azathioprine treatments or in the presence of severe uveitis showing a decrease in visual acuity, macular edema, and/or retinal vasculitis, interferon-alpha or anti-TNF drugs are indicated [12–14]. There is no definite consensus on whether interferon-alpha or anti-TNF agents should be prioritized in these patients, and the decision should be made considering patient characteristics [12]. Infliximab, a chimeric TNF-alpha antibody, has been shown to be effective in recurring or refractory uveitis cases [12, 24, 25]. Similarly, adalimumab, a fully recombinant human immunoglobulin G1 monoclonal antibody, is effective in the treatment of anterior and posterior uveitis [26]. In cases of primary or secondary unresponsiveness, or the development of side effects, a switch between these two anti-TNF agents is mentioned in the EULAR recommendations [12]. Unlike adalimumab and infliximab, etanercept, a soluble TNF receptor fusion protein, is not indicated for uveitis treatment [13]. Interferon-alpha has long been used as an effective alternative in the treatment of resistant uveitis cases instead of anti-TNF agents [14, 27]. The most common side effects of interferon treatment are flu-like symptoms, local reactions, and alopecia. It has been recommended as an effective and safe alternative to conventional drugs for the treatment of sight-threatening uveitis in EULAR recommendations [12, 14]. Several studies have shown that interferon-alpha treatment is more effective and better tolerated than cyclosporin treatment, and it has similar efficacy to infliximab treatment in Behçet's disease-associated uveitis [14, 28, 29]. The reduction/discontinuation of immunomodulatory/immunosuppressive treatment in Behçet's disease-associated uveitis should be considered on a case-by-case basis at least after 2 years of remission [13].

Studies are insufficient to provide solid recommendations regarding the effectiveness of anti-IL1, anti-IL6, and JAK inhibitors in the treatment of Behçet's disease-associated uveitis.

25.2.3 Vascular Involvement

Behçet's disease-associated thrombosis is primarily attributed to vascular inflammation; therefore, similar to other systemic involvements of the disease, immunosuppression is the main treatment approach for acute venous thrombosis [12, 14]. In addition to steroids, immunosuppressive agents such as azathioprine, cyclosporin-A, and cyclophosphamide can be used in the treatment of acute venous thrombosis [12]. There is no reliable data or guideline recommendation demonstrating the superiority of one of these agents over the others. Due to potential side effects, cyclophosphamide may be considered for use in more severe cases [12]. Several studies suggest that monoclonal anti-TNF agents are an effective option in the treatment of refractory venous thrombosis [30, 31]. Moreover, in recent years, tocilizumab has been proposed as an effective and tolerable alternative in severe and/or refractory vascular Behçet's disease cases [32].

The use of anticoagulant therapy in the treatment of Behçet's disease-associated thrombosis is a subject of debate. A meta-analysis study compiled from studies on adult Behçet's patients showed that the use of anticoagulant therapy in conjunction with immunosuppressive treatment did not provide additional benefits in reducing relapse rates [12]. In another retrospective study evaluating adult Behçet's patients showed that the nonuse of anticoagulants increased the risk of post-thrombotic syndrome. In light of these data, the EULAR recommendations for Behçet's disease management do not express a contrary opinion on anticoagulant therapy, stating that they can be added to the treatment in refractory thrombosis cases after considering the risk of bleeding and ruling out the presence of arterial aneurysms [12]. The French guidelines for Behçet's disease management, providing recommendations for both adult and pediatric cases, suggest initiating curative anticoagulant treatment in cases of deep vein thrombosis [13].

In cases with arterial involvement, high-dose steroids and cyclophosphamide are recommended as the primary treatment approach. Anti-TNF agents (such as infliximab) are encouraged as alternative agents in all guidelines since they have been shown to be effective in refractory cases [12, 13].

Surgical interventions and radiological interventional procedures should be limited, especially in cases with a high risk of bleeding or symptomatic cases [12, 13]. Steroid and immunosuppressive treatment should be initiated before interventions to reduce postoperative complications. However, in symptomatic cases, intervention should not be delayed for the initiation of immunosuppressive treatment [12]. For symptomatic cases, invasive radiological interventions are recommended over open surgery [12, 13].

25.2.4 Neurological Involvement

Behçet's disease neurological involvement can be divided into two main groups: parenchymal and non-parenchymal involvement [33]. In children with Behçet's disease, parenchymal neuro-Behçet's form is reported to be more common. Acute parenchymal form of neurologic involvement of Behçet's disease generally responds well to high-dose steroid treatment. The recommended treatment for this form is to initiate treatment with a 3–7 day course of high-dose steroids, then continue treatment with methylprednisolone at a dose of 1 mg/kg/day for at least 1 month, followed by tapering [12, 13]. In the treatment of parenchymal form of neurologic involvement of Behçet's disease, an immunomodulatory/immunosuppressive agent such as azathioprine or methotrexate should be added to steroid therapy [13]. In severe, chronic, progressive, and refractory cases, the addition of anti-TNF agents or cyclophosphamide to the treatment is recommended [12, 13]. A restricted number of studies have suggested tocilizumab as a viable alternative for refractory parenchymal neurologic involvement in Behçet's disease [12]. Isolated meningitis cases can be managed with steroid therapy alone [13]. Due to potential neurotoxic effects, the use of cyclosporine in the management of parenchymal neurologic involvement of Behçet's disease should be avoided [12, 13]. Additionally, it should be kept in mind that anti-TNF agents may increase the risk of demyelinating events [14, 34].

Behçet's disease-associated acute cerebral thrombophlebitis is treated similarly to parenchymal disease with 3 days of high-dose steroid therapy, followed by treatment with methylprednisolone at a dose of 1 mg/kg/day for 3–4 weeks. The addition of immunosuppressive drugs to the treatment has not shown additional benefits in the first attack of cerebral vein thrombosis. In relapsed cases, immunosuppressive drugs should be added to the treatment [12, 13]. The addition of anticoagulants to the treatment is recommended in the management of cerebral thrombophlebitis [13].

25.2.5 Gastrointestinal Involvement

Gastrointestinal involvement in Behçet's disease should be confirmed through endoscopy and imaging, and mimickers such as ulcers associated with nonsteroidal drugs or inflammatory bowel disease should be ruled out. Considering the risk of gastrointestinal bleeding associated with steroids, their use is preferred in acute attacks, early stages of induction, and severe disease involvement [12, 13]. For cases with mild to moderate gastrointestinal involvement without small bowel involvement, 5-aminosalicylates (mesalazine, mesalamine, sulfasalazine) are appropriate treatment options [12, 13]. Similarly, azathioprine therapy is recommended as an effective alternative in moderate to severe cases [12, 13]. There is ample evidence showing the effectiveness of anti-TNF agents (especially infliximab and adalimumab) in refractory cases to azathioprine therapy [35, 36]. With increasing evidence regarding the efficacy of monoclonal anti-TNF agents, especially in the treatment of severe cases, they have become the main players. Additionally, real-world data suggest that switching between anti-TNF agents may be beneficial in cases unresponsive to the first-used anti-TNF agent [37]. While data on the use of methotrexate alone in Behçet's disease-associated gastrointestinal involvement are limited, combining it with anti-TNF agents has been shown to reduce their immunogenicity [14]. The potential need for surgical intervention in cases of severe gastrointestinal involvement should be kept in mind, and patients should be followed with a multidisciplinary approach.

25.2.6 Articular Involvement

Behçet's disease-associated arthritis is initially treated with colchicine. In cases with limited involvement of a few large joints, intra-articular steroids can be beneficial. For refractory and recurrent cases, methotrexate, azathioprine, or anti-TNF agents may be preferred [13].

25.3 Course of the Disease and Prognosis

The disease follows a course characterized by periods of remission and relapse [14]. There is limited and conflicting data in the literature regarding the impact of the age at onset on the course and prognosis of the disease. In a recent study comparing juvenile-onset and adult-onset Behçet's disease cases, it was reported that the clinical spectrum of the disease is similar, but the risk of major organ involvement is lower in pediatric-onset cases, leading to a better prognosis for these patients [10]. Similarly, in a study comparing 19 pediatric and 34 adult-onset patients with Behçet's disease, a less severe disease course was reported in pediatric cases [11].

In another study, it was reported that the occurrence of the complete symptom complex is delayed in pediatric-onset cases, and the frequency of serious complications is lower [38] Contrary to these studies, there are also studies reporting that the onset of the disease does not alter the prognosis or that an early onset age worsens the prognosis [39, 40]. Similarly, a recent study reported a comparable risk of major organ involvement and a similar clinical course in both juvenile and adult-onset cases of Behçet's disease [41].

Eye disease and neurological involvement are the most significant contributors to morbidity [14, 42]. Neurological and vascular involvement are often cited as the primary causes of mortality. [14]. In a pediatric-onset Behçet's disease cohort, it was found that eye involvement and vascular involvement are more common in males [43]. In a study evaluating neurological involvement in pediatric-onset Behçet's disease, 17% developed permanent neurological sequelae [42, 44]. The mortality rate was reported as 3% in an international pediatric-onset Behçet's disease cohort published in 1998, and it was associated with large vessel involvement [45].

In conclusion, Behçet's disease is a multifaceted condition that can affect individuals of all ages, including children. Although it is generally seen in adults, approximately one-fourth of cases begin during childhood. The prognosis for pediatric Behçet's disease is a subject of discussion, with differing reports on the effect of the age at which the disease starts on its course and severity. Nonetheless, it is clear that detecting and addressing the issue early on can reduce the likelihood of significant organ involvement and complications. This review emphasizes the diverse clinical manifestations and unique challenges associated with pediatric Behçet's disease, stressing the importance of tailored treatment strategies and a multidisciplinary care team. Although evidence-based treatment recommendations are available for adult Behçet's disease, there is a scarcity of sufficient studies on pediatric cases, necessitating the adaptation of adult guidelines for managing young patients. Additional research is necessary to better understand the genetic and immunological characteristics of pediatric Behçet's patients, to establish early diagnosis and prognosis, and to develop optimal treatment approaches for children.

References

1. Behcet H. Uber rezidivierende, aphtose, durch ein virus verursachte geschrwre am mund, am auge und an den genitalien. Dermatol Wochenschr. 1937;105:1152–7.
2. Jennette JC, Falk RJ, Bacon PA, Basu N, Cid MC, Ferrario F, et al. 2012 revised International Chapel Hill consensus conference nomenclature of Vasculitides. Arthritis Rheum. 2013;65(1):1–11.
3. Yıldız M, Köker O, Adrovic A, Şahin S, Barut K, Kasapçopur Ö. Pediatric Behçet's disease—clinical aspects and current concepts. Eur J Rheumatol. 2019;7(Suppl 1):1–10.
4. Yildiz M, Haslak F, Adrovic A, Sahin S, Koker O, Barut K, et al. Pediatric Behçet's disease. Front Med (Lausanne). 2021;8:627192.
5. Akkoç N. Update on the epidemiology, risk factors and disease outcomes of Behçet's disease. Best Pract Res Clin Rheumatol. 2018;32(2):261–70.
6. Verity DH, Marr JE, Ohno S, Wallace GR, Stanford MR. Behçet's disease, the Silk Road and HLA-B51: historical and geographical perspectives. Tissue Antigens. 1999;54(3):213–20.
7. Karincaoglu Y, Borlu M, Toker SC, Akman A, Onder M, Gunasti S, et al. Demographic and clinical properties of juvenile-onset Behçet's disease: a controlled multicenter study. J Am Acad Dermatol. 2008;58(4):579–84.
8. Kone-Paut I. Behcet's disease in children, an overview. Pediatr Rheumatol Online J. 2016;14(1):10.
9. Gallizzi R, Pidone C, Cantarini L, Finetti M, Cattalini M, Filocamo G, et al. A national cohort study on pediatric Behçet's disease: cross-sectional data from an Italian registry. Pediatr Rheumatol. 2017;15(1):84.
10. Sota J, Rigante D, Lopalco G, Emmi G, Gentileschi S, Gaggiano C, et al. Clinical profile and evolution of patients with juvenile-onset Behçet's syndrome over a 25-year period: insights from the AIDA network. Intern Emerg Med. 2021;16(8):2163–71.
11. Krause I, Uziel Y, Guedj D, Mukamel M, Harel L, Molad Y, et al. Childhood Behçet's disease: clinical features and comparison with adult-onset disease. Rheumatology (Oxford). 1999;38(5):457–62.
12. Hatemi G, Christensen R, Bang D, Bodaghi B, Celik AF, Fortune F, et al. 2018 update of the EULAR recommendations for the management of Behçet's syndrome. Ann Rheum Dis. 2018;77(6):808–18.
13. Kone-Paut I, Barete S, Bodaghi B, Deiva K, Desbois AC, Galeotti C, et al. French recommendations for the management of Behçet's disease. Orphanet J Rare Dis. 2021;16(Suppl 1):352.
14. Giani T, Luppino AF, Ferrara G. Treatment options in pediatric Behçet's disease. Paediatr Drugs. 2023;25(2):165–91.
15. Dalessandri D, Zotti F, Laffranchi L, Migliorati M, Isola G, Bonetti S, et al. Treatment of recurrent aphthous stomatitis (RAS; aphthae; canker sores) with a barrier forming mouth rinse or topical gel formulation containing hyaluronic acid: a retrospective clinical study. BMC Oral Health. 2019;19(1):153.
16. Alpsoy E, Er H, Durusoy C, Yilmaz E. The use of sucralfate suspension in the treatment of oral and genital ulceration of Behçet disease: a randomized, placebo-controlled, double-blind study. Arch Dermatol. 1999;135(5):529–32.
17. Yazici H, Pazarli H, Barnes CG, Tüzün Y, Ozyazgan Y, Silman A, et al. A controlled trial of azathioprine in Behçet's syndrome. N Engl J Med. 1990;322(5):281–5.
18. Hatemi G, Melikoglu M, Tunc R, Korkmaz C, Turgut Ozturk B, Mat C, et al. Apremilast for Behçet's syndrome--a phase 2, placebo-controlled study. N Engl J Med 2015;372(16):1510–8.
19. Mirouse A, Barete S, Monfort JB, Resche-Rigon M, Bouyer AS, Comarmond C, et al. Ustekinumab for Behçet's disease. J Autoimmun. 2017;82:41–6.
20. Fagni F, Bettiol A, Talarico R, Lopalco G, Silvestri E, Urban ML, et al. Long-term effectiveness and safety of secukinumab for treatment of refractory mucosal and articular Behçet's phenotype: a multicentre study. Ann Rheum Dis. 2020;79(8):1098–104.
21. Dincses E, Yurttas B, Esatoglu SN, Melikoglu M, Hamuryudan V, Seyahi E. Secukinumab induced Behçet's syndrome: a report of two cases. Oxf Med Case Rep. 2019;2019(5):omz041.
22. BenEzra D, Cohen E, Chajek T, Friedman G, Pizanti S, de Courten C, et al. Evaluation of conventional therapy versus cyclosporine A in Behçet's syndrome. Transplant Proc. 1988;20(3 Suppl 4):136–43.
23. Grekas D, Nikolaidis P, Karamouzis M, Alivanis P, Tourkantonis A. Effects of azathioprine on ciclosporin metabolism. Nephron. 1992;60(4):489.
24. Tugal-Tutkun I, Mudun A, Urgancioglu M, Kamali S, Kasapoglu E, Inanc M, et al. Efficacy of infliximab in the treatment of uveitis that is resistant to treatment with the combination of azathioprine, cyclosporine,

and corticosteroids in Behçet's disease: an open-label trial. Arthritis Rheum. 2005;52(8):2478–84.
25. Sfikakis PP, Theodossiadis PG, Katsiari CG, Kaklamanis P, Markomichelakis NN. Effect of infliximab on sight-threatening panuveitis in Behçet's disease. Lancet (London, England). 2001;358(9278):295–6.
26. Vallet H, Riviere S, Sanna A, Deroux A, Moulis G, Addimanda O, et al. Efficacy of anti-TNF alpha in severe and/or refractory Behçet's disease: multicenter study of 124 patients. J Autoimmun. 2015;62:67–74.
27. Alpsoy E, Durusoy C, Yilmaz E, Ozgurel Y, Ermis O, Yazar S, et al. Interferon alfa-2a in the treatment of Behçet disease: a randomized placebo-controlled and double-blind study. Arch Dermatol. 2002;138(4):467–71.
28. Qian Y, Qu Y, Gao F, Pei M, Liang A, Xiao J, et al. Comparison of the safety and efficacy of interferon alpha-2a and cyclosporine-a when combined with glucocorticoid in the treatment of refractory Behçet's uveitis: a randomized controlled prospective study. Front Pharmacol. 2021;12:699903.
29. De Simone L, Invernizzi A, Aldigeri R, Mastrofilippo V, Marvisi C, Gozzi F, et al. Effectiveness of infliximab and interferon alpha-2a for the treatment of Behçet's uveitis: customizing therapy according to the clinical features. Ocul Immunol Inflamm. 2022;30(2):506–14.
30. Desbois AC, Addimanda O, Bertrand A, Deroux A, Pérard L, Depaz R, et al. Efficacy of anti-TNFα in severe and refractory neuro-Behcet disease: an observational study. Medicine (Baltimore). 2016;95(23):e3550.
31. Aksoy A, Yazici A, Omma A, Cefle A, Onen F, Tasdemir U, et al. Efficacy of TNFα inhibitors for refractory vascular Behçet's disease: a multicenter observational study of 27 patients and a review of the literature. Int J Rheum Dis. 2020;23(2):256–61.
32. Ding Y, Li C, Liu J, Yu X, Wang Y, Shi J, et al. Tocilizumab in the treatment of severe and/or refractory vasculo-Behçet's disease: a single-centre experience in China. Rheumatology (Oxford). 2018;57(11):2057–9.
33. Uluduz D, Kürtüncü M, Yapıcı Z, Seyahi E, Kasapçopur Ö, Özdoğan H, et al. Clinical characteristics of pediatric-onset neuro-Behçet disease. Neurology. 2011;77(21):1900–5.
34. Kemanetzoglou E, Andreadou E. CNS demyelination with TNF-α blockers. Curr Neurol Neurosci Rep. 2017;17(4):36.
35. Hatemi I, Hatemi G, Pamuk ON, Erzin Y, Celik AF. TNF-alpha antagonists and thalidomide for the management of gastrointestinal Behçet's syndrome refractory to the conventional treatment modalities: a case series and review of the literature. Clin Exp Rheumatol. 2015;33(6 Suppl 94):S129–37.
36. Tanida S, Inoue N, Kobayashi K, Naganuma M, Hirai F, Iizuka B, et al. Adalimumab for the treatment of Japanese patients with intestinal Behçet's disease. Clin Gastroenterol Hepatol. 2015;13(5):940–8.e3.
37. Sugimura N, Mizoshita T, Sugiyama T, Togawa S, Miyaki T, Suzuki T, et al. Real-world efficacy of adalimumab and infliximab for refractory intestinal Behçet's disease. Dig Liver Dis. 2019;51(7):967–71.
38. Treudler R, Orfanos CE, Zouboulis CC. Twenty-eight cases of juvenile-onset Adamantiades-Behçet disease in Germany. Dermatology (Basel, Switzerland). 1999;199(1):15–9.
39. Hamzaoui A, Jaziri F, Ben Salem T, F SIBG, Lamloum M, Smiti Khanfir M, et al. Comparison of clinical features of Behcet disease according to age in a Tunisian cohort. Acta med. Iran. 2014;52(10):748–51.
40. Alpsoy E, Donmez L, Onder M, Gunasti S, Usta A, Karincaoglu Y, et al. Clinical features and natural course of Behçet's disease in 661 cases: a multicentre study. Br J Dermatol. 2007;157(5):901–6.
41. Boyvat A, Oktem A, Kalay Yildizhan I, Ates A, Yalcindag N, Koksoy C, et al. A comparison of adult and juvenile Behcet patients and a look at clinical trends: retrospective data from a Turkish follow-up cohort study. Dermatology (Basel, Switzerland). 2023;239(6):958–65.
42. Pain CE. Juvenile-onset Behçet's syndrome and mimics. Clinical immunology (Orlando, Fla). 2020;214:108381.
43. Koné-Paut I, Shahram F, Darce-Bello M, Cantarini L, Cimaz R, Gattorno M, et al. Consensus classification criteria for paediatric Behçet's disease from a prospective observational cohort: PEDBD. Ann Rheum Dis. 2016;75(6):958–64.
44. Mora P, Menozzi C, Orsoni JG, Rubino P, Ruffini L, Carta A. Neuro-Behçet's disease in childhood: a focus on the neuro-ophthalmological features. Orphanet J Rare Dis. 2013;8:18.
45. Koné-Paut I, Yurdakul S, Bahabri SA, Shafae N, Ozen S, Özdogan H, et al. Clinical features of Behçet's disease in children: an international collaborative study of 86 cases. J Pediatr. 1998;132(4):721–5.
46. Petty RE, Laxer RM, Lindsley CB, Wedderburn L, Fuhlbrigge RC, Mellins ED. Textbook of pediatric rheumatology e-book. Philadelphia: Elsevier Health Sciences; 2020.

Treatment Algorithms in Patients with Behçet's Disease During Pregnancy and Lactation

26

Göknur Kalkan

Contents

26.1 Behçet's Disease During Pregnancy

Behçet's disease poses significant concerns during pregnancy, especially considering the reproductive age of many affected patients. Existing literature on the impact of Behçet's disease on pregnancy is limited and characterized by conflicting data. Various studies, including case reports and retrospective analyses, have presented mixed findings on disease activity during pregnancy, contributing to an ambiguous understanding of its effects. The disease course varies among individuals and even within the same woman across different pregnancies. Past retrospective studies suggest a tendency for Behçet's

G. Kalkan (✉)
Department of Dermatology, School of Medicine, Ankara Yıldırım Beyazıt University, Ankara, Türkiye

E. Alpsoy et al. (eds.), *Behçet's Disease: An Integrated Approach*,
https://doi.org/10.1007/978-3-031-77251-1_26

disease activity to recede or stabilize during pregnancy, possibly influenced by the immunomodulatory effects of elevated estrogen and progesterone. While some studies found no increase in pregnancy-related complications, others reported higher risks of maternal and fetal complications. Notably, active Behçet's disease may heighten the risk of obstetric complications. To mitigate risks to both mother and fetus, vigilant pregnancy monitoring is crucial. A local multicenter study revealed that Behçet's disease patients, compared to healthy controls, had lower birth weight and higher miscarriage rates, with a connection to placental vasculitis [1–8].

26.2 Maternal-Paternal Approach Before Pregnancy

Research on the long-term effects of medications during pregnancy and breastfeeding on child health is limited and often of low quality. While there is no specific guideline dedicated to treatments for pregnancy and breastfeeding in Behçet's disease, international guidelines for rheumatic diseases provide guidance for those with inflammatory/autoimmune rheumatic conditions. Recommendations outlining key considerations for the use of antirheumatic drugs before, during, and after pregnancy and breastfeeding are presently guided by the European League Against Rheumatism (EULAR) 2016, the American College of Rheumatology (ACR) 2020, and the British Society for Rheumatology/British Health Professionals in Rheumatology (BSR/BHPR) 2016. The utilization of drugs in the treatment of Behçet's disease during pregnancy and breastfeeding will be examined in alignment with these established guidelines [9–11].

In patients with autoimmune rheumatic diseases, pregnancy planning aligns with inactive or stable disease periods, as recommended by the EULAR 2016, specifying a 6- to 12-month window of inactive or moderately stable disease based on maternal factors [9–12]. Similarly, Behçet's disease mandates the management of active disease before pregnancy, aiming for clinical remission and minimized disease activity. The treatment guideline from a French research group briefly notes in a subsection on pregnancy and breastfeeding that, particularly in severe forms of Behçet's disease like vascular and neurological involvement, pregnancy is not contraindicated if Behçet's disease has been in remission for at least 12 months [13].

Monitoring drug usage before and during pregnancy is crucial, emphasizing the significance of pre-pregnancy counseling and birth control. Adapting treatments to pregnancy and educating patients on medication usage are vital aspects. Both male and female patients of reproductive age should be informed about medications before starting treatment due to potential effects on fertility and increased risks of miscarriage/congenital anomalies. Consequently, unplanned pregnancies, particularly while receiving teratogenic drugs, are discouraged. Ideally, pre-pregnancy planning should ensure conception at the optimal time, with decisions on pregnancy timing and suitable contraceptive methods made collaboratively between clinician and patient. Patients not planning for pregnancy or requiring teratogenic drugs should be guided to appropriate contraceptive methods. In planned pregnancies, drugs with teratogenic effects should be discontinued at least 3 months before conception and replaced with low-risk alternatives. In unplanned pregnancies involving teratogenic drugs, immediate cessation is recommended, managed through collaborative physician–patient efforts. The Behçet's disease treatment guideline from the French research group also highlights that, especially in Behçet's disease patients with vascular involvement, estrogens should be avoided, favoring progestin and mechanical contraceptives [9–13].

In this chapter, the use of main drug groups proven to be compatible with pregnancy according to current guidelines in Behçet's disease will be discussed sequentially. Additionally, contraindicated drug groups, which are teratogenic and should not be used during pregnancy, will be addressed. The section will also cover the use of biological agents during pregnancy, treatment during the lactation period, and paternal drug usage. The initial group of medications discussed comprises those identified as compatible with pregnancy and breastfeeding, as per the EULAR 2016 recommendations, receiving a recommendation level B. This category encompasses glucocorticoids, sulfasalazine, azathioprine, colchicine, cyclosporine, and tacrolimus. The guidelines stress the continuity of these drugs during pregnancy for individuals with inflammatory/autoimmune rheumatic diseases, either for sustaining remission or managing flare-ups [9].

26.3 Colchicine

Colchicine serves as a prominent anti-inflammatory agent in the first-line treatment of Behçet's disease and various rheumatological conditions. Its anti-mitotic properties raise concerns about its use during pregnancy, warranting evaluation for potential teratogenic effects. A prospective comparative study involving 238 pregnancies exposed to colchicine found no significant increase in teratogenicity or congenital abnormalities, aligning with previous research emphasizing its safety during pregnancy at clinically recommended doses [14]. Systematic meta-analyses of four studies, primarily involving Familial Mediterranean Fever (FMF) patients but including Behçet's disease patients in one instance, indicated that colchicine did not significantly increase the risk of fetal malformations or miscarriage throughout pregnancy. Notably, when addressing untreated FMF with risks of recurrence and systemic amyloidosis, discontinuing colchicine during pregnancy is not recommended due to an increased teratogenic risk [15].

Despite animal studies suggesting an elevated risk of congenital malformations, human studies show no adverse outcomes. Both ACR 2020 and EULAR recommendations strongly endorse colchicine use during pregnancy and breastfeeding. EULAR highlights that evidence supports its continued use throughout pregnancy at doses up to 1 mg/day, with compatibility observed during breastfeeding [9, 10]. The Behçet's disease treatment guide from the French research group concurs, emphasizing that colchicine is not contraindicated during pregnancy and breastfeeding, advocating for its uninterrupted use at standard doses in these periods [13].

26.4 Glucocorticoids

Glucocorticoids play a pivotal role in managing both cutaneous and mucosal symptoms as well as organ involvement in Behçet's disease. While studies indicate a slight increase in miscarriage rates during pregnancy, current evidence does not associate their use with elevated congenital malformation rates compared to control groups. Although not deemed teratogenic, exposure during intrauterine development (average 20 mg/day) has been linked to growth retardation. To mitigate potential risks, glucocorticoids should be utilized at the lowest effective dose and for the shortest duration feasible during pregnancy. ACR guidelines conditionally recommend tapering nonfluorinated glucocorticoids to <20 mg daily of prednisone by incorporating pregnancy-compatible immunosuppressants [10].

In the context of Behçet's disease, glucocorticoids are advised at the lowest effective dose and for a limited duration, particularly in severe mucocutaneous symptoms or exacerbation scenarios. Nonfluorinated prednisone, with its short half-life and efficient placental metabolism by 11-β-hydroxy-steroid, is the preferred steroid due to low placental transfer. Fluorinated glucocorticoids, metabolized less by the placenta, should be cautiously administered. However, the use of glucocorticoids during pregnancy heightens the risk of pregnancy-related hypertension, gestational diabetes, and osteoporosis. Prolonged use of glucocorticoids can increase the risk of premature and low birth weight infants. Prophylactic measures are recommended to prevent osteoporosis and it is crucial to plan for adequate intake of calcium and vitamin D throughout this process [9–11, 16, 17].

26.5 Azathioprine and Sulfasalazine

Azathioprine and sulfasalazine, as outlined in the ACR 2020 guidelines, are deemed suitable for administration throughout pregnancy, strongly endorsed for maintaining remission/exacerbation treatment. Current evidence negates an elevated risk of congenital malformations for either drug. Azathioprine administration during pregnancy is considered acceptable at doses up to 2 mg/kg/day, with the potential for mitigating transient lymphopenia and immune insufficiency by adhering to this daily limit.

Sulfasalazine, a key treatment for gastrointestinal involvement, is recommended for use throughout pregnancy and is highly endorsed. Its administration during pregnancy, coupled with concurrent folic acid supplementation up to 2 g/day, is considered compatible. While sulfasalazine crosses the placenta, extensive studies have not identified any teratogenic effects associated with its use [9–11].

26.6 Calcineurin Inhibitors (Tacrolimus and Cyclosporine)

The ACR 2020 guidelines conditionally recommend the use of calcineurin inhibitors, specifically tacrolimus and cyclosporine, during pregnancy. These inhibitors can be continued at the lowest effective dose throughout pregnancy, as indicated by current evidence showing no increase in congenital malformation rates. The EULAR 2016 recommendations also align with this, categorizing them as drugs compatible for use throughout pregnancy [9, 10].

26.7 Methotrexate, Cyclophosphamide, Mycophenolate Mofetil, and Thalidomide

Methotrexate, cyclophosphamide, mycophenolate mofetil, and thalidomide are identified as teratogenic drugs, presenting an increased risk of congenital malformations. These agents, acting as DNA mutagens, also induce irreversible azoospermia. Discontinuation of these drugs three months before conception is strongly advised. Specifically, for methotrexate, it is recommended to cease usage 1–3 months before conception, accompanied by folic acid supplementation throughout pregnancy to prevent neural tube defects. Cyclophosphamide should be discontinued 3 months before conception, with conditional approval for use during the second or third trimester in life-threatening situations. Mycophenolate mofetil is contraindicated during pregnancy and should be halted 6 weeks before planned conception. In cases of inadvertent exposure to teratogenic drugs, a thorough assessment by relevant specialists is imperative [9–11, 16, 17]. Preconception, a strong recommendation advocates transitioning from potentially teratogenic drugs to pregnancy-compatible alternatives or adopting drug-free monitoring to ensure disease stability.

26.8 Biologics During Pregnancy

The utilization of biologics during pregnancy presents a challenge due to limited experiential data stemming from observational studies. These studies, particularly those exploring TNF-α inhibitors, reveal insights into placental transference and fetal impact. The most extensive knowledge originates from cases of inflammatory bowel disease (IBD) treated with TNF-α inhibitors, during pregnancy, with TNF inhibitors being the most scrutinized among biologics. TNF-α inhibitors particularly certolizumab exhibit notable safety during pregnancy, with minimal placental transfer attributed to its absence of an Fc chain. ACR 2020 guidelines strongly recommend the uninterrupted use of certolizumab throughout pregnancy. Biologic treatments exhibit variable placental transfer and fetal exposure during pregnancy stages. Those designed for rheumatic diseases, characterized by an Fc IgG1 structure, attain significant fetal circulation only from the second trimester onward. In the third trimester, TNF-α inhibitors (infliximab, etanercept, adalimumab, and golimumab) with the IgG1 Fc structure result in notable placental transfer and considerable drug levels in newborns. Guidelines recommend conditionally continuing TNF-α inhibitor therapies, such as infliximab, etanercept, or adalimumab, both pre-pregnancy and throughout, with advice to persist during the first and second trimesters, followed by discontinuation a few half-lives before the third trimester delivery [9–11, 16, 18, 19]. This tailored strategy seeks to balance therapeutic efficacy with minimizing fetal exposure during critical gestational periods.

Limited data exists on the compatibility of other biologics with pregnancy. IgG-based molecules, excluding TNF-α inhibitors, are conditionally regarded as compatible during the periconception period, with discontinuation advised upon pregnancy confirmation. Anakinra, belimumab, abatacept, tocilizumab, secukinumab, and ustekinumab can be conditionally continued for those attempting conception, ceasing upon pregnancy confirmation. If disease control requires noncompatible drugs, a thorough discussion between physician and patient regarding potential risks is essential [9–11, 16, 18, 19]. There are no current recommendations regarding the safety or usage of small-molecule agents like tofacitinib and baricitinib during pregnancy due to insufficient evidence. While the likelihood of placental transfer is acknowledged, specific guidance awaits further research [10, 18].

26.9 Rituximab

Rituximab, designated pregnancy category C, exhibits transplacental transfer, impacting fetal B-cells and potentially inducing newborn lymphopenia. In Behçet's disease, it serves as a therapeutic option for severe ocular and treatment-resistant neuro-Behçet cases. Contrarily, it is deemed contraindicated during pregnancy due to heightened risks of maternal–fetal and newborn infections. Yet, conditional recommendations allow continued use for women attempting conception and during pregnancy when facing severe, life-threatening disease. Transplacental passage is minimal in the first trimester, increasing moderately in the second, and peaking in the third trimester. Planning pregnancies with a 12-month post-infusion interval is crucial. Contraception is advised for a year post-treatment. Limited safety data indicates potential newborn hematological abnormalities, primarily mild and transient, resolving spontaneously within weeks to months [10, 18–21]. This nuanced approach balances therapeutic necessities with pregnancy-related precautions in managing Behçet's disease with rituximab [10, 18–21].

26.10 Apremilast

Apremilast, a selective phosphodiesterase-4 inhibitor, stands as a noteworthy option for treating mucocutaneous involvement, demonstrating efficacy in reducing oral and genital ulcers. Classified under pregnancy category C, its use has not shown a risk of major birth defects, miscarriage, or adverse maternal/fetal outcomes. However, limited data necessitates caution, lacking sufficient well-controlled studies during pregnancy. Recommendations advise discontinuation 2 days before conception, emphasizing reproductive planning for women of childbearing age. The presence of apremilast or its metabolites in human milk remains uncertain, warranting avoidance during breastfeeding. Animal studies suggest dose-dependent miscarriages and low birth weights, indicating potential risks that require careful consideration in clinical practice [10, 18, 22, 23].

26.11 The Other Agents

For patients with a history of vascular involvement or deep vein thrombosis in Behçet's disease, a potential heightened risk of obstetric complications, including miscarriages, has been suggested. The vasculitic process, endothelial dysfunction, and increased hypercoagulability during pregnancy are proposed contributors to these complications [24, 25]. Management of deep vein thrombosis and pulmonary embolism in Behçet's disease during pregnancy lacks a clear consensus. Typically, anticoagulation with

Table 26.1 Treatment of Behçet's disease during pregnancy

During pregnancy
Drugs proven to be compatible with pregnancy
Glucocorticoids, sulfasalazine, azathioprine, colchicine, cyclosporine, and tacrolimus
Continuation of sulfasalazine, azathioprine, and colchicine is strongly recommended, while continuation of cyclosporine and tacrolimus is conditionally recommended.
Glucocorticoids
Use lowest effective dose (<20 mg/day) for mucocutaneous symptoms; consider adding pregnancy-compatible immunosuppressant; reduce high-dose corticosteroid in organ involvement (strong recommendation).
TNF inhibitors
Certolizumab strongly recommended; others conditionally recommended.
Continue in first and second trimesters; discontinue a few half-lives before third trimester delivery.
Teratogenic drugs
Methotrexate, cyclophosphamide, mycophenolate mofetil, and thalidomide
Strongly advised for discontinuation three months before conception due to the increased risk of congenital malformations and irreversible azoospermia.

These recommendations follow the ACR guideline development process, using a systematic literature review and Grading of Recommendations Assessment, Development and Evaluation methodology [9, 10]

aspirin and low-molecular-weight heparin is employed due to pregnancy-associated hypercoagulability. However, discontinuation of immunosuppressive treatment may lead to nonresponsiveness or relapse. Recommendations favor the compatibility of low-molecular-weight heparin throughout pregnancy. Warfarin, associated with heightened fetal risk, is considered only in exceptional cases. Low-dose aspirin can be continued throughout pregnancy, with its use recommended until delivery for pregnancy-related hypertension prophylaxis [11, 26].

Treatment of Behçet's disease during pregnancy has been summarized in Table 26.1.

26.12 Drug Utilization During the Breastfeeding Period

Encouraging breastfeeding is considered standard clinical practice for Behçet's disease patients. It is recommended to maintain disease control with drugs compatible with breastfeeding, necessitating an individualized assessment of the benefit-risk ratio for each patient. Generally, drugs compatible with pregnancy are also deemed compatible with breastfeeding, although the evidence levels for most drugs remain low due to limited studies often based on single-dose or short-term treatment.

According to both ACR 2020 and EULAR 2016 recommendations, anti-inflammatory drugs suitable for breastfeeding, such as colchicine, sulfasalazine, rituximab, and TNF inhibitors, are strongly advised and should be continued during the breastfeeding period. TNF inhibitors, including infliximab, adalimumab, etanercept, and certolizumab, exhibit low transfer to breast milk, supporting their compatibility with breastfeeding. Prednisone at daily doses <20 mg is considered compatible, but doses ≥20 mg/day necessitate delayed breastfeeding or discarding milk produced within 4 h post-administration. Azathioprine, calcineurin inhibitors, and non-TNF biologics (anakinra, belimumab, abatacept, tocilizumab, secukinumab, and ustekinumab) are conditionally recommended during breastfeeding. Conversely, strongly discouraging recommendations apply to the use of cyclophosphamide, mycophenolate mofetil, and thalidomide during breastfeeding, given their limited safety data. Conditional discouragement is also advised for methotrexate, as weekly use may lead to its accumulation in the newborn despite minimal transfer to breast milk. Drugs lacking breastfeeding data, such as anakinra, belimumab, ustekinumab, tocilizumab, and abatacept, should be avoided during the breastfeeding period if alternative treatments are available for disease control. If no alternatives exist, breastfeeding may continue

Table 26.2 Treatment of Behçet's disease during breastfeeding period

Breastfeeding period
Drugs proven to be compatible with the breastfeeding period Glucocorticoids, sulfasalazine, azathioprine, colchicine, cyclosporine, and tacrolimus
Colchicine, sulfasalazine, rituximab, and TNF inhibitors are strongly recommended for compatibility with breastfeeding.
Glucocorticoids Daily doses of prednisone <20 mg (or equivalent nonfluorinated glucocorticoid) are compatible. For daily doses ≥20 mg, it is strongly recommended to either delay breastfeeding or discard milk produced within 4 h post-administration.
Azathioprine, calcineurin inhibitors, and *non-TNF biological agents* (such as *anakinra, belimumab, abatacept, tocilizumab, secukinumab, and ustekinumab*) are conditionally recommended.
The use of *cyclophosphamide, mycophenolate mofetil, and thalidomide* during the breastfeeding period is strongly discouraged. The use of *methotrexate* during breastfeeding is conditionally discouraged since there is minimal transfer into breast milk, with weekly administration.

These recommendations follow the ACR guideline development process, using a systematic literature review and Grading of Recommendations Assessment, Development and Evaluation methodology [9, 10]

cautiously, considering the pharmacological properties of these agents [9–11, 13, 16, 18, 19, 21, 22]. Treatment of Behçet's disease during breastfeeding period has been summarized in Table 26.2.

26.13 Paternal Drug Use

Addressing paternal drug use is imperative, recognizing its potential impact on male fertility and the risk of fetal teratogenicity. Although the available data on this matter is constrained, a judicious evaluation of an individual's disease activity should prompt considerations for drug discontinuation. The presence of drugs in seminal fluid introduces the possibility of traversing the vaginal mucosa and reaching the placenta, thereby posing a potential for teratogenic effects. Importantly, the limited seminal concentrations of drugs and transferred volumes suggest that postconception exposure to the embryo or fetus is likely minimal. It is advisable for men to refrain from the preconception use of cyclophosphamide and thalidomide due to their adverse effects on spermatogenesis and high teratogenicity, respectively. Cyclophosphamide, with its potential disruption of spermatogenesis and mutagenic properties, should be discontinued at least 3 months before attempting conception. Likewise, thalidomide, detectable in seminal fluid and highly teratogenic, should be ceased at least 1 month before conception. Conversely, the continuous use of azathioprine, colchicine, and TNF-α inhibitors is strongly recommended. However, limited evidence prompts a conditional recommendation for the use of methotrexate, mycophenolate mofetil, leflunomide, sulfasalazine, calcineurin inhibitors, and nonsteroidal anti-inflammatory drugs during preconception periods [10, 11].

References

1. Iskender C, Yasar O, Kaymak O, Yaman ST, Uygur D, Danisman N. Behçet's disease and pregnancy: a retrospective analysis of course of disease and pregnancy outcome. J Obstet Gynaecol Res. 2014;40:1598–602. https://doi.org/10.1111/jog.12386.
2. Uzun S, Alpsoy E, Durdu M, Akman A. The clinical course of Behçet's disease in pregnancy: a retrospective analysis and review of the literature. J Dermatol. 2003;30:499–502. https://doi.org/10.1111/j.1346-8138.2003.tb00423.x.
3. Ben-Chetrit E. Behçet's syndrome and pregnancy: course of the disease and pregnancy outcome. Clin Exp Rheumatol. 2014;32:S93–8.
4. Noel N, Wechsler B, Nizard J, Costedoat-Chalumeau N, Boutin du Tremblay LT, Dommergues M, et al. Behçet's disease and pregnancy. Arthritis Rheum. 2013;65:2450–6. https://doi.org/10.1002/art.38052.
5. Merlino L, Del Prete F, Lobozzo B, Priori R. Behcet's disease and pregnancy: a systematic review. Minerva Ginecol. 2020;72(5):332–8. https://doi.org/10.23736/S0026-4784.20.04564-5. Epub 2020 May 13

6. Barros T, Braga A, Marinho A, Braga J. Behçet's disease and pregnancy: a retrospective case-control study. Yale J Biol Med. 2021;94(4):585–92. PMID: 34970095; PMCID: PMC8686781
7. Orgul G, Aktoz F, Beksac MS. Behcet's disease and pregnancy: what to expect? J Obstet Gynaecol. 2018;38(2):185–8. https://doi.org/10.1080/01443615.2017.1336614. Epub 2017 Aug 17
8. Gungor AN, Kalkan G, Oguz S, Sen B, Ozoguz P, Takci Z, Sacar H, Dogan FB, Cicek D. Behcet disease and pregnancy. Clin Exp Obstet Gynecol. 2014;41(6):617–9.
9. Götestam Skorpen C, Hoeltzenbein M, Tincani A, Fischer-Betz R, Elefant E, Chambers C, et al. The EULAR points to consider for use of antirheumatic drugs before pregnancy, and during pregnancy and lactation. Ann Rheum Dis. 2016;75(5):795–810. https://doi.org/10.1136/annrheumdis-2015-208840. Epub 2016 Feb 17
10. Sammaritano LR, Bermas BL, Chakravarty EE, Chambers C, Clowse MEB, Lockshin MD, et al. 2020 American College of Rheumatology guideline for the management of reproductive health in rheumatic and musculoskeletal diseases. Arthritis Rheumatol. 2020;72(4):529–56. https://doi.org/10.1002/art.41191. Epub 2020 Feb 23
11. Flint J, Panchal S, Hurrell A, van de Venne M, Gayed M, Schreiber K, et al. BSR and BHPR guideline on prescribing drugs in pregnancy and breastfeeding-part I: standard and biologic disease modifying anti-rheumatic drugs and corticosteroids. Rheumatology (Oxford). 2016;55(9):1693–7. https://doi.org/10.1093/rheumatology/kev404. Epub 2016 Jan 10
12. Fischer-Betz R, Späthling-Mestekemper S. Pregnancy and rheumatic diseases. Z Rheumatol. 2020;79(1):55–73.
13. Kone-Paut I, Barete S, Bodaghi B, Deiva K, Desbois AC, Galeotti C, et al. French recommendations for the management of Behçet's disease. Orphanet J Rare Dis. 2021;16(Suppl 1):352. https://doi.org/10.1186/s13023-020-01620-4. PMID: 33622338; PMCID: PMC7903591
14. Diav-Citrin O, Shechtman S, Schwartz V, Avgil-Tsadok M, Finkel-Pekarsky V, Wajnberg R, et al. Pregnancy outcome after in utero exposure to colchicine. Am J Obstet Gynecol. 2010;203(2):144.e1–6. https://doi.org/10.1016/j.ajog.2010.02.063. Epub 2010 Jul 1
15. Indraratna PL, Virk S, Gurram D, Day RO. Use of colchicine in pregnancy: a systematic review and meta-analysis. Rheumatology (Oxford). 2018;57(2):382–7. https://doi.org/10.1093/rheumatology/kex353.
16. Murase JE, Heller MM, Butler DC. Safety of dermatologic medications in pregnancy and lactation: part I. Pregnancy. J Am Acad Dermatol. 2014;70(3):401.e1–14.; quiz 415. https://doi.org/10.1016/j.jaad.2013.09.010.
17. Brzezińska-Wcisło L, Zbiciak-Nylec M, Wcisło-Dziadecka D, Salwowska N. Pregnancy: a therapeutic dilemma. Postepy Dermatol Alergol. 2017;34(5):433–8. https://doi.org/10.5114/ada.2017.71108. Epub 2017 Oct 31. PMID: 29507557; PMCID: PMC5831277
18. Beltagy A, Aghamajidi A, Trespidi L, Ossola W, Meroni PL. Biologics during pregnancy and breastfeeding among women with rheumatic diseases: safety clinical evidence on the road. Front Pharmacol. 2021;12:621247. https://doi.org/10.3389/fphar.2021.621247. PMID: 34122062; PMCID: PMC8189556
19. Birru Talabi M, Clowse MEB. Antirheumatic medications in pregnancy and breastfeeding. Curr Opin Rheumatol. 2020 May;32(3):238–46. https://doi.org/10.1097/BOR.0000000000000710.
20. Perrotta K, Kiernan E, Bandoli G, Manaster R, Chambers C. Pregnancy outcomes following maternal treatment with rituximab prior to or during pregnancy: a case series. Rheumatol Adv Pract. 2021;5(1):rkaa074. https://doi.org/10.1093/rap/rkaa074. PMID: 33521513; PMCID: PMC7819866
21. Dobson R, Rog D, Ovadia C, Murray K, Hughes S, Ford HL, Pearson OR, White S, Bonham N, Mathews J, Nelson-Piercy C, Brex P. Anti-CD20 therapies in pregnancy and breast feeding: a review and ABN guidelines. Pract Neurol. 2023;23(1):6–14. https://doi.org/10.1136/pn-2022-003426. Epub 2022 Jul 8
22. Ibarra Barrueta O, García Martín E, López Sánchez P, Ramírez Herráiz E, Merino Bohórquez V, Ais Larisgoitia A. Biological and immunosuppressive medications in pregnancy, breastfeeding and fertility in immune mediated diseases. Farm Hosp. 2023;47(1):39–49. https://doi.org/10.1016/j.farma.2022.12.005. English, Spanish. Epub 2023 Jan 27
23. Nassim D, Alajmi A, Jfri A, Pehr K. Apremilast in dermatology: a review of literature. Dermatol Ther. 2020;33(6):e14261. https://doi.org/10.1111/dth.14261. Epub 2020 Sep 27
24. Noel N, Wechsler B, Nizard J, Costedoat-Chalumeau N, Boutin LT, Dommergues M, et al. Behçet's disease and pregnancy. Arthritis Rheum. 2013;65(9):2450–6.
25. Jadaon J, Shushan A, Ezra Y, Sela HY, Ozcan C, Rojansky N. Behçet's disease and pregnancy. Acta Obstet Gynecol Scand. 2005 Oct;84(10):939–44.
26. Daughety MM, Zilberman-Rudenko J, Shatzel JJ, McCarty OJT, Raghunathan V, DeLoughery TG. Management of anticoagulation in pregnant women with mechanical heart valves. Obstet Gynecol Surv. 2020;75(3):190–8.

Prognosis in Behçet's Disease: What to Expect?

27

Seçil Vural

Contents

27.1 Introduction

Behçet's disease (BD), a complex and chronic condition, necessitates a nuanced understanding of its prognosis. The prognosis of BD exhibits considerable variability. At one end of the spectrum are cases characterized by mucocutaneous manifestations, where disease intensity tends to diminish with advanced age. In contrast, at the other end of the spectrum are instances marked by vascular involvement, impacting critical organ systems and posing a potential threat to mortality. Prognosis serves as a compass, guiding individuals and healthcare providers through the intricate landscape of this disease. It illuminates the potential course of BD, providing critical insights into the challenges that lie ahead. By elucidating the

S. Vural (✉)
Department of Dermatology and Venereology, Koç University School of Medicine, Istanbul, Türkiye

E. Alpsoy et al. (eds.), *Behçet's Disease: An Integrated Approach*,
https://doi.org/10.1007/978-3-031-77251-1_27

factors that contribute to prognosis this chapter seeks to equip readers with a profound understanding of the variables shaping BD trajectories. In this chapter, we delve into the understanding BD prognosis, recognizing it as a cornerstone for informed decision-making and proactive management.

27.2 Factors Influencing Prognosis Associated with Patient Characteristics

The research has highlighted several factors that significantly impact the prognosis of BD. The genetic risk is higher in male patients. Specifically, the presence and severity of ocular manifestations, vascular involvement, and heightened mortality are unequivocally linked to male gender and younger age [1–12]. A worse prognosis is associated with male gender, as male patients often exhibit major organ involvement, including vascular disease, eye involvement leading to blindness, and neurological issues, which are linked to increased morbidities [1–10].

Studies conducted in the UK and Korea reveal a higher prevalence of BD in females. However, interestingly, even in these countries, the hazard ratio for mortality is significantly lower among female patients [13, 14]. Yazici and Kural-Seyahi et al. reported that a younger age at disease onset is associated with a less favorable outcome [9]. In their comprehensive 20-year study involving 387 patients, they observed that major vessel involvement, particularly pulmonary artery aneurysm, was the primary cause of mortality in BD [9, 15]. CNS involvement, heart involvement, renal involvement were leading causes of mortality following pulmonary artery aneurysms (PAA) [3, 9, 15–17]. Immunosuppressive treatment with early recognition of vascular involvement is associated with a more positive outcome. Neoplasms were identified as additional contributing factors to mortality and morbidity in BD [3, 14, 16]. Studies conducted by the Pediatric Behçet Disease Study Group and Italian investigators concurred that ocular and neurological involvements are major factors contributing to both mortality and morbidity [18–20].

27.3 Prognosis Related to Disease Severity

The severity of BD significantly influences prognosis, with distinct implications across various age groups. The long-term outcomes and mortality rates differ significantly between patients with only-mucocutaneous symptoms who have a benign course and patients with large vessel and/or major organ involvement. To enhance long-term prognosis and decrease mortality, physicians face the critical challenge of identifying individuals at higher risk for vascular, primarily arterial, involvement. Additionally, they need to pinpoint eye involvement and conduct thorough assessments to detect signs of systemic involvement in patients. A comprehensive study revealed a significantly increased risk of ischemic heart disease, venous thrombosis, and pulmonary embolism in patients with BD [17].

While mucocutaneous symptoms negatively impact the quality of life, their control through treatment is notable, and lesions, particularly in cases of genital ulcers, may heal but not without leaving scars [12]. Conversely, erythema nodosum and papulopustular lesions tend to resolve without long-term consequences [21].

Ophthalmic involvement introduces additional challenges, leading to vision loss and blindness, constituting a major source of morbidity. The outlook for vision has notably advanced in individuals with uveitis due to the introduction of more potent therapeutic options [22]. However, there remains a considerable risk of blindness within the first 5 years, affecting up to 25% of cases [7, 23–25]. Factors associated with an unfavorable visual prognosis include an early onset of the disease, male gender, the presence of skin lesions or arthritis, neurological involvement, vascular thrombosis, recurrent episodes of posterior uveitis (more than three per year dense vitreous opacities, and the existence of retinal infiltrates) [25–27].

Individuals younger than 45 years of age, face a marked excess mortality linked to cardiovascular events (observed/expected = 6.25, $p < 0.001$) highlighting the critical importance of early disease management [14]. These findings underscore the multifaceted nature of BD, emphasizing the importance of tailored analyses of patients considering the varied risks and outcomes associated with different early but severe manifestations of the disease. Physicians should be vigilant about the increased risk of developing stroke/transient ischemic attack, ischemic heart disease, deep venous thrombosis, and pulmonary vascular complications in patients with BD.

27.4 The Course of Behçet's Disease Activity Over Time

Studies indicate that disease activity tends to decrease with advanced age [9]. Particularly those patients presenting with cutaneous and mucosal manifestations, the ailment often exhibited a diminishing trajectory over time [9, 28, 29]. Frequent attacks in the early years of the disease and slowing of disease after 3–7 years is also reported by Shimuzi et al. [30]. This is supported by the 20-year survey of BD patients which indicated that, by the end of the study, 59% of patients did not fulfill the criteria for BD, as the disease naturally fades away over the years [9]. Several outcome surveys demonstrate a trend of declining mortality as time progresses [9, 29]. Interestingly, a recent study reported significant mortality due to hematologic malignancies for patients who died over 65 years of age [14]. Hematologic malignancies are also reported in studies investigating mortality as a cause of death [9, 29].

27.5 Emphasis on the Variation in Prognosis Based on Specific Organ Manifestations

27.5.1 Prognosis in Eye Involvement

Eye involvement is a prevalent aspect of BD and poses a significant threat to vision causing disability and dependency in affected patients. BD-related uveitis is a major contributor to cases of blindness or low vision in regions with a high prevalence of BD. Onset of eye disease occurs within the initial years of the disease and exhibits its most severe progression during this period. Poor prognostic factors, including male gender, posterior segment involvement, strong vitreous opacity, and the presence of exudates alongside retinal vascular arcades, have been identified [24, 27, 31].

While early studies conducted before the 1980s indicated a very poor visual prognosis, recent data suggest an improvement in the visual outcomes of treated patients. Total blindness is often considered the eventual outcome within an average of 3 years after the onset of ocular symptoms [32]. In Japan, about 12% of acquired visual loss in adulthood was attributed to BD and over half of Japanese BD patients lost their sight within 5 years of disease onset [33]. A study from Israel found that 75% of treated patients had lost useful vision 6–10 years after the onset of uveitis [34].

In a review of patient records from 1990 to 1994 and from 2000 to 2004, the authors observed that visual acuity at the latter 3 years significantly improved, with 43/156 [27.6%] eyes having a visual acuity of 20/200 or worse in the first group compared to 26/201 [12.9%] eyes in the second group ($p < 0.001$) [24]. This improvement was attributed to earlier and more aggressive therapeutic approaches, particularly the use of conventional disease-modifying antirheumatic drugs and biologics [23]. However, based on the most recent series, the rate of blindness has persisted, ranging between 11% and 25% [10]. Notably, the bilateral vision loss occurs either during the initial years of follow-up or within the first 5 years following inception, with a substantial decrease thereafter [9].

Several studies have reported a more favorable outcome in recent patient cohorts, possibly attributed to milder disease manifestations and more aggressive and effective treatment involving conventional immunosuppressives, interferon, and biologic therapies such as infliximab and adalimumab [35–38].

27.5.2 Prognosis in Vascular Disease

Vascular involvement in disease is observed in approximately 25–49% of individuals, with a pronounced prevalence in males [1–4, 9–11, 14, 15, 17, 29, 30, 33, 39–43]. Venous involvement is seen more commonly than arterial disease with lower extremity deep vein thrombosis [DVT being the most prevalent manifestation [44]. Other manifestations include vena cava thrombosis, PAA, Budd–Chiari syndrome (BCS), peripheral artery aneurysms, dural sinus thrombosis, and abdominal aorta aneurysms.

DVT typically occurs in the initial years of disease onset, while PAA and BCS are also reported early [44]. Arterial aneurysms, except for PAA, which may be present at disease onset, tend to appear later, with abdominal aorta and peripheral arterial aneurysms developing over a median of 7 years [9, 17]. Relapses are common in DVT patients. Desbois et al. reported long-term outcomes for 296 patients with venous thrombosis, showing that 34% experienced at least one DVT recurrence, and the mortality rate was 6.4% after a median follow-up of 4.75 years [43]. It is noteworthy that in this study, mortality was statistically significantly associated with cardiac involvement and BCS. Moreover, the utilization of immunosuppressants was linked to a reduced recurrence of DVT.

Tascilar et al. analyzed the clinical course of vascular involvement in 882 patients registered between 1977 and 2006, revealing that DVT was the most frequent type of vessel pathology (67.1%) [44]. Recurrent DVT may lead to venous insufficiency and leg ulcers associated with vascular insufficiency.

BCS exhibited the worst outcome among vascular involvement types in BD [45–47]. In a substantial series on 61 BD patients with BCS, the onset of the first symptom and the median age of diagnosis were earlier than BD patients without BCS ($p = 0.005$ and $p = 0.007$) Lower extremity DVT and inferior vena cava (IVC) thrombosis were more common in patients with BCS (all; $p < 0.01$) compared to the control group. Mortality associated with BCS is higher in BD-BCS patients with IVC thrombosis.

PAA represent a serious complication, potentially causing death by massive hemoptysis and reported in mortality studies as the leading cause of death in BD patients. Hamuryudan et al. initially reported that half of the 24 patients PAA died after a mean of 10 months, with a 5-year survival rate of 62% after a 10-year follow-up [15, 48]. However, a later update in 2004 showed significantly fewer deaths [23%] in a group of 26 patients, attributed mainly to earlier recognition and prompt and effective treatment [49]. The researchers emphasized that initiating treatment at an earlier stage could lead to a more positive outcome.

Aortic and peripheral arterial aneurysms are significant causes of death due to the risk of rupture. Tüzün et al. identified 24 male patients with abdominal aorta or peripheral artery aneurysms between 1977 and 1996, with a mortality rate of 17% [40]. Saadoun et al. reported the clinical characteristics and outcome of 101 BD patients with arterial involvement, combining both pulmonary and peripheral arterial aneurysms [42]. After a median follow-up of 7.6 years, 39% achieved complete remission, 28% had a relapsing course. The mortality rate was 14%. A multivariate analysis revealed that the co-presence of venous involvement and arterial thrombosis were negative prognostic factors, while the use of effective immunosuppressant therapy was positively associated with remission in BD. The two decade survival rate was significantly lower in patients with arterial involvement than in those without arterial lesions [42]. Recent studies indicate improved morbidity and mortality rates, underscoring a more favorable prognosis for individuals with vascular involvement. The utilization of effective immunosuppressive therapies has contributed positively to patient outcomes. This underscores the crucial significance of prompt and efficient treatment in enhancing the prognosis of individuals affected by vascular complications.

27.5.3 Prognosis in Cardiac Involvement

Cardiac irregularities observed in individuals with BD encompass pericarditis, myocarditis, endocarditis leading to valvular regurgitation, intracardiac thrombosis, endomyocardial fibrosis, coronary arteritis with or without myocardial infarction, and the development of aneurysms in the coronary arteries or sinus of Valsalva [50–54]. Asymptomatic coronary aneurysms may be detected in the angiography, or may be symptomatic with acute coronary syndrome [50–54]. Aneurysms are usually single, often coexisting with coronary stenosis and occasionally accompanying multiple arterial aneurysms. The most commonly reported cardiac complications in BD involve sinus of Valsalva aneurysms which may lead to chronic aortic failure and aortitis, with a particular predilection for the aortic root [40, 52, 55–57]. The aneurysms may lead to or myocardial infarctions or rupturing of an aneurysm may cause cardiac tamponade [52, 53].

Cardiac involvement in BD may progress through various manifestations, including endocarditis, myocarditis, pericarditis, intracardiac thrombosis, endomyocardial fibrosis, and valve diseases. Among those pericarditis is reported to be the most common cardiac manifestation in some series [51]. The clinical presentation of pericardial involvement varies, encompassing acute pericarditis, hemorrhagic pericardial tamponade, constrictive pericarditis, recurrent pericarditis, or even a small, asymptomatic pericardial effusion [58]. Geri et al. investigated 52 BD patients with cardiac complications for a median follow-up of 3.0 years. At the end of 3 years 15% had died, and the 5-year survival rate was significantly lower among BD patients with cardiac involvement compared to those without [50].

27.5.4 Prognosis in Neuro-Behçet's Disease

Neurological involvement is a major cause of mortality and dependency in BD patients. Studies measuring the outcome of neuro-Behçet's disease (NBD) suggest that 35–45% of patients become disabled over time [6, 51–53]. CNS involvement occurs in 5–25% of individuals with BD, with varying prevalence reported in different studies. Serdaroğlu et al. reported that 5.3% of 323 patients exhibited neurological symptoms within a 1-year follow-up period [54].

BD affects both the central and peripheral nervous systems, leading to parenchymal or nonparenchymal lesions and a wide variety of symptoms associated with the affected region. A recent study of 208 NBD patients revealed that higher initial modified Rankin score and the progressive parenchymal NBD type were the indicators of a poor outcome in this cohort [55]. Parenchymal syndrome can manifest as brain stem symptoms, cranial neuropathy, cerebellar or pyramidal dysfunction, spinal cord involvement, myelopathy, optic neuropathy, and cerebral symptoms like encephalopathy, hemiparesis, hemisensory loss, seizures, dysphasia, and cognitive and mood disturbances. Nonparenchymal syndrome involves vascular manifestations, especially cerebral venous thrombosis, intracranial hypertension, and acute meningeal syndrome [6, 51, 52, 56].

Adult neurological symptoms typically emerge 3–5 years after the systemic onset [2, 3, 18, 31, 33]. Talarico et al. demonstrated in their 117-patient retrospective analysis that CNS involvement usually begins within the first 10 years, with a higher incidence rate in the initial 5 years [57]. Akman-Demir et al. conducted a review involving 200 patients, and among the 110 with a follow-up period of 3 years or more, 28 individuals became either physically or mentally dependent, and 22 succumbed, resulting in a mortality rate of 20% [6]. In Siva et al.'s retrospective assessment spanning 15 years, the mortality ratio was 5.5% [51]. The three patients who died had cerebellopyramidal syndrome, and 45.1% of patients exhibited moderate to severe disability a decade after the disease onset [51]. A Kaplan–Meier analysis revealed survival rates of 95% at 1 year, decreasing to 40% at 10 years [51].

27.5.5 Prognosis in Gastrointestinal Disease

Involvement of BD in the gastrointestinal tract, referred to as "intestinal BD," is characterized by distinctive deep ulcerative lesions in the region of the ileocecal valve, as observed through colonoscopy. Individuals with intestinal BD may experience notable gastrointestinal symptoms like abdominal pain, diarrhea, and gastrointestinal bleeding. However, some patients may be asymptomatic, indicating a dormant disease state. A Korean study tracking the medical records of 130 BD patients with gastrointestinal involvement over at least 5 years revealed the majority (71.5%) experienced remission or mild clinical activity, while the remaining 28.5% had a relapsing course [58]. While intestinal BD is rare, it exhibits a higher prevalence in East Asia, particularly in countries like Korea and Japan, compared to other regions [30]. Gastrointestinal manifestations can lead to severe complications, such as perforation or extensive gastrointestinal bleeding, necessitating intestinal resection. Importantly, intestinal BD is significantly linked to increased morbidity and mortality among patients with BD. A retrospective Turkish study covering 60 patients with a mean follow-up of 7.5 years reported that 80% were in remission, 5% had died from non-gastrointestinal-related causes, 7% were lost to follow-up, and the remaining 8% were still active at the last visit. During follow-up, 20% a relapsing course. Mortality resulting from gastrointestinal involvement is relatively uncommon [59].

27.6 Mortality Trends in Behçet's Disease Over the Years

Mortality is a significant aspect of BD, and Table 27.1 provides a comprehensive overview of key outcome studies. The studies consistently show that male BD patients experience an even higher risk for mortality.

The mortality study by Sadoon et al. reported that 5% of BD patients faced mortality outcomes after a median follow-up of 7.7 years (41/8179) [29]. The average age at the time of death stood at 34.6 ± 11.5 years, with a vast majority, 95.1%, being male. Leading causes of death encompassed major vessel disease, notably arterial aneurysms (26.8%) (pulmonary, thoracic aorta and cerebral arteries) and venous aneurysms

Table 27.1 Mortality patterns and reported death outcomes in Behçet's disease studies

References	Patients (n)	Follow-up (mean years)	Mortality	Comments
Yamamoto et al. [11]	2031	1	1%	
Chajek et al. [39]	41	8	2%	One patient died due to diabetic hyperosmolar coma
Benamour et al. [1]	316	ND	3.2%	
Park et al. [2]	2200	ND	0.3%	85.7% of deaths in this study belong to male patients
Yazıcı et al. [3]	152	10	5%	All of deaths in this study belong to male patients
Seyahi et al. [9]	428	20	10%	92% of deaths in this study belong to male patients
Saadoun et al. [29]	817	7.7	7%	95.1% of deaths in this study belong to male patients
Savey et al. [10]	769	15	5.2%	Male patients have higher hazards ratio: 5.1/1 Mortality rate according to ethnicity: Sub-Saharan African BD 19% North African BD 9% European BD 6%
Lee et al. [13]	19,937	6.06	2.85%	Male-specific mortality: 4.3%
Thomas et al. [17]	1281	5.32	8.5%	Male patients have higher hazards ratio (1.55/1)
David et al. [14]	328 BD associated deaths out of 20,460,583 deaths between 1979 and 2016		0.15/1,000,0000 person-years standardized mortality rate Main causes were arterial (n = 73, 22%) infections (n = 69, 21%) Mean age at death for men: 52.8 (±11.3), women: 58.4 (±16.5) (versus 71.2 and 79.8 in the general population)	

(17.1%) including BCS and PAA, solid organ and hematologic malignancies (14.6%), and CNS involvement (12.2%) and sepsis (12.2%). The mortality rate at 5 years was 3.3%. Of significance, there was an escalated mortality rate within the 15–24-year age group (standardized mortality ratio (SMR) with a 95% confidence interval, 2.99 (1.54–5.39)) and the 25–34-year age group (SMR 2.90 (1.80–4.49)), in comparison to age- and sex-matched healthy controls. The mortality trend exhibited a decrease in patients aged over 35 years (SMR, 1.23 (0.75–1.92)). In a multivariate analysis, male gender (hazard ratio (HR): 4.94, CI: 1.53–16.43), arterial involvement (HR: 2.51, CI: 1.07–5.90), and a high frequency of BD flares (HR: 2.37, CI: 1.09–5.14) were identified as independent factors associated with mortality. It is crucial to emphasize that the reported neurological involvement rate (26.9%) and the arterial involvement rate (13.9%) in this cohort exceeds the expected ratios in a general BD cohort. The elevated mortality rates observed are primarily attributed to patients with significant organ involvement.

Yazıcı et al. reported a 5% mortality rate in a 10-year survey involving 152 patients. The data on outcomes is available for 120 patients, and within this study, six patients, all male, succumbed [3]. The causes of death were diverse, including PAA (n = 3), gastrointestinal hemorrhage (potentially BCS) (n = 1), NBD (n = 1), and cerebrovascular events (n = 1) [3].

In another study by Park et al. among 2200 registered BD patients, seven deaths were reported, resulting in a mortality rate of 0.3% in the cohort [2]. The mean follow-up until death was 6.5 years, with the average age of death being 39.1. The causes of death mirrored those observed in previous studies, including bowel perforation, large vessel diseases, NBD, and sepsis due to immunosuppression [2].

In the two-decade outcome hospital-based survey of Kural-Seyahi et al. 42 patients (39 males and 3 females constituting 10% of the cohort) had succumbed by the conclusion of the study period [9]. Notably, the mortality rate exhibited a notable gender disparity, with males experiencing a significantly higher rate compared to females (39/286 vs. 3/142, $p = 0.001$). SMRs were particularly elevated among young males in the 14–24 and 25–34 age groups, while older males (35–50 age group and females demonstrated a life span consistent with the general population. Additionally, the mortality rate exhibited a peak within the initial 7 years of disease onset, subsequently demonstrating a tendency to decrease over time [9]. Deceased patients exhibited a higher incidence of major organ involvement, including ocular, large vessel, and CNS manifestations at disease onset, compared to their surviving counterparts. Probable causes of mortality associated with BD encompassed large vessel disease, particularly PAA (n = 17), parenchymal CNS disease (n = 5), neoplasms (n = 4), chronic renal failure (n = 4), ischemic heart disease (n = 3), and congestive heart failure/stroke (n = 3) [9]. This cohort originates from a tertiary rheumatology center in Türkiye, where a notable prevalence of major organ involvement is common. It is essential to acknowledge that this characteristic might have influenced the observed mortality outcomes, as the high rate of major organ involvement in this specific cohort could contribute to an atypical mortality pattern (n = 3) [9].

Several outcome surveys exhibit the pattern of decreasing mortality over time [9, 29]. However, one particular study from South Korea, utilizing the National Health Insurance Service database, presented contradictory results [13]. In their cohort (n = 19,937) with female predominance (female: 13,435) a total of 570 deaths occurred after a mean follow-up of 6.06 years. The mortality rate was elevated with advanced age [13]. This observation persisted even after adjusting for age, sex, diabetes mellitus, hypertension, dyslipidemia status, household income, and habitat. Discrepancies in these results may be attributed to methodological differences, the diagnostic criteria and clinical recognition of the disease, the retrospective nature of the analyses, the variations in disease expression in different countries.

In 2020, a comprehensive analysis involving 1281 patients diagnosed with BD was conducted, comparing them with 5124 controls carefully matched for age and gender [17]. The findings revealed a significantly heightened risk of ischemic heart disease (adjusted hazard ratio (aHR)

3.09 (1.28–7.44)), venous thrombosis (aHR 4.80 (2.42–9.54)), and overall mortality (aHR 1.40 (1.07–1.84 in BD patients compared to their corresponding controls. Moreover, BD patients demonstrated an elevated risk of pulmonary embolism at baseline (adjusted odds ratio 4.64 (2.66–8.09 $P < 0.0001$) [17]. The authors also reported elevated risk of developing ischemic heart disease, stroke, transient ischemic attacks, and deep vein thrombosis at an earlier age in patients with BD compared with the population. It is important to highlight that pulmonary embolism is infrequently reported in BD due to tightly adherent thrombosis. The authors propose that pulmonary thrombosis may occur in situ as a result of localized endothelial dysfunction or pulmonary vasculitis, rather than manifesting as pulmonary embolism.

In 2022, BD related mortality was investigated using multiple cause of death analysis [14]. Between 1979 and 2016, 328 death certificates out of 20,460,583 recorded deaths mentioned BD as either the underlying cause of death in 171 cases or a non-underlying cause of death in 157 cases. The average age at death was notably lower for both men and women, standing at 52.8 years for men and 58.4 years for women. This contrasted sharply with the general population's average life expectancy of 71.2 years for men and 79.8 years for women. Additionally, the study revealed that 64% of the deceased individuals were males. BD-related deaths showed distinct patterns: individuals younger than 45 years old were more likely to die from cardiovascular events (observed/expected = 6.25, $p < 0.001$), while those older than 45 years of age were more prone to die from infections (observed/expected = 9.69, $p < 0.001$) [14].

These studies indicate that despite the application of advanced therapies and the use of biologic treatments, mortality remains a substantial concern in individuals with BD.

27.7 Prognostic Indicators, Regular Check-Ups, and Monitoring

In geographical regions with a high prevalence of BD it is crucial to inform patients experiencing recurrent aphthous stomatitis about BD and its associated symptoms. Oral aphthous ulcers often serve as the initial manifestation of the disease, preceding the fulfilment of full diagnostic criteria by approximately to 6 years [12].

Limtong et al. suggest that the location of oral aphthous lesions may be associated with the disease activity. The buccal location of oral aphthae suggests a lower disease activity, whereas minor oral ulcers arising on the tonsils may signal a higher disease activity or an attack [60].

The 2020 UK study shows that the majority of patients experiencing pulmonary vascular complications and subsequently diagnosed with BD had pulmonary thrombosis before the BD diagnosis was made (n = 28/32, 87.5%) [17]. This data underscores the critical significance of early detection of life-threatening symptoms in patients, beginning from the onset of the disease.

The clinical prognostic factors outlined in prior studies predominantly include male gender, young age, and the occurrence of frequent and severe attacks. Figure 27.1 illustrates the causes of mortality and organ-specific morbidities observed in individuals with BD based on the extent of organ involvement. Special attention can be directed towards male patients in the age range of 20–40 years and the first 5 years of the disease onset. Another noteworthy information is that the onset of eye involvement typically manifests within the initial 5 years of the disease.

Patients diagnosed with BD should undergo regular monitoring, including physical examinations and blood tests assessing acute phase reactants. Physicians need to inquire about symptoms indicating major organ involvement, such as bloody stool, hemoptysis, and balance difficulties. In follow-up sessions, it is essential to inquire about headaches, as they emerge as the predominant neurological symptom in NBD patients. Additionally, patients should be examined for skin lesions, collateral veins at the posterior of the legs, variations in leg circumference, and the presence of collateral veins in the abdominal wall, inguinal area, and chest. Routine ophthalmic examinations every 6 months during the first 5 years is recommended even in BD patients who do not report significant eye symptoms in follow-up.

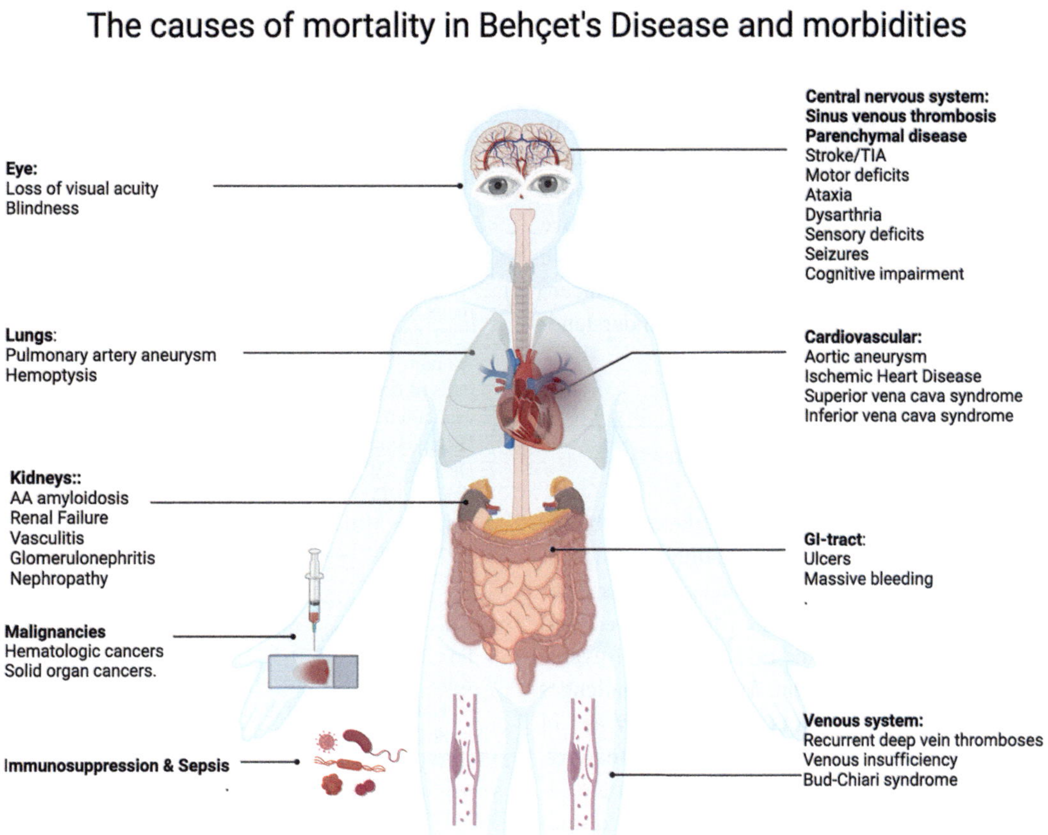

Fig. 27.1 The causes of mortality in Behçet's Disease and morbidities. (Created with BioRender.com)

During follow-up, caution is essential as studies suggest an elevated risk of hematologic malignancies in BD patients, particularly those aged over 65 [14]. Additionally, the effective utilization of immunosuppressants results in chronic immunosuppression, heightening the vulnerability of patients to infections. It is crucial to ensure proper vaccination recommendations are provided to mitigate these risks effectively.

This comprehensive approach aims to ensure early detection of symptoms, prompt intervention, and effective management for individuals affected by BD.

27.8 Patient Education on Recognizing and Reporting Symptoms

Effective management of BD relies significantly on patient education regarding symptom recognition and reporting. Achieving remission hinges on patient adherence to therapy, a factor underscored by a prior study revealing that roughly half of BD patients were non-adherent to prescribed treatments [37]. Predictors of nonadherence included male sex, low income, and a lack of awareness regarding the consequences of BD. This shows that patients need to be made aware of the severe complications and the associated risk of mortality.

Patients should receive comprehensive education about the broad spectrum of potential signs of BD, ranging from mucocutaneous symptoms, and eye involvement to systemic symptoms such as vascular complications. Additionally, they should be informed about the possible constitutional symptoms that may arise during attacks. For example patients should understand that prolonged headaches, dizziness and any kind of a new neurological symptom may signal neurological involvement. Edema or pain in one leg or the development of new visible collateral veins could be associated with BD. Eye symptoms such as pain, blurry vision, and redness should alert patients to seek medical attention.

By fostering awareness and understanding, individuals afflicted with BD can play an active role in monitoring their health, promptly identifying emerging symptoms, and reporting changes to their healthcare providers. This proactive approach empowers patients and contributes to a more collaborative and responsive healthcare journey, ensuring a comprehensive understanding of their condition.

27.9 Conclusion

In conclusion, BD presents a multifaceted clinical landscape with diverse manifestations that significantly impact prognosis. Advances in therapeutic interventions have contributed to improved outcomes, particularly in the management of uveitis and systemic involvement. However, challenges persist, and certain factors, such as early age of onset, male gender, and specific clinical features, continue to pose risks for adverse prognosis. Studies consistently underscore an elevated mortality rate, particularly among males.

Vascular complications and systemic involvement contribute substantially to the mortality risk, emphasizing the need for targeted interventions. While advancements in treatment have positively influenced outcomes, challenges remain in mitigating mortality risks, necessitating a nuanced understanding of contributing factors. Vigilant monitoring, timely intervention, and patient education play pivotal roles in enhancing long-term outcomes. The identification of high-risk individuals, recognition of varied symptoms, and addressing potential complications, such as vascular involvement, remain essential components of a comprehensive approach to BD management.

References

1. Benamour S, Zeroual B, Bennis R, Amraoui A, Bettal S. Behcet's disease. 316 cases. Presse Med. 1990;19(32):1485–9.
2. Park KD, Bang D, Lee ES, Lee SH, Lee S. Clinical study on death in Behcet's disease. J Korean Med Sci. 1993;8(4):241–5.
3. Yazici H, Basaran G, Hamuryudan V, Hizli N, Yurdakul S, Mat C, et al. The ten-year mortality in Behcet's syndrome. Br J Rheumatol. 1996;35(2):139–41.
4. Yazici H, Tuzun Y, Pazarli H, Yurdakul S, Ozyazgan Y, Ozdogan H, et al. Influence of age of onset and patient's sex on the prevalence and severity of manifestations of Behcet's syndrome. Ann Rheum Dis. 1984;43(6):783–9.
5. Leccese P, Padula MC, Lascaro N, Padula AA, D'Angelo S. Clinical phenotypes of Behcet's syndrome in a large cohort of Italian patients: focus on gender differences. Scand J Rheumatol. 2021;50(6):475–8.
6. Akman-Demir G, Serdaroglu P, Tasci B. Clinical patterns of neurological involvement in Behcet's disease: evaluation of 200 patients. The Neuro-Behcet Study Group Brain. 1999;122(Pt 11):2171–82.
7. Desbois AC, Terrada C, Cacoub P, Bodaghi B, Saadoun D. Ocular manifestations in Behcet's disease. Rev Med Interne. 2018;39(9):738–45.
8. Serpa Pinto L, Xavier Pires S, Silva B, Farinha F, Vasconcelos C, Araujo CJ. Predictive factors of severe Behcet's disease: a longitudinal, prospective cohort followed between 1981-2020. Reumatol Clin (Engl Ed). 2022;18(7):410–5.
9. Kural-Seyahi E, Fresko I, Seyahi N, Ozyazgan Y, Mat C, Hamuryudan V, et al. The long-term mortality and morbidity of Behcet syndrome: a 2-decade outcome survey of 387 patients followed at a dedicated center. Medicine (Baltimore). 2003;82(1):60–76.
10. Savey L, Resche-Rigon M, Wechsler B, Comarmond C, Piette JC, Cacoub P, Saadoun D. Ethnicity and association with disease manifestations and mortality in Behcet's disease. Orphanet J Rare Dis. 2014;9:42.
11. Yamamoto S-i. A nation-wide survey of Behcet's disease in Japan-1-epidemiological survey. Jpn J Ophthalmol: the Official International Journal of the Japanese Ophthalmological Society. 1974;18(3):282–90.
12. Gurler A, Boyvat A, Tursen U. Clinical manifestations of Behcet's disease: an analysis of 2147 patients. Yonsei Med J. 1997;38(6):423–7.
13. Lee YB, Lee SY, Choi JY, Lee JH, Chae HS, Kim JW, et al. Incidence, prevalence, and mortality of Adamantiades-Behcet's disease in Korea: a nation-wide, population-based study (2006-2015). J Eur Acad Dermatol Venereol. 2018;32(6):999–1003.
14. David E, Fauvernier M, Saadoun D, Gerfaud-Valentin M, Maurcort-Boulch D, Seve P, Jamilloux Y. Mortality associated with Behcet's disease in France assessed by multiple-cause-of-death analysis. Clin Rheumatol. 2022;41(6):1749–58.
15. Hamuryudan V, Yurdakul S, Moral F, Numan F, Tuzun H, Tuzuner N, et al. Pulmonary arterial aneurysms in Behcet's syndrome: a report of 24 cases. Br J Rheumatol. 1994;33(1):48–51.
16. Yazici H, Esen F. Mortality in Behcet's syndrome. Clin Exp Rheumatol. 2008;26(5 Suppl 51):S138–40.
17. Thomas T, Chandan JS, Subramanian A, Gokhale K, Gkoutos G, Harper L, et al. Epidemiology, morbidity and mortality in Behcet's disease: a cohort study

using The Health Improvement Network (THIN). Rheumatology (Oxford). 2020;59(10):2785–95.
18. Li C, Li L, Wu X, Shi J, Liu J, Zhou J, et al. Clinical manifestations of Behcet's disease in a large cohort of Chinese patients: gender- and age-related differences. Clin Rheumatol. 2020;39(11):3449–54.
19. Gallizzi R, Pidone C, Cantarini L, Finetti M, Cattalini M, Filocamo G, et al. A national cohort study on pediatric Behcet's disease: cross-sectional data from an Italian registry. Pediatr Rheumatol Online J. 2017;15(1):84.
20. Kone-Paut I, Shahram F, Darce-Bello M, Cantarini L, Cimaz R, Gattorno M, et al. Consensus classification criteria for paediatric Behcet's disease from a prospective observational cohort: PEDBD. Ann Rheum Dis. 2016;75(6):958–64.
21. Vural S, Boyvat A. The skin in Behçet's disease: mucocutaneous findings and differential diagnosis. JEADV Clinical Practice. 2022;1(1):11–20.
22. Abolhasani S, Khabbazi A, Hosseini F, Gholizadeh-Ghaleh Aziz S, Alipour S. Effects of anti-TNF biologic drugs on uveitis severity in Behcet patients: systematic review and meta-analysis. Int J Ophthalmol. 2022;15(5):813–9.
23. Saadoun D, Cassoux N, Wechsler B, Boutin D, Terrada C, Lehoang P, et al. Ocular manifestations of Behcet's disease. Rev Med Interne. 2010;31(8):545–50.
24. Cingu AK, Onal S, Urgancioglu M, Tugal-Tutkun I. Comparison of presenting features and three-year disease course in Turkish patients with Behcet uveitis who presented in the early 1990s and the early 2000s. Ocul Immunol Inflamm. 2012;20(6):423–8.
25. Tugal-Tutkun I, Onal S, Altan-Yaycioglu R, Huseyin Altunbas H, Urgancioglu M. Uveitis in Behcet disease: an analysis of 880 patients. Am J Ophthalmol. 2004;138(3):373–80.
26. Ksiaa I, Abroug N, Kechida M, Zina S, Jelliti B, Khochtali S, et al. Eye and Behcet's disease. J Fr Ophtalmol. 2019;42(6):626–41.
27. Takeuchi M, Hokama H, Tsukahara R, Kezuka T, Goto H, Sakai J, Usui M. Risk and prognostic factors of poor visual outcome in Behcet's disease with ocular involvement. Graefes Arch Clin Exp Ophthalmol. 2005;243(11):1147–52.
28. Uskudar Cansu D, Korkmaz C. Age-related immunosenescence in Behcet's disease. Rheumatol Int. 2022;42(9):1513–22.
29. Saadoun D, Wechsler B, Desseaux K, Le Thi HD, Amoura Z, Resche-Rigon M, Cacoub P. Mortality in Behcet's disease. Arthritis Rheum. 2010;62(9):2806–12.
30. Shimizu T, Ehrlich GE, Inaba G, Hayashi K. Behcet disease (Behcet syndrome). Semin Arthritis Rheum. 1979;8(4):223–60.
31. Sakamoto M, Akazawa K, Nishioka Y, Sanui H, Inomata H, Nose Y. Prognostic factors of vision in patients with Behcet disease. Ophthalmology. 1995;102(2):317–21.
32. Mamo JG, Baghdassarian A. Behcet's disease; a report of 28 cases. Arch Ophthalmol. 1964;71:4–14.
33. Mishima S, Masuda K, Izawa Y, Mochizuki M, Namba K. The eighth Frederick H. Verhoeff lecture. Presented by Saiichi Mishima, MD Behcet's disease in Japan: ophthalmologic aspects. Trans Am Ophthalmol Soc. 1979;77:225–79.
34. Benezra D, Cohen E. Treatment and visual prognosis in Behcet's disease. Br J Ophthalmol. 1986;70(8):589–92.
35. Tugal-Tutkun I, Mudun A, Urgancioglu M, Kamali S, Kasapoglu E, Inanc M, Gul A. Efficacy of infliximab in the treatment of uveitis that is resistant to treatment with the combination of azathioprine, cyclosporine, and corticosteroids in Behcet's disease: an open-label trial. Arthritis Rheum. 2005;52(8):2478–84.
36. Diwo E, Gueudry J, Saadoun D, Weschler B, LeHoang P, Bodaghi B. Long-term efficacy of interferon in severe uveitis associated with Behcet disease. Ocul Immunol Inflamm. 2017;25(1):76–84.
37. Alizadegan F, Yalcinbayir O, Ucan Gunduz G, Pehlivan Y. Infliximab therapy in Behcet's uveitis. J Fr Ophtalmol. 2022;45(9):1036–41.
38. Tugal-Tutkun I. Uveitis in Behcet disease—an update. Curr Opin Rheumatol. 2023;35(1):17–24.
39. Chajek T, Fainaru M. Behcet's disease. Report of 41 cases and a review of the literature. Medicine (Baltimore). 1975;54(3):179–96.
40. Tuzun H, Besirli K, Sayin A, Vural FS, Hamuryudan V, Hizli N, et al. Management of aneurysms in Behcet's syndrome: an analysis of 24 patients. Surgery. 1997;121(2):150–6.
41. Seyahi E, Melikoglu M, Akman C, Hamuryudan V, Ozer H, Hatemi G, et al. Pulmonary artery involvement and associated lung disease in Behcet disease: a series of 47 patients. Medicine (Baltimore). 2012;91(1):35–48.
42. Saadoun D, Asli B, Wechsler B, Houman H, Geri G, Desseaux K, et al. Long-term outcome of arterial lesions in Behcet disease: a series of 101 patients. Medicine (Baltimore). 2012;91(1):18–24.
43. Desbois AC, Wechsler B, Resche-Rigon M, Piette JC, Huong Dle T, Amoura Z, et al. Immunosuppressants reduce venous thrombosis relapse in Behcet's disease. Arthritis Rheum. 2012;64(8):2753–60.
44. Tascilar K, Melikoglu M, Ugurlu S, Sut N, Caglar E, Yazici H. Vascular involvement in Behcet's syndrome: a retrospective analysis of associations and the time course. Rheumatology (Oxford). 2014;53(11):2018–22.
45. Akyol L, Toz B, Bayindir O, Zengin O, Cansu D, Yigit M, et al. Budd-Chiari syndrome in Behcet's disease: a retrospective multicenter study. Clin Rheumatol. 2022;41(1):177–86.
46. Seyahi E, Caglar E, Ugurlu S, Kantarci F, Hamuryudan V, Sonsuz A, et al. An outcome survey of 43 patients with Budd-Chiari syndrome due to Behcet's syndrome followed up at a single, dedicated center. Semin Arthritis Rheum. 2015;44(5):602–9.
47. Sakr MA, Reda MA, Ebada HE, Abdelmoaty AS, Hefny ZM, Ibrahim ZH, Aboelmaaty ME. Characteristics and outcome of primary Budd-

Chiari syndrome due to Behcet's syndrome. Clin Res Hepatol Gastroenterol. 2020;44(4):503–12.
48. Hamuryudan V, Er T, Seyahi E, Akman C, Tuzun H, Fresko I, et al. Pulmonary artery aneurysms in Behcet syndrome. Am J Med. 2004;117(11):867–70.
49. Hamuryudan V, Seyahi E, Ugurlu S, Melikoglu M, Hatemi G, Ozguler Y, et al. Pulmonary artery involvement in Behcet's syndrome: effects of anti-Tnf treatment. Semin Arthritis Rheum. 2015;45(3):369–73.
50. Geri G, Wechsler B, Thi Huong DL, Isnard R, Piette JC, Amoura Z, et al. Spectrum of cardiac lesions in Behcet disease: a series of 52 patients and review of the literature. Medicine (Baltimore). 2012;91(1):25–34.
51. Siva A, Kantarci OH, Saip S, Altintas A, Hamuryudan V, Islak C, et al. Behcet's disease: diagnostic and prognostic aspects of neurological involvement. J Neurol. 2001;248(2):95–103.
52. Sorgun MH, Kural MA, Yucesan C. Clinical characteristics and prognosis of neuro-Behcet's disease. Eur J Rheumatol. 2018;5(4):235–9.
53. Yan D, Liu J, Zhang Y, Yuan W, Xu Y, Shi J, et al. The clinical features and risk factors of parenchymal neuro-Behcet's disease. J Immunol Res. 2019;2019:7371458.
54. Serdaroglu P, Yazici H, Ozdemir C, Yurdakul S, Bahar S, Aktin E. Neurologic involvement in Behcet's syndrome. A prospective study. Arch Neurol. 1989;46(3):265–9.
55. Sahin Eroglu D, Torgutalp M, Yucesan C, Sezer S, Yayla ME, Boyvat A, Ates A. Prognostic factors for relapse and poor outcome in neuro-Behcet's syndrome: results from a clinical long-term follow-up of a single centre. J Neurol. 2022;269(4):2046–54.
56. Noel N, Bernard R, Wechsler B, Resche-Rigon M, Depaz R, D LTHB, et al. Long-term outcome of neuro-Behcet's disease. Arthritis Rheumatol. 2014;66(5):1306–14.
57. Talarico R, d'Ascanio A, Figus M, Stagnaro C, Ferrari C, Elefante E, et al. Behcet's disease: features of neurological involvement in a dedicated centre in Italy. Clin Exp Rheumatol. 2012;30(3 Suppl 72):S69–72.
58. Jung YS, Cheon JH, Park SJ, Hong SP, Kim TI, Kim WH. Clinical course of intestinal Behcet's disease during the first five years. Dig Dis Sci. 2013;58(2):496–503.
59. Hatemi I, Esatoglu SN, Hatemi G, Erzin Y, Yazici H, Celik AF. Characteristics, treatment, and long-term outcome of gastrointestinal involvement in Behcet's syndrome: a strobe-compliant observational study from a dedicated multidisciplinary center. Medicine (Baltimore). 2016;95(16):e3348.
60. Limtong P, Chanprapaph K, Vachiramon V, Ngamjanyaporn P. Cutaneous and extracutaneous manifestations of Behcet's disease linked to its disease activity and prognosis. Clin Cosmet Investig Dermatol. 2020;13:639–47.

Future Directions of Behcet's Disease

28

Haner Direskeneli

Contents

As with any disease with a chronic, multisystemic course with multifactorial etiology, Behcet's disease has numerous areas requiring further definition and understanding. In this section, we will discuss some of the areas that need further research.

28.1 Clarifying Epidemiology—Changing Trends

The epidemiology of Behcet's disease seems to be changing in recent years [1]. Data from countries with reliable registries and a high prevalence of BD (Japan and Korea) suggest a decreasing incidence of BD [2, 3]. Several factors may contribute to this decrease including triggering factors (such as decreasing infections or increasing allergies and changes in diet, etc.), disease modulation with early diagnosis and treatment and shifts in demographics such as immigration or an increase in the elderly populations. However, similar observations are lacking from other countries with a high prevalence of BD such as Middle Eastern countries or southern Europe. Nevertheless, differences in the prevalence of BD is reported in immigrant populations (among citizens of Turkish ethnicity in Türkiye vs Germany) [4]. Further studies utilizing comprehensive country-wide registries such as in East Asia might enable investigators to determine whether these epidemiological trends are present worldwide with potential implications for understanding disease pathogenesis and for health economics.

H. Direskeneli (✉)
Division of Rheumatology, Department of Internal Medicine, Marmara University, School of Medicine, Istanbul, Türkiye
e-mail: haner@marmara.edu.tr

E. Alpsoy et al. (eds.), *Behçet's Disease: An Integrated Approach*,
https://doi.org/10.1007/978-3-031-77251-1_28

Another crucial observation is the change in disease clusters/subtypes. Studies, especially from Japan, suggest that ocular BD is decreasing among patients with noninfectious uveitis whereas gastrointestinal manifestations, incomplete BD, and HLA-B51* negativity are increasingly reported [5]. Again, the reasons are not clear; however, this trend might be explained with the microbial dysbiosis discussed in other chapters, as an increase in inflammatory bowel disease is also observed in Japan due to Western-type diet habits. Changes in milder phenotypes such as mucocutaneous BD can also be expected due to earlier use of immunosuppressive treatments, although other contributing factors warrant exploration.

28.2 Pathogenesis

Recent advances in understanding the pathogenesis of BD have provided insights into immune mechanisms and the classification of BD among immune-mediated inflammatory diseases (IMIDs). BD is first thought to be an "autoimmune" disorder with limited number of autoantibodies and CD4+ T-cell responses [6]. Clinical responses to T-cell suppressive agents such as calcineurin inhibitors supported this hypothesis. However, anti-nuclear antibodies, the hallmark of autoimmunity, are lacking and autoantibodies shown are usually nonspecific or nonpathogenic (anti-endothelial cell, anti-phospholipid antibodies). Classical associations of MHC class II are also not present in BD.

Recent studies shed some light on the role of the genetic association of BD with HLA-B*51 allele [7]. As an MHC class-I allele, B*51 should interact with CD8+ T-cells with short-length (8–9 amino acids) peptides and HLA-B51*/ERAP1/hap 10+ cells are shown to stimulate CD8+ T-cell responses [8]. Naïve/effector CD8+ T-cell shifts in affected carriers provided evidence of the biological relevance of *ERAP1-Hap10/HLA-B*51* at the cellular level pointing to an HLA-B*51-restricted process. MHC-I-associated disorders are not classified as autoimmune, and the term "MHC-I-opathy" is offered for spondyloarthritis-group disorders such as ankylosing spondylitis, psoriasis, inflammatory bowel disease, and BD, all with separate MHC Class I associations [9]. Among the immune mechanisms leading to pathogenesis, local mechanical stress factors (skin trauma, tendon stress, etc.), and IL-23/IL-17 immune signaling seem more prominent in MHC-I-opathy-associated disorders.

BD is also classified among "autoinflammatory" disorders with augmented innate-immune responses. The ever-increasing number of innate-immune activation mechanisms such as inflammasome/interferonopathies and NfKB pathway responses seem to be important especially in the early activation of BD [10].

The classification of BD among IMIDs is important to understand the possible therapeutic role of currently increasing number of biological agents (anti-cytokine, anti-cell therapies, or signal inhibitors). Further studies in BD will clarify the role of HLA-B*51/ERAP1/hap 10 restricted CD8+ T-cell responses and other possible B-51*-associated immune activations such as NK/ILC cell/HLA interactions. Role of autoinflammation will be better understood in BD with possible neutrophil/monocyte activation mechanisms linked to autoinflammatory gene/signal transduction pathways.

BD also extensively involves the venous vascular system including the central nervous system and ocular veins as well as similar structures such as pulmonary arteries [11, 12]. Both tissue studies and noninvasive imaging methods such as Doppler US and MR venography will further demonstrate the role of venous inflammation in BD pathogenesis in the future [13, 14].

Although males are known to have a more severe disease course in BD, this also has never been fully understood. Immune factors such as augmented innate immune responses as well as suppression of T-cell responses with estrogen (and vice versa with testosterone) are previously shown [15]. Recently, the genetic load is also shown to be higher in males [16]. However, the number of studies is limited and further research is warranted.

28.2.1 Diagnosis of BD

Diagnosing BD remains problematic due to few pathognomonic clinical features, serum/transcriptomic/genetic biomarkers, or diagnostic imaging. The dominant role of "expert opinion" is reflected in the so-called BD diagnostic criteria (though they would be more accurately defined as classification criteria for clinical studies). Except for the pathergy (skin prick) reaction, all other items are clinically defined organ manifestations in the most commonly used International Study Group (ISG) criteria, International Criteria for BD (ICBD), or Japanese diagnostic criteria of BD sets. As expected, increasing the number of organ manifestations in these criteria improves sensitivity but at the cost of specificity compared to expert opinion for diagnosing BD in routine practice.

Although expert opinion is still the gold standard, the unmet need of less-experienced clinicians for diagnostic tools will possibly stimulate further research in this field. One of the prominent developments in this area comes from the efforts to improve the sensitivity of pathergy reaction with immune-triggering stimuli such as bacterial antigens. Pneumococcal vaccine is the most promising of these agents for standardization and validation [17]. Another approach is using a cost-effective, fast, and practical imaging method such as ultrasound and recent demonstration of increased "venous-wall thickness" in common femoral vein of BD patients with Doppler US is an important new step [13, 18]. Further studies will show the feasibility of these methods in routine practice with validation studies in multiethnic cohorts.

28.3 Disease Assessment

Disease assessment in BD requires a multisystemic approach to different organ manifestations. Typically each organ manifestation is evaluated through patient and physician global assessments based on expert opinion in routine practice. For mucocutaneous lesions, oral and genital ulcer numbers, duration of ulcers, and pain are assessed, with new oral ulcer numbers considered the primary outcome in clinical trials. Similarly, the number, duration, and pain associated with nodular lesions are determined. Major organ manifestations are usually evaluated using activity and relapse/flare numbers. Although previously validated ocular scores such as standardization of uveitis nomenclature (SUN), neurological disability scores for multiple sclerosis, and vascular post-thrombotic scores are helpful, they are primarily used in clinical trials [19]. Future studies will clarify the use of these scoring systems, as well as multisystemic BD-specific tools such as the Behçet's Disease Current Activity Form (BDCAF) and Behçet's Disease Activity Index (BDAI). A BD-specific damage score is also validated in different studies and will help to assess disease and treatment-related long-term damage in BD.

A new approach to disease assessment is pursued by OMERACT (outcome measures in clinical trials) BD study interest group. A set of core outcomes for clinical trials in BD are defined by OMERACT including five domains mandatory for study in all trials in BD (disease activity, new organ involvement, quality of life, adverse events, and death) with additional subdomains mandatory for study of specific organ systems [20]. OMERACT BD Study interest group now aims to develop and validate instruments for each organ manifestation such as a mucocutaneous index, an ocular score, or a vascular tool. A minimal clinically acceptable state for oral ulcers is also studied. As patient input is increasingly required both for routine practice and clinical trials, several generic tools such as SF-36, fatigue, or sleep scales are studied in BD. However, disease-specific patient-reported outcome tools are insufficiently studied in clinical trials and not used in routine practice. However, patient and physicians-based tools possibly measure different aspects of disease state and have a limited effect on each other in BD [21].

28.4 Future Approach to Therapeutic Aspects in BD

Primary outcomes for the therapeutic aims in BD still needs further studies. Most studies aim to prevent relapse/flares of different organ manifestations; however, whether all relapses lead to organ damage is not clear. Some aggressive regimens such as "treat-to-target" approaches aim "complete remission" which is both difficult to attain and require extensive immune-suppressive use which might lead to increased side effects such as infections or malignancies [22]. A recent study demonstrated that aggressive cyclophosphamide use in young males for vascular or neurological disease have caused significant infertility in BD patients [23]. Although current regimens for refractory major organ disease with more biological use such as anti-TNF agents have less side effects such as infections or infertility compared to high-dose glucocorticosteroids or cyclophosphamide, there is still an unmet need to better understand the disease course for each different manifestation of BD. In the opposite side, mucocutaneous lesions such as oral ulcers are usually insufficiently treated in BD patients as they do not cause organ damage. However, oral quality-of-life (QoL) studies with patient-reported outcomes (PROs) demonstrated poor oral QoL of BD patients with difficulty due to oral ulcers in such daily activities as talking, chewing, etc. [24]. Although immunosuppressive drugs usually suppress mucocutaneous lesions, reluctance of clinicians to use them for mucocutaneous lesions is understandable as they increase infection risk. Agents such as apremilast have a better efficacy/safety ratio; however, their use is currently limited by reimbursement issues due to high cost.

In this context, non-pharmacological approaches such as dental/periodental care to decrease oral ulcers are also underused in BD. As a healthy dental/periodental mouth leads to less oral ulcers, oral medicine approaches should be better incorporated into clinical practice and take part in clinical research spectrum [25]. Similarly, prevention and protection against severe post-thrombotic syndrome require more than just immunosuppressive or anti-coagulant treatments. Compression socks and exercise should be a part of clinical approach to patients with recurrent deep venous thrombosis (DVT) and post-thrombotic syndrome (PTS). Finally, psychosocial support is a crucial part of rare and chronic diseases such as BD. Patients usually describe unexpected fatigue, musculoskeletal pains, and depressive symptoms even with only mild mucocutaneous disease. The broader health issues of BD patients should be better explored with patient-reported outcome tools in-person/group meetings, support groups, and personal approach to individual psycosocial problems.

As a rare disease (<1:2000) especially in Caucasian populations, the research efforts for BD are hampered by low patient numbers, limited clinician interest, or funding problems from governmental agencies or pharmaceutical industry. Better collaboration between all stakeholders (physicians, patients, health professionals, basic and clinical scientists, and Pharma) is required for a better future for our patients.

References

1. Direskeneli H, Mumcu G. A possible decline in the incidence and severity of Behcet's disease: implications for an infectious etiology and oral health. Clin Exp Rheumatol. 2010;28(4 Suppl 60):S86–90.
2. Iwata D, Namba K, Yamamoto T, Mizuuchi K, Saito W, Ohno S, et al. Recent clinical features of intraocular inflammation in Hokkaido, Japan—comparison with the previous decade. Ocul Immunol Inflamm. 2022;30(4):848–54.
3. Jun JB, Kim HJ, Kazmi SZ, Kang T, Kim KB, Kang MJ, Ahn HS. Significant decline in the incidence of Behcet's disease in South Korea: a Nationwide population-based study (2004–2017). Arthritis Care Res (Hoboken). 2021;73(11):1689–96.
4. Papoutsis NG, Abdel-Naser MB, Altenburg A, Orawa H, Kotter I, Krause L, et al. Prevalence of Adamantiades-Behcet's disease in Germany and the municipality of Berlin: results of a nationwide survey. Clin Exp Rheumatol. 2006;24(5 Suppl 42):S125.
5. Soejima Y, Kirino Y, Takeno M, Kurosawa M, Takeuchi M, Yoshimi R, et al. Changes in the proportion of clinical clusters contribute to the phenotypic evolution of Behcet's disease in Japan. Arthritis Res Ther. 2021;23(1):49.

6. Direskeneli H. Autoimmunity vs autoinflammation in Behcet's disease: do we oversimplify a complex disorder? Rheumatology (Oxford). 2006;45(12):1461–5.
7. Ortiz Fernandez L, Coit P, Yilmaz V, Yentur SP, Alibaz-Oner F, Aksu K, et al. Genetic association of a gain-of-function IFNGR1 polymorphism and the intergenic region LNCAROD/DKK1 with Behcet's disease. Arthritis Rheumatol. 2021;73(7):1244–52.
8. Cavers A, Kugler MC, Ozguler Y, Al-Obeidi AF, Hatemi G, Ueberheide BM, et al. Behcet's disease risk-variant HLA-B51/ERAP1-Hap10 alters human CD8 T cell immunity. Ann Rheum Dis. 2022;81(11):1603–11.
9. McGonagle D, Aydin SZ, Gul A, Mahr A, Direskeneli H. 'MHC-I-opathy'-unified concept for spondyloarthritis and Behcet disease. Nat Rev Rheumatol. 2015;11(12):731–40.
10. Seyahi E, Ugurlu S, Amikishiyev S, Gul A. Behcet disease, familial Mediterranean fever and MEFV variations: more than just an association. Clin Immunol. 2023;251:109630.
11. Bettiol A, Alibaz-Oner F, Direskeneli H, Hatemi G, Saadoun D, Seyahi E, et al. Vascular Behcet syndrome: from pathogenesis to treatment. Nat Rev Rheumatol. 2023;19(2):111–26.
12. Kutlug Agackiran S, Sunbul M, Dogan Z, Kocakaya D, Kayaci S, Direskeneli H, Alibaz-Oner F. Pulmonary arterial wall thickness increased in Behcet's disease patients with major organ involvement: is it a sign of severity? Rheumatology (Oxford). 2023;62(3):1238–42.
13. Alibaz-Oner F, Ergelen R, Yildiz Y, Aldag M, Yazici A, Cefle A, et al. Femoral vein wall thickness measurement: a new diagnostic tool for Behcet's disease. Rheumatology (Oxford). 2021;60(1):288–96.
14. Karadeniz H, Ucar M, Mammadov T, Mirzayeva LS, Guler AA, Kardas RC, et al. Diffuse generalized venulitis as the primary pathology of Behcet's disease: a comprehensive magnetic resonance venography study. Semin Arthritis Rheum. 2023;62:152246.
15. Yavuz S, Ozilhan G, Elbir Y, Tolunay A, Eksioglu-Demiralp E, Direskeneli H. Activation of neutrophils by testosterone in Behcet's disease. Clin Exp Rheumatol. 2007;25(4 Suppl 45):S46–51.
16. Jo YG, Ortiz-Fernandez L, Coit P, Yilmaz V, Yentur SP, Alibaz-Oner F, et al. Sex-specific analysis in Behcet's disease reveals higher genetic risk in male patients. J Autoimmun. 2022;132:102882.
17. Deniz R, Emrence Z, Yalcinkaya Y, Artim Esen B, Inanc M, Ocal ML, Gul A. Improved sensitivity of the skin pathergy test with polysaccharide pneumococcal vaccine antigens in the diagnosis of Behcet disease. Rheumatology (Oxford). 2023;62(5):1903–9.
18. Alibaz-Oner F, Direskeneli H. Update on the diagnosis of Behcet's disease. Diagnostics (Basel). 2022;13(1)
19. Hatemi G, Yazici Y. Outcome measures in Behcet syndrome. Clin Immunol. 2023;251:109341.
20. Hatemi G, Meara A, Ozguler Y, Direskeneli H, Mahr A, Shea B, et al. Core set of domains for outcome measures in Behcet's syndrome. Arthritis Care Res (Hoboken). 2022;74(4):691–9.
21. Floris A, Espinosa G, Serpa Pinto L, Kougkas N, Lo Monaco A, Lopalco G, et al. Discordance between patient and physician global assessment of disease activity in Behcet's syndrome: a multicenter study cohort. Arthritis Res Ther. 2020;22(1):278.
22. Fragoulis GE, Bertsias G, Bodaghi B, Gul A, van Laar J, Mumcu G, et al. Treat to target in Behcet's disease: should we follow the paradigm of other systemic rheumatic diseases? Clin Immunol. 2023;246:109186.
23. Gurcan M, Esatoglu SN, Hamuryudan V, Saygin D, Ugurlu S, Seyahi E, et al. Long term follow-up of Behcet's syndrome patients treated with cyclophosphamide. Rheumatology (Oxford). 2020;59(9):2264–71.
24. Mumcu G, Karacayli U, Yay M, Aksoy A, Tas MN, Armagan B, et al. Oral ulcer activity assessment with the composite index according to different treatment modalities in Behcet's syndrome: a multicentre study. Clin Exp Rheumatol. 2019;37 Suppl 121(6):98–104.
25. Karacayli U, Mumcu G, Simsek I, Pay S, Kose O, Erdem H, et al. The close association between dental and periodontal treatments and oral ulcer course in Behcet's disease: a prospective clinical study. J Oral Pathol Med. 2009;38(5):410–5.

Index

E. Alpsoy et al. (eds.), *Behçet's Disease: An Integrated Approach*,
https://doi.org/10.1007/978-3-031-77251-1

GPSR Compliance

The European Union's (EU) General Product Safety Regulation (GPSR) is a set of rules that requires consumer products to be safe and our obligations to ensure this.

If you have any concerns about our products, you can contact us on ProductSafety@springernature.com

In case Publisher is established outside the EU, the EU authorized representative is:

Springer Nature Customer Service Center GmbH
Europaplatz 3
69115 Heidelberg, Germany

Batch number: 10731385

Printed by Printforce, the Netherlands